Handbook of Ambulatory Anesthesia

Second Edition

MW00986826

Handbook of Ambulatory Anesthesia

Second Edition

Rebecca S. Twersky, MD, MPH
Beverly K. Philip, MD

Editors

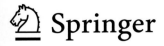 Springer

Editors

Rebecca S. Twersky, MD, MPH
Professor and Vice Chair for Research
Department of Anesthesiology
SUNY Downstate Medical Center at
  Brooklyn
Medical Director—Ambulatory Surgery
  Unit
Long Island College Hospital
Brooklyn, NY, 11203 USA

Beverly K. Philip, MD
Professor of Anaesthesia
Harvard Medical School
Director, Day Surgery Unit
Brigham and Women's Hospital
Boston, MA 02115 USA

ISBN: 978-0-387-73328-9   e-ISBN: 978-0-387-73329-6
DOI: 10.1007/978-0-387-73329-6

Library of Congress Control Number: 2007930546

Printed on acid-free paper

9 8 7 6 5 4 3 2 1

springer.com

*To our loving, supportive,
and understanding families*

*David, Baila, Ari, Yitzy, Nomi and Yitzchak Jim,
Ben, Noah and Shara*

Preface

The practice of medicine has changed dramatically over the past quarter century. These changes have often wedged physicians into situations in which clinical practice is being shaped by the competing quest for optimum outcomes built on evidence-based practice and the pressure of economic forces. Influenced by the same factors, ambulatory surgery and anesthesia have also undergone major changes, even since the *Ambulatory Anesthesia Handbook* (Mosby, 1995) was first published. Key examples are the number of surgical procedures that now can be performed on an ambulatory basis due to improved surgical technology; the exponential growth in the number of ambulatory surgery centers, particularly in the U.S.; and advances in anesthesia with drugs that produce shorter emergence and fewer postoperative adverse reactions, enabling more rapid patient discharge. The health industry in the U.S. is at a crossroads, shifting to ambulatory surgery as the primary mode of surgical care. The number of ambulatory surgery centers nears or surpasses the number of hospitals. This continued shift is also apparent in the rapid growth of office-based surgery. An increasing number of complex procedures are moving from the inpatient to the outpatient environment, out of hospital-based settings into freestanding ambulatory surgery centers, and to physicians' offices and diagnostic facilities. As ambulatory surgery pushes to expand the scope of procedures and increase the quality of care provided, anesthesia practices will continue to play a pivotal role. Additionally, the push for patient-centered care and measurements of performance will greatly influence the ways that hospitals, ambulatory surgery centers, office-based surgical practices, and their anesthesiologists approach patient selection, sedation, anesthesia, pain management, and postoperative recovery.

It is no coincidence that this updated *Ambulatory Anesthesia Handbook* is being published now. The intention of this handbook is to address the clinical and administrative concerns that have arisen from the expanding daily practice of ambulatory surgery and anesthesia. The handbook is directed to anesthesiologists both in training and in practice as well as other physicians, nurses, health care professionals, ancillary providers, and administrators involved in the care of ambulatory surgery patients. Practical approaches to the common problems encountered in this continually growing field, including recommendations and guidelines for actual practice, are addressed. This book is intended to guide these individuals through the steps of treating the ambulatory surgery patient.

The authors of this handbook are acknowledged and respected authorities in the field of ambulatory surgery and anesthesia and have elegantly provided both state-of-the-art and cutting-edge information for clinical practice. Although this book is multi-authored, we as editors have standardized the format for each chapter, providing a brief outline with text materials accompanied by succinct illustrative and tabular enhancements and key references. The handbook covers the spectrum of care, starting with preoperative evaluation (Chapter 1) and anesthesia considerations for cutting-edge, minimally invasive ambulatory surgery procedures (Chapter 2). Extensive discussions of the management of common clinical conditions and considerations for the perioperative physician for treating both adult and pediatric patients are provided (Chapters 3 and 4). The preoperative preparation of pediatric and adult patients is covered in Chapters 5 and 6, and specific anesthesia techniques—sedation, regional, and general—are addressed in Chapters 7 through 9. Anesthesia outside the operating room (Chapter 10) and office-based anesthesia (Chapter 11) are clearly growing segments of clinical practice, and an especially in-depth discussion of office-based anesthesia practice is provided. The success of ambulatory anesthesia is also measured in the safe recovery and discharge of the patient, as is illustrated in Chapters 12 and 13. Quality measures, pay for performance, and economic and administrative aspects are no less important than the anesthesia techniques, and Chapters 14 through 16 provide an excellent overview for both administrative and nonclinical management personnel. In keeping with the format of a handbook, we have attempted to provide the most relevant and up-to-date information; readers are referred to basic texts for more in-depth discussions.

We sincerely acknowledge the scholarly efforts of all the contributing authors, our colleagues in our respective departments, and the members of our families, who appreciated the importance of this undertaking and permitted us to dedicate our time and energy needed to complete this task.

Rebecca S. Twersky, MD, MPH
Beverly K. Philip, MD

Contents

Contributors

Shireen Ahmad, MD
Associate Professor, Department of Anesthesiology, Northwestern University Feinberg School of Medicine, Chicago, IL, USA

Tom Archer, MD, MBA
Department of Anesthesiology, University of Texas Health Science Center, San Antonio, TX, USA

William H. Beeson, MD
Medical Director, Beeson Aesthetic Surgery Institute, Clinical Professor, Departments of Dermatology and Otolaryngology, Indiana University School of Medicine, Carmel, IN, USA

Sorin J. Brull, MD
Professor of Anesthesiology, Mayo Clinic College of Medicine, Jacksonville, FL, USA

Frances Chung, MD, FRCPC
University of Toronto, Toronto Western Hospital, Department of Anesthesia, University Health Network, Toronto, ON, Canada

Jerry A. Cohen, MS, MD
Associate Professor of Anesthesiology, University of Florida, College of Medicine, Gainesville, FL, USA

Meena S. Desai, MD
President and CEO, Nova Anesthesia Professionals, Villanova, PA, USA

Holly C. L. Evans, MD, FRCP(C)
Assistant Professor, Department of Anesthesiology, University of Ottawa, Ottawa, ON, Canada

Lucinda L. Everett, MD
Chief, Pediatric Anesthesia, Associate Professor, Harvard Medical School, Anesthesia and Critical Care, Massachusetts General Hospital, Boston, MA, USA

Gennadiy Fuzaylov, MD
Assistant in Anesthesia, Harvard Medical School, Anesthesia and Critical Care, Massachusetts General Hospital, Boston, MA, USA

Tong J. Gan, MB, BS, FRCA
Professor, Department of Anesthesiology, Duke University Medical Center, Duke North Hospital, Durham, NC, USA

Ralph Gertler, MD
Staff Anesthesiologist, Technical University of the State of Bavaria, German Heart Centre, Munich, Germany

Steven C. Hall, MD
Anesthesiologist-in-Chief, Arthur C. King Professor of Pediatric Anesthesia, Children's Memorial Hospital, Feinberg School of Medicine, Northwestern University, Chicago, IL, USA

Raafat S. Hannallah, MD
Professor of Anesthesiology and Pediatrics, The George Washington University Medical Center, Division of Anesthesiology, Children's National Medical Center, Washington, DC, USA

Girish P. Joshi, MB, BS, MD, FFARCSI
Professor of Anesthesiology and Pain Management, University of Texas Southwestern Medical Center at Dallas, Dallas, TX, USA

Patricia A. Kapur, MD
Professor and Chair, Department of Anesthesiology, The David Geffen School of Medicine, UCLA Medical Center, Los Angeles, CA, USA

Jeremy Lermitte, BM, FRCA
University of Toronto, Toronto Western Hospital, University Health Network, Toronto, ON, Canada

J. Lance Lichtor, MD
Professor, Department of Anesthesiology and Pediatrics, University of Massachusetts Medical School, Worcester, MA, USA

Alex Macario, MD, MBA
Professor of Anesthesia and Health Research and Policy, Department of Anesthesia, Stanford University Medical Center, Stanford, CA, USA

Steve Mannis, MD, MBA
Anesthesiologist, Sacramento, CA, USA

Donald M. Mathews, MD
Associate Professor of Clinical Anesthesiology, New York Medical
College, Department of Anesthesiology, St. Vincent Catholic Medical
Centers—St. Vincent's Manhattan, New York, NY, USA

Walter G. Maurer, MD
Associate Chief of Staff for Quality Management, Department of Anesthesiology, Cleveland Clinic Foundation, Cleveland, OH, USA

Rafael V. Miguel, MD
Professor, Department of Anesthesiology, University of South Florida,
Moffitt Cancer Center, Tampa, FL, USA

Karen C. Nielsen, MD
Assistant Professor of Anesthesiology, Duke University Medical Center,
Durham, NC, USA

L. Reuven Pasternak, MD, MPH, MBA
Adjunct Clinical Professor of Anesthesiology, University of Cincinnati
College of Medicine, Cincinnati, OH, USA

Beverly K. Philip, MD
Professor of Anaesthesia, Harvard Medical School, Director, Day
Surgery Unit, Brigham and Women's Hospital, Boston, MA, USA

Johnathan L. Pregler, MD
Clinical Professor, The David Geffen School of Medicine, UCLA
Medical Center, Los Angeles, CA, USA

Susan M. Steele, MD
Professor of Anesthesiology, Duke University Medical Center, Durham,
NC, USA

Rebecca S. Twersky, MD, MPH
Professor and Vice Chair for Research, Department of Anesthesiology,
SUNY Downstate Medical Center at Brooklyn, Medical Director—
Ambulatory Surgery Unit, Long Island College Hospital, Brooklyn, NY,
USA

Hector Vila, Jr., MD
Assistant Professor, University of South Florida, Department of Anesthesiology, Moffitt Cancer Center and Research Institute, Inc., Tampa, FL, USA

1. Preanesthesia evaluation and testing

L. Reuven Pasternak, MD, MPH, MBA

The explosive growth of ambulatory surgical programs has been one of the most formidable changes in the practice of medicine in the past 30 years. Few other events have affected so many patients in such a fundamental fashion. It has been estimated that approximately more than 80% of all surgical procedures performed in the United States are now being done on an ambulatory basis. Ambulatory surgery continues to diffuse to include a wider range of procedures, involving higher risk patients in more diverse environments increasingly removed from the traditional hospital setting.

Conventional wisdom holds that complications in ambulatory surgery are relatively uncommon. This situation reflects the not-uncommon phenomenon of rapid diffusion of a technology without an evidence-based analysis to determine appropriate risk factors for analysis. Nonetheless, ambulatory surgery is a common medical practice that is fraught with the potential for uncommon events. The assessment of patients for appropriate management requires no less diligence than assessment for procedures that are more invasive. This often-overlooked aspect of the patient's management is the first step in the process of reducing the risk for adverse events for the patient and ensuring an optimal outcome for both the patient and the system.

2   L.R. Pasternak

American Society of Anesthesiologists physical status classification

The first attempt to quantify risks associated with surgery and anesthesia was undertaken by Meyer Saklad[1] in 1941 at the request of the American Society of Anesthesiologists (ASA). This effort was the first by any medical specialty to stratify risk for its patients. Saklad's system was based on mortality secondary to anesthesia due to associated preoperative medical conditions. Type of anesthesia and nature of surgery were not considerations in this system, and the divisions were based on empirical experience rather than on specific sets of data and reflect the techniques and standards of practice of 50 years ago. Four preanesthesia risk categories ranging from category 1 (least likely to die) to category 4 (highest expectation of mortality) were established.

The current ASA system (Table 1-1) is a modification of this work, adding an additional fifth category for moribund patients undergoing surgery in a desperate attempt to preserve life. Numerous studies have demonstrated an association of mortality with ASA class independent of anesthetic technique.[1–10] However, most of this information has limited application as it relates to mortality as its sole outcome and is based on anesthetic techniques as practiced more than 20 years ago. Apfelbaum[2] and Meridy[3], for example, have noted a lack of correlation between ASA status and cancellations, unplanned admissions, and other perioperative complications in ambulatory surgery. It should also be noted that the original study of Saklad[1] and subsequent derivations were not based on actual determinations of mortality and associated morbidity and mortality, either

Table 1-1. American Society of Anesthesiologists (ASA) physical status classification system

ASA status	Description	Example
P1	A normal, healthy patient	Healthy adult with no medical problems, no medications
P2	Patient with mild systemic disease	Well-controlled hypertension
P3	Patient with severe systemic disease	Angina pectoris without congestive heart failure, reactive airway disease regularly requiring inhalers
P4	Patient with severe systemic disease that is a constant threat to life	Severe congestive heart failure
P5	A moribund patient who is not expected to survive without the operation	Severe trauma, end-stage terminally ill

Examples are provided by author. Adapted from http://www.asahq.org/clinical/physicalstatus.htm. Used with permission. The designation E after the status refers to emergency operation and generally would not apply to the ambulatory surgical patient.

retrospectively or prospectively. Thus, while useful as a broad assessment of preoperative medical status, the current ASA classification is limited in its ability to truly establish risk or serve as a basis for formulating clinical guidelines without an associated risk index for the surgical procedure.

Surgical risk classification

The Johns Hopkins risk classification system[4] was one of the first attempts to formulate a multifactorial risk assessment system by adding the invasiveness of the surgical procedure as a function of risk along with the more traditional preoperative medical condition. The Johns Hopkins surgical risk classification system (Table 1-2) is based on the well-established assumption that the nature of the surgery is clearly a major determinant of risk and needs to be coordinated

Table 1-2. Johns Hopkins surgery risk classification system (JHSRCS)

JHSRCS status	Description	Example
1	Noninvasive procedure with minimal blood loss and minimal risk to the patient independent of medical conditions and anesthesia	Breast biopsy, carpal tunnel repair, cataract surgery
2	Procedures limited in their invasive nature, usually with minimal to mild blood loss and only mild associated risk to the patient independent of medical conditions and anesthesia	Diagnostic laparoscopy, arthroscopy, rhinoplasty, inguinal hernia repair
3	More invasive procedures and/or those involving moderate blood loss with moderate risk to the patient independent of medical conditions and anesthesia	Open abdominal procedures, major joint replacement
4	Procedures posing significant risk to the patient independent of medical conditions and anesthesia	Planned postoperative intensive care, open thoracic procedure, intracranial procedure, major vascular/skeletal or neurological repair

Adapted from Pasternak RL.[4] Used with permission.

with medical status in determining preoperative risk assessment. This system is predicated on the assumption that patients of identical medical status undergoing minor office procedures are at less risk of adverse events and in need of less preparation than those undergoing surgery that entails blood loss, fluid shifts, or other significant physiologic intervention and compromise. Although various systems exist for stratifying surgical and medical risk in an intensive care setting, these have several drawbacks when applied in a general preoperative setting, especially for ambulatory procedures.

The Johns Hopkins system was built upon the observations of the confidential inquiry into perioperative deaths in Great Britain as reported in 1987.[9] In that retrospective study, it was determined that surgical condition was most frequently cited as the cause of death, followed by medical status and then anesthesia. It was also proposed that mortality was most often due to a combination of factors rather than to a single specific cause. The nature of surgical causation was not established with regard to invasiveness, site of surgery, or other factors. The Johns Hopkins risk classification system proposed that the risk of surgery is a combination of several factors, including invasiveness, associated blood loss and fluid shift, entry into specific body areas (e.g., intrathoracic and intracranial), postoperative anatomic and physiologic alterations, and the need for postoperative intensive care monitoring. Procedures were assigned to the various categories in consultation with the surgical, anesthesia, medical, and nursing staffs who manage these patients. Though broad in their scope and subject to potential variations in interpretation, the five categories may provide a reasonable basis for use in the practice environment, pending further verification. However, like the ASA classification, this system is based on assumptions and presumptions rather than actual fact.

Outcome

The ability to determine risk by using measures of admission and death for ambulatory surgery is difficult due to the low frequency of events. Such a study would most certainly have to be multi-institutional and, perhaps, national in scope to capture the relevant variables to allow for a true determination of the appropriate risks associated with this endeavor. To add to the complexity of such an analysis, additional factors have come into play as confounding variables in this enterprise. Beyond the issue of medical status and type of surgery, the concern of site of surgery has now come forward. As with the issue of the proliferation of procedures done in the absence of controlled studies to assess outcome, ambulatory surgery locations have expanded beyond the traditional hospital to freestanding multispecialty surgery centers, single-specialty centers, and physician offices. The often-cited episodic cases of deaths in physician office locations for cosmetic procedures have brought much attention but little objective insight into the issue of the extent to which the factors of type of surgery, medical status, anesthesia, and location of procedure interact to create a true risk assessment structure for the tens of millions of ambulatory procedures performed annually in North America alone. During the late 1990s, office-based surgical procedures became much more common, with an estimated 5% to 8% of procedures being performed in the office in the year 2000.

A study by Fleisher et al.[11] was one of the first to address this issue. The authors used a 5% sample of Medicare beneficiaries from 1994 to 1999, matching part A and part B data to obtain both facilities and medical provider data. Patients undergoing any one of 16 surgical procedures were identified with outcome of death, hospital admission, or emergency room (ER) visit measured. The selection of surgical procedures was based upon their prevalence in the ambulatory setting and their rapid diffusion from the inpatient to ambulatory setting in the last 10 years. Death, hospitalizations, and ER visits on the day of surgery (calendar day), within 7 days, and within 30 days of the procedure were the three outcome variables. The authors identified 564,267 surgical procedures that were further stratified by site of surgery: hospital-based outpatient (64%), freestanding ambulatory surgical center (ASC) (31%), and office-based (5%) (Table 1-3).

Table 1-3. Rate of adverse events per day (per 100,000 procedures) by site of care for 16 procedures performed in Medicare beneficiaries from 1994 to 1999

Adverse events	Outpatient hospital	ASC	Office	Overall outpatient	P value
Death same calendar day as procedure	2.5	2.3	0	2.3	NS
Death 0–7 days	6.2	3.1*	4.4	5.1	
Death 8–30 days	7.3	5.6	5.2	6.6	
Death 0–30 days	7.0	4.9	5.1	6.3	
ER visit, 0–7 days	259.1†	103.6†	109.9	203.3	
ER visit, 8–30 days	106.6	79.6	60.3	95.9	
ER visit 0–30 days	139.0	82.9	69.9	118.1	
Inpatient admission, 0–7 days	432.7‡	91.3‡	226.5‡	316.3	
Inpatient admission, 8–30 days	115.3	74.0	74.3	100.4	
Inpatient admission 0–30 days	174.5	70.2	101.0	138.4	
Total procedures	360,780	175,288	28,199	564,267	

*$p < 0.05$ ASC versus outpatient hospital.
†$p < 0.05$ outpatient hospital versus ASC or office.
‡$p < 0.05$ all groups.
ASC, ambulatory surgery center; ER, emergency room; NS, not significant. Adapted from Fleisher et al.[11] Used with permission.

For the 16 procedures, there was a trend toward increasing frequency in the outpatient setting from 1994 to 1999, except for cataract surgery, which was already performed in the outpatient setting 98.6% of the time in 1994.

Table 1-3 shows the rates of death, ER visits, and inpatient admissions at 7 and 30 days postsurgery. The rate of deaths per day was lower during the first 7 days after surgery compared with the subsequent days, and the rates of ER visits and inpatient hospital admissions per day were greatest during the first 7 days. There were no significant differences based on site of surgery for deaths on day of surgery. Within 7 days of surgery, the death rate was significantly lower in ASCs compared to the outpatient hospital. The number of ER visits within 7 days of surgery was greater for outpatient hospital compared to either ASC or office. The number of patients admitted to an inpatient hospital within 7 days was different among all three sites.

Estimates of operative mortality associated with anesthesia and surgery in the ambulatory setting have ranged from 1 in 200,000 to 1 in 400,000 procedures. Although these statistics are often cited, they are not based on large, rigorous studies of ambulatory surgery mortality and morbidity, especially with regard to the rapidly expanding geriatric population. The study by Fleisher et al.[11] calculated the same-day mortality rate in a population over age 65 to be 2.5 per 100,000 or 5 to 10 times greater than these estimates. Furthermore, as seen in Table 1-4, age alone does not appear to be an independent risk factor once the patient population enters into the geriatric grouping until age 85.

The influence of location of care varied by procedure. For those models with sufficient sample size, the risk-adjusted odds ratio for hospitalization and death within 7 days for office-based care is shown in Table 1-5. Hemorrhoidectomy in the office was associated with a significantly lower risk-adjusted rate of

Table 1-4. Event rates and total cases for basic demographic and location of care factors for Medicare beneficiaries undergoing 15 procedures during 1995–1999

	Inpatient admission rate per 100,000	ER visit rate per 100,000	Death rate per 100,000
	Procedures 0–7 days	Procedures 0–7 days	Procedures 0–7 days
Male	3,043	2,061	56
Female	2,187	1,577	34
70–74	2,426	1,712	37
75–79	2,345	1,648	42
80–84	2,440	1,714	42
85+	2,837	1,936	64
Office	1,727	900	34
Outpatient hospital	3,385	2,102	51
ASC	703	834	24

ASC, ambulatory surgery center; ER, emergency room. Adapted from Fleisher et al.[11] Used with permission.

Table 1-5. Increased risk associated with office care compared to the ASC for a given procedure when each risk procedure was evaluated individually

Effect	Increased risk of confidence limits office care compared to ASC	Odds ratio for 95%
Hemorrhoidectomy	0.146	0.076–0.281
Cataract extraction	1.555	1.288–1.877
Hysteroscopy	2.313	1.094–4.890
Inguinal hernia repair	3.818	2.335–6.243
A-V graft placement	4.046	1.580–10.361
Knee arthroscopy	4.718	2.472–9.005
TURP	7.491	4.162–13.481
Umbilical hernia repair	10.79	0.731–31.223

Adjusted for age, gender, race, and prior admission history.
ASC, ambulatory surgery center; A-V, arterio-venous; TURP, transurethral resection of the prostate. Adapted from Fleischer et al.[11] Used with permission.

adverse events compared to ASCs, whereas cataract surgery, inguinal hernia repair, arteriovenous graft placement, knee arthroscopy, and transurethral procedures of the prostate were associated with higher rates of adverse events in the office. Hysteroscopy and umbilical hernia repair did not have significant variance between sites. Given these considerations, site alone does not constitute the basis of risk but is likely a combination of factors about the procedure and the patient's associated medical status.

American Society of Anesthesiologists Practice Advisory for Preanesthesia Evaluation

Time of assessment

When the ASA Task Force on Preanesthesia Evaluation began its deliberations in 1994, it affirmed that the purpose of the "preanesthesia" assessment[12] was to address strategies designed to reduce the risk associated with elective surgical procedures. Furthermore, it was determined to do so on an evidence-based strategy that included interventions (including testing) only on the assumption that information would be obtained that was not previously known and that may affect the perioperative management of the patient (Box 1-1).

By means of this approach, the ability to determine appropriate risk, for purposes of patient testing and consultation, needed to include medical condition and the nature of the surgical procedure. The task force determined that an algorithm that fit most situations relating to the timing of the preanesthesia evaluation could be used (Figure 1-1). The system includes two levels of stratification for the medical status and three for the nature of the surgical procedure. In doing so, it was using an algorithm based on the same type of flow as that

Box 1-1. American Society of Anesthesiologists practice advisory for preanesthesia evaluation[12]

- All patients should have information made available to anesthesia providers prior to the day of surgery.
- It is the responsibility of the system in which the anesthesia staff operate to ensure the receipt of that information.
- It is the responsibility of the anesthesia staff to review and act upon that data in a timely fashion.
- In some, but not most, circumstances preoperative evaluation may require a visit with anesthesia staff prior to the day of surgery.
- Consultations should be obtained only on the basis of a reasonable expectation that the information may change the nature of perioperative care.
- Consultants provide information used by anesthesia staff to asses the patient; they do not "clear for anesthesia" or dictate type of anesthesia or agents to be used—only anesthesiologists may do that.
- Laboratory testing is obtained only on the reasonable expectation that the test results may be abnormal and change the nature of perioperative care.

adopted by the American Heart Association/American College of Cardiology guidelines.[13] On the basis of this algorithm, it was determined that healthy patients undergoing procedures of minor or intermediate complexity or stable patients with significant medical issues but with procedures of low risk or complexity may have their evaluation on the day of surgery with the caveat that appropriate information be available for review prior to surgery to provide reasonable assurance of a patient who is sufficiently prepared for surgery or anesthesia. This recommendation did not preclude the possible benefit of a preanesthesia evaluation prior to the day of surgery for such purposes as education, allaying anxiety, or prevention of day-of-surgery delays associated with last-minute evaluation. It simply referred to the safety of this timing of the evaluation if that were the preference of the physician and patient.

Conversely, patients with high medical risk having complex procedures were believed to benefit from a preanesthesia evaluation prior to the day of surgery. Exceptions to this mandate were to be made on the basis of the anesthesiologist's comfort with the nature of information provided prior to the day of surgery and the ability to appropriately prepare the patient without such a visit. However, again, this system represented a consensus of opinion rather than an actual evidence-based model of appropriate risk factors and outcomes. In fact, the ASA in its report noted the paucity of appropriate data on which to base such a system and strongly advocated for studies that were more definitive.

Scientific basis for testing

Preoperative testing of the patient undergoing elective surgical procedures has been the focus of several specialty societies, regulatory agencies, and clinical

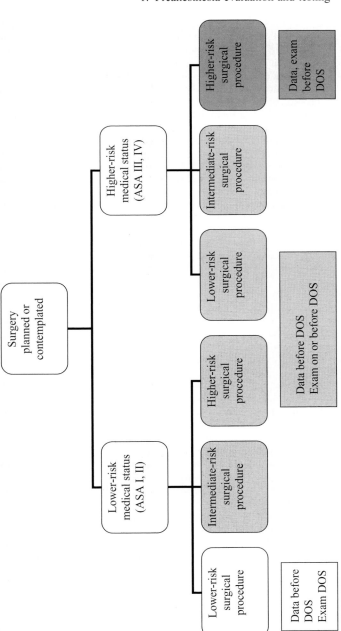

Figure 1-1. Sample timing of the preoperative assessment. ASA, American Society of Anesthesiologists; DOS, date of surgery. Adapted from the American Society of Anesthesiologists Task Force on Pre-anesthesia Evaluation.[12] Used with permission.

researchers during the past 20 years, and despite much interest in this area, it can best be described as dynamic and subject to continual change that mirrors much of the history of testing throughout health care. It is difficult to attach a precise dollar cost on the preoperative evaluation activity. In the past, there existed an assumption that all elective surgical procedures must be preceded by a series of comprehensive tests, regardless of the patient's age, health status, or planned procedure. The traditional system of the protocol "battery of tests" evolved from a lack of clear definition of their role in preoperative screening, insufficient information on their utility, and a mistaken belief that voluminous information, no matter how extraneous, enhanced the safety of care and reduced physician liability for adverse events. Protocol testing relieved physicians and their associates of the responsibility of decision-making, with an easier, though more costly, test battery as the alternative to selective tests based on patients' individual health profiles.

The issue of testing as a method of screening for diseases actually occurred as an early attempt to enhance the efficiency of managed health care systems, especially early health maintenance organizations, during the 1960s and 1970s. The practice evolved from an assumption that by early and frequent testing medical conditions could be detected in their preclinical phase and allow for earlier and more effective, and less expensive, intervention. In one of the first studies to debunk this association between testing and improved health outcomes, Olsen et al.[14] looked at 574 families randomly assigned for care with and without automated multiphasic health testing. After 1 year of assessment, there was no difference between the two groups with regard to physician visits, hospital admission or length of stay for those admitted, health status index, or total days lost from work. Despite this study (in 1976), the testing mythology lived on and awaited more concerted efforts for better assessment.

Now, when the cost of care and the convenience of patients are major concerns, the role of tests as a screening device is rightfully diminishing. The patient history, physical examination, and judgment of the physician are replacing protocols as the basis for testing. Although information about other aspects of the preoperative evaluation may be ambiguous, there are extensive literature and experience to support the selective use of testing and the finding that the use of broad testing panels has a strong tendency to result in excessive testing. Laboratory testing, like all areas of medical intervention, should be undertaken on a "value-added" basis: a reasonable expectation that a potential issue exists that is relevant to anesthesia.

The usefulness of the preanesthesia test is based on several key considerations. The first issue is relevance. Although some abnormalities are clearly of concern (e.g., cardiac and respiratory), others may have little or no effect on anesthetic plan and outcome and thus do not warrant thorough investigation in this format. The second issue is the prevalence of the condition in both symptomatic and asymptomatic patients. A low prevalence in asymptomatic patients would indicate that screening is of little use. The third issue is that of sensitivity and specificity. Low sensitivity permits false-negative results, and patients at risk undergo anesthesia without appropriate preparation. Low specificity causes many false-positives with patients being subjected to additional testing with their coincident inconvenience, costs, and potential morbidity. Testing, therefore, should be done for conditions that are medically relevant and with tests of high sensitivity and specificity. A final consideration is cost. Selection of alternative testing modalities should also take into consideration the financial and nonfinancial costs of testing, with selection of the less costly approach when it does not compromise the quality of the information desired. Testing in the asymptomatic population should be carried out only in patients for whom the potential condition is significant and of reasonable prevalence with tests of reasonable sensitivity.

The intersection of these considerations has been addressed in several studies over the past 30 years. It has been established in the medical, surgical, and anesthesia literature that the use of screening tests without a specific indication is not appropriate. In a study of 19,980 tests on 1,000 medical patients, Korvin et al.[15] encountered 2,223 abnormal values, of which 993 were initially considered to be unanticipated. Of these, 223 led to further evaluation and new diagnoses; in only one case, the diagnosis was unrelated to other known medical issues and resulted in new patient care. This involved elevated liver function studies in a man who had received halothane anesthesia and for whom the recommendation was made that this agent be avoided.

In the surgical population, two seminal studies have evaluated the utility of routine testing batteries. In the first, Kaplan et al.[16] (Table 1-6) reviewed the records of 2,000 patients undergoing elective surgery who received a routine battery of complete blood cell count, differential cell count, prothrombin time, partial thromboplastin time, platelet count, glucose level, and six chemistries. They found that 60% of these tests would not have been performed had they been done only on the basis of clinical indication and that of these only 22% revealed abnormalities that might have affected perioperative management. Of

Table 1-6. Preoperative screening battery tests

Test	Normal	Not indicated (NI)	Abnormal (AB)	NI + AB	NI + AB and significant
Prothrombin time	201	154	2	0	0
Partial thromboplastin time	199	154	1	0	0
Platelet count	407	366	3	2	1
Complete blood count	61	293	22	2	0
White blood count with differential	390	324	2	1	0
Chemistry 6 panel	514	176	41	1	1
Glucose	464	361	25	4	2
Total	2,236	1,828	96	10	4

Adapted from Kaplan et al.[16] Used with permission.

Table 1-7. Preoperative testing: battery testing

	Arthroscopy		Level 1 laparoscopy		Level 2 laparoscopy	
	Outpatient	Inpatient	Outpatient	Inpatient	Outpatient	Inpatient
X-ray	12%	30%	24%	58%	0%	79%
Electro-cardiogram	11%	30%	12%	50%	2%	83%
Chemistry panel	3%	92%	0%	75%	2%	86%

Outpatient testing: ordered by anesthesia staff on the day of surgery. Inpatient testing: ordered by surgical staff prior to the day of surgery without anesthesia guidelines. Adapted from Kitz et al.[18] Used with permission.

the 96 abnormal test results, only 10 were in patients who did not have an indication by exam or clinical history; of these 10, only 4 were of actual clinical significance. These findings were replicated by Turnbull and Buck,[17] who in a review of 1,010 otherwise-healthy patients undergoing cholecystectomy, discovered 225 abnormal results in 5,003 tests, of which 104 were judged to be important and for whom only 4 patients might have derived some benefit.

Similarly, Kitz et al.[18] (Table 1-7) revealed that among patient populations undergoing minor procedures, testing varied considerably depending on the specialty of the physician doing the testing. Among a patient population undergoing knee arthroscopy and diagnostic laparoscopy or laparoscopic tubal ligation, surgeons ordered chest x-rays, electrocardiograms, and chemistry panels at several multiples of the anesthesiologists because of their concern about potential cancellations and disruption to their schedule. This study demonstrated the need for the development of some standardization among physicians of testing protocols and guidelines in an environment where practices varied widely without scientific rationale. Fischer,[19] using a system that reviewed all patients undergoing elective surgery regardless of ASA status and intensity of the procedure, was able to prospectively replicate the findings of the previously mentioned retrospective studies. In his results (Table 1-8), he was able to achieve a reduction in overall testing of 55%, ranging from an 89% reduction in urinalyses to a 17% reduction in the complete blood count. It is now believed that using the patient-focused criteria mentioned earlier, an even greater reduction might be possible. Therefore, although more ambiguous than would be preferred by many, the new testing advisory does allow for significant streamlining of the testing process. More recent studies have confirmed that despite extensive efforts to address this issue, preoperative testing continues to be inconsistent with established guidelines and varies extensively within the same regions with little utility.[20–23]

Subsequent studies of specific tests have also confirmed the use of the history and physical as the optimal basis for intervention. Urinalysis, long a mainstay of testing and (until recently) required by law in some states, has been found to be of limited use in patients without a pre-existing medical condition or positive physical findings.[24,25] Rucker et al.,[26] in a review of 905 routine chest x-rays for elective surgical procedures, determined that 40.6% (368) had no risk factors by

Table 1-8. Reduction in testing with a preoperative evaluation center (PEC)

Test	Surgical service	PEC	Percentage reduction
Number of patients	3,576	4,313	
Complete blood count	3,417	3,395*	17.7%
Platelet count	3,207	2,620*	32.3%
PT/PTT	2,703	578*	82.3%
Urinalysis	2,489	309*	89.7%
General survey panel	2,199	811*	69.4%
Electrolytes	1,775	739*	65.5%
Renal panel	1,402	1,022*	39.5%
Electrocardiograms	2,202	1,362*	48.7%
Chest x-rays	2,510	1,026*	66.1%
Total preoperative tests	21,904	11,862*	45.8%
Tests per patient	6.13	2.75*	55.1%

*$p < 0.001$.
PT/PTT, prothrombin time/partial thromboplastin time. Adapted from Fischer SP.[19] Used with permission.

history and physical and that only one had an abnormality (and even that was minor in nature). Only 12.6% (114) had serious abnormalities, virtually all of which would have been anticipated by the history and physical examination. Charpak et al.,[27] in a retrospective review of postoperative complications, found no circumstances in which absence of a chest x-ray in patients without prior pulmonary disease would have altered outcome or management, even when the complications were respiratory in nature. In both studies, there was no correlation between age and occurrence of positive chest x-rays in patients independent of coexisting positive history or physical examination. Similar findings are available for hemoglobin determinations,[22,28,29] serum chemistries,[30] and pulmonary function testing.[31]

In one of the most widely cited studies on this subject, Schein et al.[32] looked at testing associated with patients undergoing cataract surgery and adverse outcomes. In this analysis, even among an elderly patient population with considerable medical comorbidity, there was no demonstrated association between testing and outcomes of surgery. It should be remembered that despite the widespread use of this study to justify the denial of tests to all patients having elective surgery, the investigators intended this to apply only to the more limited universe of patients undergoing this minimally invasive surgery with light sedation.

In accordance with the philosophy that a test should be undertaken only if there is a realistic possibility of adding valuable information, protocol screening without specific indication is not appropriate. In addition to a lack of usefulness for the physician, such testing may in fact do harm to patients through unnecessary and potentially invasive interventions, heightened anxieties, and markedly increased costs that may place the physician in a position of having to explain proceeding with surgery in the face of incomplete or irrelevant data. As observed in the literature, there is little rationale for testing other than on the basis of specific indicators. Testing should be carried out only with an expectation of a finding that might have reasonable relevance for anesthesia and surgery based on:

- Presence of a positive finding on the history or physical examination
- Need of the surgeon or other clinician for baseline values in anticipation of significant changes caused by surgery or other medical interventions (e.g., chemotherapy)
- The patient's inclusion in a population at higher risk for the presence of a relevant condition even though they may exhibit no individual signs of that condition.

As noted by Guyatt et al.,[33] evidence-based practice "de-emphasizes intuition, unsystematic clinical experience and stresses the examination of evidence from clinical research." The evidence-based model thus provides a basis for guideline development based on empiric science rather than individual experience and has been adopted by numerous professional, academic, and governmental bodies as the basis for guideline and advisory development. Under such a format, there are three potential outcomes: definitive findings with firm and consistent scientific data, marginal findings with trends of a limited number of appropriate studies that agree with consensus opinion, and no guidance when the literature does not provide an adequate number of studies that meet methodological standards. In its Task Force on Preanesthesia Evaluation,[12] the ASA panel found that of more than 1,200 articles reviewed, only 163 qualified as original studies and that, of these, only 11 satisfied criteria for inclusion. As a result, the ASA Practice Advisory notes that there is insufficient evidence to support any form of protocol testing in patients other than that which is prompted by specific aspects of the patient's history and physical examination that are of direct concern to the surgical procedure and anesthesia.

Preanesthesia evaluation

The preparation of the patient for surgery and anesthesia involves multiple health care providers, starting with the primary care provider and then including associated medical specialists, surgeons, anesthesiologists, and, often, additional specialists who are asked to address issues specifically related to the process. Information provided to anesthesiologists by surgeons, primary care providers, and specialists does not constitute "clearance for anesthesia" but is used by anesthesia staff for assessment of the patient by means of criteria developed and used by anesthesiologists. The full scope of the elements of the preanesthesia assessment are included in Box 1-2. These form the critical elements of any aspect of the assessment, whether done in person or on the basis of written or electronic information provided by the various sources.

The challenge of this process has been increased during the past 20 years because now fewer than 30% of patients undergoing surgery are admitted to the hospital before the day of surgery. Even with the advent of formal preoperative systems in many institutions, many patients do not have a definitive preoperative visit with anesthesia staff before the day of surgery. Thus, anesthesia teams are

Box 1-2. Components of the preanesthesia assessment
- Physical examination
  - Heart
  - Lungs
  - Airway
  - Baseline neurological function
  - Intravenous access
  - Anatomy of area where regional anesthesia may be indicated
  - Other (based on medical issues, type of surgery, and anesthetic technique)
- Vital signs
  - Height and weight
  - Blood pressure
  - Pulse
- Medications
- Allergies
- Medical problems
- Past surgical and anesthesia history
- Primary care and specialty care providers
- Responsible individual who will accompany patient to and from the procedure

dependent on other providers to provide appropriate data to best judge who is an appropriate candidate for anesthesia. This issue is becoming all the more difficult because the acuity of patients and complexity of procedures being managed on an ambulatory (or same-day admission) basis increases.

Despite the temptation to use the preanesthesia evaluation process as a vehicle for managing several patient issues, this evaluation should be a focused assessment of issues associated with safety and efficiency of the surgical process. The evaluation, and associated testing, is a focused effort to address these clinical conditions of relevance to the safety of anesthesia and is not designed to be a comprehensive assessment of all medical issues. When concerns arise about the management of chronic health issues or the workup of new problems, patients should be referred back to their primary care provider or their specialist. Thus, testing should not be an open-ended issue but one that is designed to assess whether the medical conditions in question are as optimally managed as possible.

Though routine for the operating room practitioner, any surgical procedure is a departure from the usual health routine of a patient and warrants appropriate preparation. At a minimum, as recommended by the ASA, patients undergoing ambulatory anesthesia should have their medical history, medications, and overall risk issues identified and optimally managed prior to the day of surgery. In its advisory, the ASA also advises that anesthesia staff alone may "clear" patients for anesthesia and that it is the responsibility of the system in which this staff operates to provide a support structure to allow these functions to be done in a methodical and comprehensive method.

Box 1-3. Preoperative evaluation of the airway
- Mallampati classification (ability to view posterior pharynx)
- Mentum-to-thyroid distance
- Mandible-to-hyoid bone distance
- Oral opening
- Nares
- Quality of dentition (teeth, gum, and dentures)
- Intraoral structures (tonsils, uvula, and palates)
- Mask fit (e.g., facial anatomy and beard)
- Range of motion of neck
- Obesity

History and physical examination

The examination of the patient prior to anesthesia should include at least the critical elements cited in Box 1-2. Perhaps the most difficult to convey to those not practicing anesthesia is the importance of the airway (Box 1-3). Instruction in the Mallampati classification system[34] may be time-consuming but represents the simplest method of conveying to nonanesthesia staff a basis for assessing potential difficulties in airway management (Table 1-9).

Laboratory and ancillary testing

As noted in the discussion of the ASA Practice Advisory,[12] there is no indication for "routine" testing. Tests should be obtained on the basis of demonstrated need. On this basis, testing is an individualized function based on the patient's history, physical examination, and planned procedure. This author's recommendations for preanesthesia laboratory testing in ambulatory surgery patients are noted in Table 1-10. For example, a healthy individual less than 50 years of age undergoing an elective ambulatory procedure would likely need no preoperative tests at all, as none would change perioperative management. At times, physicians and staff have been anxious about so significant a change in testing practice, fearing that past precedent had established a standard that could

Table 1-9. Mallampati classification for airway evaluation

The patient is asked to open the mouth and protrude the tongue maximally while in the sitting position.

Class 1	Soft palate and uvula can be visualized.
Class 2	Soft palate can be visualized, but uvula is obstructed by the base of the tongue.
Class 3	Only the soft palate can be visualized.

Table 1-10. Recommended laboratory testing for patients having ambulatory surgery

---

Age less than 50 years, Healthy
- No tests unless specified by surgeon for specific surgical issues

Electrocardiogram
- Age 50 or older
- Hypertension
- Current or past significant cardiac disease
- Current or past circulatory disease
- Cardiothoracic procedure

Chest x-ray
- Major respiratory condition with change of symptoms or acute episode within past 6 months
- Cardiothoracic procedure

Serum chemistries
- Renal disease
- Adrenal, thyroid, or other major metabolic disorders
- Diuretic therapy

Urinalysis
- Genito-urological procedure

Complete blood count
- Hematological disorder
- Vascular procedure
- Chemotherapy

Coagulation studies
- Anticoagulation therapy
- Vascular procedure

Pregnancy testing
- Patients for whom pregnancy might complicate the surgery or anesthesia

---

These tests may be required for administration of anesthesia and are not intended to limit those required by surgeons for issues specific to their surgical management.

not be changed. In fact, the literature as well as the national society advisory strongly support such a practice, and as long as the determination of tests is made on the basis of documented health status, proposed surgery, and examination, the anesthesia team is on solid clinical and legal ground.

One area of note is that of pregnancy testing. This has been controversial based on a number of social and perceived clinical issues and has triggered considerable distress in various clinical environments. The ASA Task Force recognized that patients may present for anesthesia with early undetected pregnancy and noted that the literature is inadequate to inform patients or physicians on whether anesthesia causes harmful effects on early pregnancy.[12] Current urine pregnancy tests are fast, inexpensive, and sufficiently sensitive to allow for testing on the day of surgery. Until such time as more definitive information is available, one of two paths may be pursued. The first calls for advising female premenopausal patients that the procedure may (or may not) pose a risk to them if they are pregnant and offer the testing as an option. One criticism of this is that adolescents may decline tests fearing their sexual activity will be discovered by parents rather than make a decision based on lack of risk. The second path calls for routine pregnancy testing. Either way, it is advised that a policy that is consistent in practice and application be adopted. Decisions as to whether to proceed may then be based on deliberation of the medical team and the patient.

Patient selection

In general, the patient for ambulatory surgery should have no unevaluated medical problems and no problems severe enough to require hospitalization after surgery. Chronic illnesses should be well controlled. Ambulatory patients may be ASA grade 3 or 4 if their disease processes are compensated and the anesthesia and surgery are tailored to the patient's medical limitations. Preanesthesia evaluation would uncover any medical condition that might influence the anesthetic or surgical course or that would preclude the performance of the procedure on an ambulatory basis (Box 1-4). A determination could be made if the existing medical condition requires further evaluation or by consultation. Specific medical problems are addressed in Chapters 3 and 4. While procedure selection is often dictated by the surgeon and third-party payers, the preanesthesia evaluation should take note of the potential for intra- and postoperative physiological consequences, such as open abdominal, thoracic, and intracranial procedures, as well as major vascular and orthopedic procedures that would not be appropriate for ambulatory surgery.

The value of educating our fellow specialists in proper patient selection is key. The surgeon or proceduralist and their office staff are the first line in patient selection and might begin to identify appropriate office and ambulatory patients versus hospital candidates.

Box 1-4. Absolute or relative contraindications for ambulatory surgery
- Procedure associated with significant blood loss or severe postoperative pain
- Acute concurrent illness
- Poorly compensated or incompletely evaluated systemic disease
- Severe systemic disease requiring invasive monitoring or intensive care follow-up
- Unstable ASA 3 or 4
- Inability or unwillingness to comply with preoperative or postoperative care instructions

Location of surgery

One of the decisions that may have to be made concerning elective procedures is to change the venue from a freestanding ambulatory facility to one that is located within a hospital or even to indicate a preference for postoperative overnight stay. There are no clear guidelines in this regard and these decisions are usually individualized based on the extent of the patient's medical status, postoperative care needs, and available support in their home environment. It is generally advised that patients with extensive and/or debilitating medical issues have their surgery done in an environment where full support, including postoperative admission, is readily available.

Logistics of the preanesthesia evaluation

Having established the need to obtain appropriate information prior to the day of surgery, the means by which this is done will vary considerably. Among the factors that govern these logistics are the nature of the medical system, the distance patients need to travel for visits, and, depending on the nature of the medical system, the extent to which patients are receiving appropriate primary and specialty care. In general, it is not necessary to require all patients to make a preoperative visit prior to the day of surgery, especially if they are healthy and having minor procedures. However, it should be remembered that while preanesthesia visits cost time and money for patients and facilities, these costs are small compared to the costs and inconvenience incurred with preventable delays and cancellations on the day of surgery. Adequate clinic staff and space should be reserved for these visits.

Information may be provided through a variety of formats. One option is a questionnaire (Table 1-11). Compliance with information requests is best obtained when the questionnaire is concise, includes check-offs, and is (preferably) no more than one page. It should be remembered that the questionnaire is an initial screen and does not have to include every aspect of the patient's past medical history; additional information can always be obtained on the basis of the screening data. Whether by questionnaire, Web-based application, or phone call, the establishment of a system will require extensive education of surgeons, primary care providers, and specialty consultants to establish familiarity and comfort with the system.

As Web-based medical informatics advances, the use of this medium will likely provide a robust area for patient-provider-system interaction.

Organizational structure

Several of the frustrations encountered in operating a preoperative center are ensuring appropriate communication about scheduling of cases, ensuring communication with patients and providers, dealing with frustrated colleagues who face a complex system, and maintaining a single set of coherent policies.

For these reasons, it is recommended that the system be organized with an identified medical director, an anesthesiologist, who assumes responsibility for the clinic. Depending on the size of the clinic, he/she should also be able to maintain a significant clinical schedule. However, it is important that hospital and facility administration and clinical staff have a point person with whom to work to ensure continuity of operations. It is also advised that the operating room and preoperative assessment system operate on a one-stop shopping model in which a single call to schedule a case for the operating room automatically

Table 1-11. An excerpt from a questionnaire used at the University of Cincinnati Medical Center

"HXPHY"

THE UNIVERSITY HOSPITAL
COMBINED SURGICAL/ANESTHESIA
PERIOPERATIVE HISTORY AND PHYSICAL
Page 2 of 4

ONGOING MEDICAL PROBLEMS / REVIEW OF SYSTEMS:

CARDIAC:

HTN	☐ Yes ☐ No	PND/Orthopnea	☐ Yes ☐ No
Hypercholesterolemia	☐ Yes ☐ No	Syncope	☐ Yes ☐ No
Angina / CAD / MI	☐ Yes ☐ No	Arrhythmia	☐ Yes ☐ No
CABG / PCI	☐ Yes ☐ No	Pacemaker	☐ Yes ☐ No
Edema	☐ Yes ☐ No	Valvular Dz:	☐ Yes ☐ No

Other/Comments:

10/05

Exercise Tolerance: (Check the appropriate level)

Mets   Activity
- ☐ 1   Eating, getting dressed, working at a desk.
- ☐ 2   Walking on a flat surface for one or two blocks.
- ☐ 4   Raking leaves, weeding or pushing a power mower.
- ☐ 5   Walking four miles per hour, social dancing, washing a car.
- ☐ 8   Moving heavy furniture, rapidly climbing stairs, carrying 20 pounds up stairs.
- ☐ 10   Brisk swimming, bicycling uphill, walking briskly uphill, jogging 6 mph (10 minute mile).
- ☐ 12   Running continuously at 8 mph (8-9 minute mile.)

Indications for subspecialty referral:

Uninvestigated new / change in SOB?	☐ Yes ☐ No
Uninvestigated new / changed PND / Orthopnea?	☐ Yes ☐ No
Uninvestigated new / changed chest pain?	☐ Yes ☐ No
Uninvestigated new / changed edema?	☐ Yes ☐ No
Uninvestigated new / changed sputum production or wheezing?	☐ Yes ☐ No
Uninvestigated syncope?	☐ Yes ☐ No
Uninvestigated significant hematologic disorder?	☐ Yes ☐ No

PULMONARY:

Asthma / COPD	☐ Yes ☐ No	Active / Recent wheezing	☐ Yes ☐ No
Home O2: 1pm	☐ Yes ☐ No	Recent URI / Bronchitis / pneumonia	☐ Yes ☐ No
Bronchodilator	☐ Yes ☐ No	Frequent cough	☐ Yes ☐ No
		Sleep apnea / Snoring	☐ Yes ☐ No
		CPAP Requiring	☐ Yes ☐ No

Other/Comments:

Source: Courtesy of Dr. Sean Josephs, Dr. Angela Bader, and Dr. Andrew Friedrich. Used with permission.

results in notification of the preoperative assessment area about the prospective patient. Such notice can be as complex as an intricate common information system or as simple as a faxed sheet for each scheduled case. Either way, physician and patient satisfaction is greatly enhanced by having a single source to go to for information.

Facilities

The space and staff committed to the appropriate preparation of patients should reflect the appropriate issues of safety and efficiency. Adequate space needs to be provided for patients to wait, be examined in a private congenial atmosphere, and receive proper education and counseling regarding their preoperative and postoperative care. Technical support with information systems and communications needs to be sufficient to handle the large volume of calls, faxed materials, and records that will inevitably flow through the system.

When possible, it is ideal to locate the preoperative screening area in close proximity to the operating suite to allow for optimal sharing of anesthesia staff and information and materials. However, if placement of the clinic compromises the clinical flow or poses an inconvenience for patients, these facilities are often located in an area of flow for the facility which allows for optimal use of laboratory and diagnostic facilities and is also close to the hospital entrance, minimizing the need for patients to interact with acute care operations.

Staff

There are as many models for staffing a preanesthesia area as there are unique environments in which they operate. The common element is that they have consistent clinical leadership and a dedicated clinical and administrative staff that understand the nuances of the process. It takes a rather large system to support a clinic where all patients are seen by anesthesiologists. Often, nurse practitioners, physician assistants, and other nursing staff can be educated about anesthesia issues to be able to successfully and efficiently screen and assess patients, with appropriate physician backup support. Over time, the personal relationships that this staff form with surgeons, other physicians, and facility staff are invaluable in the smooth and safe operation of the preoperative assessment process. Although this chapter focuses on the preanesthesia evaluation, the preoperative visit includes assessment and evaluation by nursing staff. Nursing staff use this opportunity to exchange information and to inform the patient about what to expect from the upcoming surgery, the duration of stay, the need for an adult escort for discharge, and the resources needed for postoperative care. In addition, the facility can identify special needs or potential challenges to be resolved before the day of surgery. Preoperative instructions are reviewed and often provided in writing and reinforced via telephone instructions. Regardless of the system selected, the process should be consistent in meeting the goals for quality preanesthesia evaluation and preparation.

Summary

There is a great deal of interest in safety in health care, and the surgical suite is perhaps one of the greatest areas of interest due to the potential for life-threatening risk. Nonetheless, the availability of appropriate risk assessment strategies is but in its infancy despite an exponential growth of ambulatory surgery. While there is reason to believe this growth has been conducted in a safe fashion, the increasing acuity of patients and procedures performed in a multiplicity of settings reinforce the need for a scientific determination of risk to aid clinicians and policy-makers alike in their work.

References

1. Saklad M. Grading of patients for surgical procedures. *Anesthesiology*. 1941;2:281–284.
2. Apfelbaum JL. Preoperative evaluation, laboratory screening, and selection of adult surgical outpatients in the 1990s. *Anesthesiol Rev*. 1990;17:4–12.
3. Meridy HW. Criteria for selection of ambulatory surgical patients and guidelines for anesthetic management: a retrospective study of 1553 cases. *Anesth Analg*. 1982;61: 921–926.
4. Pasternak LR. Preoperative evaluation of the ambulatory surgery patient. *Anesthesiology Report*. 1990;3:8.
5. Dripps RD, Lamont A, Eckenhoff JE. The role of anesthesia in surgical mortality. *JAMA*. 1961;178:261–266.
6. Marx GF, Mateo CV, Orkin LR. Computer analysis of postanesthetic deaths. *Anesthesiology*. 1973;39:54–58.
7. Carter DC, Campbell D. Evaluation of the risks of surgery. *Br Med Bull*. 1988;44:322–340.
8. Arens JF. Assessment and reduction of cardiovascular anesthetic risk. *Anesth Analg*. 1989:52–56.
9. Fowkes SC, Fowkes FGR, Lunn JN, Robertson IB, Samuel P. Epidemiology in anaesthesia III: factors affecting mortality in hospitals. *Br J Anaesth*. 1982; 54:811–816.
10. Grazer FM, de Jong RH. Fatal outcomes from liposuction: census survey of cosmetic surgeons. *Plast Reconstr Surg*. 2000;105:436–446.
11. Fleisher LA, Pasternak LR, Herbert R, Anderson GF. Inpatient hospital admission and death after outpatient surgery in elderly patients: importance of patient and system characteristics and location of care. *Arch Surg*. 2004;139:67–72.
12. American Society of Anesthesiologists Task Force on Preanesthesia Evaluation. Practice advisory for preanesthesia evaluation. *Anesthesiology*. 2002;96:485–496.
13. Eagle KA, Berger PB, Calkins H, et al. ACC/AHA Guideline Update for Perioperative Cardiovascular Evaluation for Noncardiac Surgery–Executive Summary. A report of the American College of Cardiology/American Heart Association Task Force on Practice Guidelines (Committee to Update the 1996 Guidelines on Perioperative Cardiovascular Evaluation for Noncardiac Surgery). *Anesth Analg*. 2002;94:1052–1064.

14. Olsen DM, Kane RL, Proctor PH. A controlled study of multiphasic screening. *N Engl J Med*. 1976;294:925–930.

15. Korvin CC, Pearce RH, Stanley J. Admissions screening: clinical benefits. *Ann Intern Med*. 1975;83:197–203.

16. Kaplan EB, Sheiner LB, Boeckmann AJ, et al. The usefulness of preoperative laboratory screening. *JAMA*. 1985;253:3576–3581.

17. Turnbull JM, Buck C. The value of preoperative screening investigations in otherwise healthy individuals. *Arch Intern Med*. 1987;147:1101–1105.

18. Kitz DS, Susarz-Ladden C, Lecky JH. Hospital resources used for inpatient and ambulatory surgery. *Anesthesiology*. 1988;69:383–386.

19. Fischer SP. Development and effectiveness of an anesthesia preoperative evaluation clinic in a teaching hospital. *Anesthesiology*. 1996;85:196–206.

20. Bryson GL, Wyand A, Bragg PR. Preoperative testing is inconsistent with published guidelines and rarely changes management. *Can J Anaesth*. 2006;53:236–241.

21. Yuan H, Chung F, Wong D, Edward R. Current preoperative testing practices in ambulatory surgery are widely disparate: a survey of CAS members. *Can J Anaesth*. 2005;52:675–679.

22. Olson RP, Stone A, Lubarsky D. The prevalence and significance of low preoperative hemoglobin in ASA 1 or 2 outpatient surgery candidates. *Anesth Analg*. 2005;101:1337–1340.

23. Fleisher LA. Routine laboratory testing in the elderly: is it indicated? *Anesth Analg*. 2001;93:249–250.

24. Zilva JF. Is unselective urine biochemical urine testing cost effective? *Br Med J (Clin Res Ed)*. 1985;291:323–325.

25. Lawrence VA, Gafni A, Gross M. The unproven utility of the preoperative urinalysis economic evaluation. *J Clin Epidemiol*. 1989;42:1185–1192.

26. Rucker L, Frye E, Staten MA. Usefulness of screening chest roentgenograms in preoperative patients. *JAMA*. 1983;250:3209–3211.

27. Charpak Y, Blery C, Chastang C, Szatan M, Fourgeaux B. Prospective assessment of a protocol for selective ordering of preoperative chest x-rays. *Can J Anaesth*. 1988;35:259–265.

28. Hackman T, Steward DJ. What is the value of preoperative hemoglobin determinations in pediatric outpatients? *Anesthesiology*. 1989;71:A1168.

29. O'Conner ME, Drasner K. Preoperative laboratory testing of children undergoing elective surgery. *Anesth Analg*. 1990;70:176–180.

30. Bold AM. Use and abuse of clinical chemistry in surgery. *Br Med J*. 1965;2:1051–1052.

31. Zibrak JD, O'Donnell CR, Marton K. Indications for pulmonary function testing. *Ann Intern Med*. 1990;112:763–771.

32. Schein OD, Katz J, Bass EB, et al. The value of routine preoperative medical testing before cataract surgery. *N Engl J Med*. 2000;342:168–175.

33. Guyatt G, Cairns J, Churchill D, et al. Evidence-based medicine. A new approach to teaching the practice of medicine. Evidence-Based Medicine Working Group. *JAMA*. 1992;268:2420–2425.

34. Mallampati SR, Gatt SP, Gugino LD, et al. A clinical sign to predict difficult tracheal intubation: a prospective study. *Can Anaesth Soc J*. 1985;32:429–434.

2. Minimally invasive and advanced ambulatory procedures

Shireen Ahmad, MD

Recent advancements in surgical techniques have resulted in shorter, less-invasive procedures, and newer anesthetic agents have facilitated rapid recovery with fewer adverse side effects. These improvements have resulted in a tremendous increase in the scope and extent of surgical procedures performed on an ambulatory basis in the last two decades. In addition, patients are better informed

Box 2-1. Factors that preclude performing advanced ambulatory surgery procedures in freestanding centers

Patient-related	Significant cardio-respiratory comorbidities: American Society of Anesthesiologists physical status III
Procedure-related	Specialized equipment Potential for major complications
Surgeon-related	Potential for extended duration of surgery

and are beginning to play an active role in their health care decisions and are demanding the type of highly efficient, streamlined care commonly associated with ambulatory facilities. Initially, only the less complex procedures were performed as ambulatory surgery, but the excellent safety record of ambulatory anesthesia has prompted surgeons to widen the range of procedures being conducted in ambulatory facilities (Box 2-1). This chapter will highlight surgical procedures not traditionally considered as ambulatory surgery and familiarize anesthesiologists with both the surgical and anesthesia considerations that will help promote and work toward safe clinical management for same-day discharge.

General surgery procedures

Biliary tract surgery

Laparoscopic cholecystectomy

The evolution of ambulatory laparoscopic cholecystectomy surgery is a good example of the process by which inpatient procedures come to be advanced and then routine ambulatory procedures. Initially, small select groups of patients were discharged home after the procedure, which has now come to be regarded as the "gold standard" for the treatment of cholelithiasis.[1,2] A prospective study of patients who had laparoscopic cholecystectomy in a simulated home setting in a hospital reported that all patients met discharge criteria within 6 hours of surgery. Ninety-four percent of patients required only oral analgesics; however, 12% of patients experienced postoperative nausea and vomiting requiring parenteral therapy and 3% required an additional day in the hospital.[3]

Considerations for ambulatory laparoscopic surgery

Preoperatively, patients must be evaluated to confirm that they are able to tolerate the cardiorespiratory effects of laparoscopy (Box 2-2). Patients must be kept warm with a heated forced-air blanket, and intravenous fluids should be warmed if needed to address hypothermia from insufflation of cold, dry gas. Local anesthetic infiltration of the laparoscopy portals will reduce somatic pain, and subdiaphragmatic injection may reduce the referred shoulder pain.

Box 2-2. Physiologic effects of laparoscopy

Effects of position	Trendelenberg: ↓ FRC, ↓ total lung capacity, ↓ compliance reverse Trendelenberg: ↓ preload, ↓ cardiac output
Ventilatory effects	Decreased FRC, FEV1, VC, compliance Increased airway pressure, alveolar-arterial O_2 gradient
Hemodynamic effects	Aortic compression: ↑ SVR, ↓ cardiac output Vena cava compression: ↓ preload, ↓ cardiac output
Vascular effects	Decreased hepatic, renal, mesenteric blood flow
Neurohumoral effects	Increased vasopressin, Renin, aldosterone, epinephrine, norepinephrine

FEV1, forced expiratory volume in 1 second; FRC, functional residual capacity; SVR, systemic vascular resistance; VC, vital capacity.

Nonsteroidal anti-inflammatory agents are routinely used as adjuncts to reduce opioid requirements. Pre-emptive multimodal antiemetic therapy will reduce the potentially high incidence of postoperative nausea and vomiting. Hemorrhage, pneumothorax, gas embolism, extra-abdominal emphysema, vascular, or visceral injury are rare complications.

Gastric surgery

Laparoscopic gastric banding

Gastric portioning procedures are devised to promote weight loss by decreasing the size of the gastric pouch and thereby limiting the amount of food ingested at one time. These patients frequently have a body mass index well in excess of $35–40 kg/m^2$, and specially sized gurneys, wheelchairs, operating tables, instrumentation, and moving devices are required to facilitate the proper care of these patients. Gastric banding has been performed in a freestanding ambulatory surgery center.[4] Patients need preoperative evaluation for cardiorespiratory and airway abnormalities associated with morbid obesity. Screening for obstructive sleep apnea is essential and these patients may not be suitable for ambulatory discharge (Figure 2-1).

Diabetes mellitus is common in obese patients, and perioperative control of blood sugar is essential. Liver function must be evaluated since it is often abnormal and results in altered drug metabolism.

An appropriately sized blood pressure cuff may provide accurate measurements, but more often optimum application is hindered by the shape of the patient's arms. A comparison of blood pressure measurement in obese patients by means of a standard-sized cuff on the forearm and upper arm revealed that the forearm blood pressure values are overestimated, but correlate, when compared to the upper arm.[5]

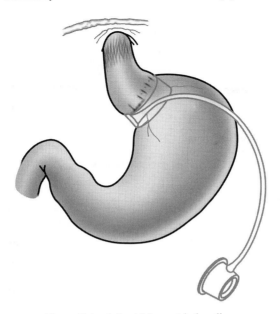

Figure 2-1. Adjustable gastric banding.

Aspiration prophylaxis is indicated and may include intravenous premedication with H_2 antagonists (ranitidine 50 mg), metoclopramide (10 mg), and sodium citrate 30 mL orally. Positioning of morbidly obese patients is essential to facilitate endotracheal intubation and ventilation. This includes elevation of the shoulders and occiput so that the head is in the "sniffing" position, and the use of a 30° reverse-Trendelenburg position will facilitate respiratory mechanics.[6] Thorough preoxygenation with attention to the expired oxygen concentration, which should be at least in the low- to mid-90% range, will prevent rapid desaturation during intubation.[7] If fiber-optic intubation is necessary, it is advisable to administer intravenous anticholinergic agents preoperatively to prevent interference with visualization due to excessive secretions. Because endotracheal tube displacement into the mainstem bronchus as a result of upward movement of the diaphragm and carina has been reported, endotracheal tube placement should be verified following insufflation of the abdomen with carbon dioxide and Trendelenberg position.[8]

Pharmacokinetics is altered in obese patients, and care must be exercised in dosing anesthetic agents (Box 2-3). Dosage based on corrected body weight (CBW) has been proposed[9] using the following calculation: CBW = ideal body weight + [0.4 × excess body weight].

Remifentanil has been shown to facilitate early recovery in obese patients undergoing laparoscopy[10] and also would be suitable for gastric banding procedures, in which postoperative pain is minimal and small doses of morphine or hydromorphone can be used following the discontinuation of the remifentanil infusion. Recovery after desflurane has also been shown to be more rapid

Box 2-3. Pharmacokinetic/pharmacodynamic alterations in obesity

Midazolam	↑ V_D, ↑ clearance	Dose by ABW
Propofol	↓ V_D, ↓ clearance	Dose by ABW
Fentanyl, sufentanil	↑ V_D, ↑ clearance	Dose by ABW
Remifentanil	↑ Clearance, ↓ V_D	Dose by IBW
Succinylcholine	↑ Plasma cholinesterase	Dose by ABW
Rocuronium	↓ V_D, ↓ clearance	Dose by IBW
Cisatracurium, atracurium	Clearance, V_D unchanged	Dose by ABW

ABW, actual body weight; IBW, ideal body weight; V_D, volume of distribution. Adapted from Casati et al.[56] © Elsevier. Used with permission.

compared to propofol or isoflurane.[11] Postoperative complications requiring hospital admission in a group of 343 ambulatory patients included nausea (1), bloody nasogastric drainage (1), and esophageal spasm (1).

Esophageal surgery

Laparoscopic fundoplication

Laparoscopic antireflux surgery is performed to relieve symptoms of gastro-esophageal reflux in patients who want to discontinue long-term medications or who get only partial relief or experience adverse side effects from the medication. The Nissen fundoplication has a greater than 80% success rate. It has been reported that the procedure has been performed on an ambulatory basis with 98% of patients being discharged 4 hours after surgery.[12] (Figure 2-2).

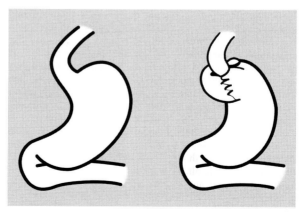

Figure 2-2. Nissen fundoplication.

Preoperatively, patients should be carefully evaluated for evidence of recurrent aspiration pneumonia. There is a risk of regurgitation and aspiration with induction of anesthesia. Intravenous premedication with H_2 antagonists (ranitidine 50 mg), metoclopramide (10 mg), and sodium citrate 30 mL orally should be considered.

The surgery is performed with general anesthesia. Due to the risk of aspiration on induction, either awake fiber-optic intubation or rapid sequence induction is employed. Postoperatively, in addition to standard discharge criteria, patients are required to demonstrate the ability to swallow sips of water without vomiting, and on the first postoperative day, patients undergo a gastrograffin swallow test to demonstrate absence of leakage.

Laparoscopic splenectomy

Splenectomy is indicated in the management of a variety of hematological diseases such as purpura, lymphoma, leukemia, sarcoidosis, or myelofibrosis. The surgery is performed laparoscopically if the spleen is of normal size or only moderately enlarged. Recently, it has been reported to have been performed successfully in a small group of ambulatory patients.[13] Patients are positioned in the left lateral decubitus position, and pressure points should be carefully padded and protected. In addition to routine complications of laparoscopy, blood loss is typically in the range of 750 to 1,000 mL, and adequate intravenous access is essential for prompt replacement.

Breast surgery

Mammoplasty

Reduction mammoplasty is performed to reduce the breast size by removal of breast tissue, usually in the range of 200 to 1,000 grams. Many of these patients are morbidly obese and should be carefully screened preoperatively for comorbidities, especially the presence of obstructive sleep apnea. Augmentation mammoplasty consists of the insertion of prosthesis above or below the pectoral muscle and may be performed for cosmetic reasons in normal patients or in patients who have undergone surgery for breast cancer. In the patient with cancer, it is important to determine the type of chemotherapeutic agents that these patients might have received. The alkylating agents are associated with pulmonary toxicity, adriamycin causes cardiomyopathy, and methotrexate may produce renal and hepatic dysfunction. Establishing intravenous access in these patients may be quite challenging since many of these agents cause thrombophlebitis and the new veins that develop are small and tortuous. Inhalation induction may be a desirable alternative in these cases.

Both general and local anesthesia have been used for these procedures. Patients are usually in the sitting position during surgery and for the application of the dressings at the end of surgery. Postoperatively, submuscular breast augmentation results in significantly more postoperative pain than subglandular insertion of the prosthesis. The pain is thought to be related to pectoralis muscle spasm, may last up to a week after surgery, and limits movement of the arm. Patients may require opioid analgesics following surgery; however, the use of continuous paravertebral catheters for infusion of local anesthetics has been shown to be an effective alternative. Patients have less postoperative pain, require less analgesics and antiemetics, have less restriction of arm movement, and can be discharged home within a few hours of the completion of surgery.[14] The complication rate following paravertebral blocks is low (in the range of 2.6% to 5%).[15] There is a potential risk of epidural spread of local anesthetic, local anesthetic toxicity, and pneumothorax. These complications, though rare, must be kept in mind in the ambulatory surgery patient who may not develop the signs and symptoms until after discharge. Therefore, this type of analgesia requires careful patient selection, preoperative education, a dedicated home caregiver, detailed written discharge instructions, ready access to the health care facility, and the ability of the patient to communicate effectively with the physician at all times.

Mastectomy

The transition to more breast-conserving procedures with less postoperative morbidity has resulted in a steady increase in ambulatory surgery for breast cancer. Procedures performed as ambulatory surgery include complete mastectomy (8%–22%), subtotal mastectomy (43%–72%), and lumpectomy (78%–88%).[16] A review of mastectomies performed in Florida in 1994 revealed that of a total of 5,418 surgeries, 1,089 had been ambulatory surgeries and the readmission rate was only 1.3%.[17] The variables that were associated with an increased odds of having mastectomy on an ambulatory basis were age (1% for each year), low incidence of comorbidities, higher level of income, nonurban (outside urban area or in rural area) residence, lack of insurance coverage, and the type of surgery. It has also been reported that patients who underwent ambulatory mastectomy manifested better emotional adjustment and fewer psychological distress symptoms than those who had been inpatients following surgery.[18]

Patients with breast cancer who have received preoperative radiation and/or chemotherapy need to be assessed preoperatively for the cardiopulmonary side effects of these treatments. Breast cancer often metastasizes to the brain, and alteration in mental status should be carefully evaluated.

Surgery may be performed with a combination of local anesthesia and intravenous sedation/analgesia, paravertebral somatic blocks, or general anesthesia. Pressure dressings are applied at the end of the procedure, and the patient may be required to sit up for the application. Due to interruption of nerves to the chest wall, postoperative pain following mastectomy may be less than expected. Axillary surgery may be more painful due to proximity to the shoulder joint and the presence of a drainage tube that moves with arm motion. Continuous paravertebral blocks with an indwelling catheter and infusion of local anesthetic (0.2% ropivacaine) offer an alternative to inpatient admission for the sole purpose of analgesic therapy.[19]

Endocrine surgery

Thyroidectomy

Thyroidectomy may be performed for benign conditions such as goiter, hyperthyroidism and benign nodules, or malignancy. Though not a common practice, ambulatory thyroidectomy was reported several years ago. Patients were discharged on the day of surgery following evaluation by the surgeon, with telephone follow-up on the evening of surgery and an office visit the next day.[20] More recently, there has been a renewed interest in performing these procedures on an ambulatory basis.[21]

Thyroid function tests need to be reviewed preoperatively for evidence of hyper- or hypothyroidism. Since myxedema coma is associated with a greater than 50% mortality rate, severely hypothyroid patients require thyroid replacement prior to surgery. Intraoperatively, thyroid storm can be mistaken for malignant hyperthermia (Box 2-4). A computed tomography (CT) scan of the neck is necessary to evaluate the airway since large goiters may give rise to tracheal compression or deviation. Vocal cord function must be evaluated prior to discharge since postoperative airway obstruction may occur due to damage to the recurrent laryngeal nerve, hematoma formation, or tracheomalacia. For this reason, this procedure is probably not suitable for freestanding facilities.

Adrenalectomy

Adrenalectomy is performed for tumors or benign hyperplasia. The extension of laparoscopic surgery to adrenalectomy has allowed the procedure to be performed on an ambulatory basis.[22] Whereas patients with pheochromocytomas are not suitable for ambulatory surgery, those with Cushing syndrome (hyperadrenocorticism) and Conn syndrome (hyperaldosteronism) may be but will need careful evaluation of their cardiac and renal function prior to surgery. Serum electrolyte levels need to be verified to rule out hypernatremia and hypokalemia which will require correction. Surgery is performed with general anesthesia, and a multimodal approach to pain and nausea and vomiting prophylaxis facilitates timely discharge.

Box 2-4. Intraoperative signs and symptoms

Thyroid storm	Malignant hyperthermia
Tachycardia	Tachycardia
Arrhythmias	$\uparrow CO_2$, $\downarrow SaO_2$
$\uparrow$ Temperature	$\uparrow$ Temperature
Sweating	Metabolic acidosis

SaO_2, oxygen saturation.

Neurosurgical procedures

Intracranial neurosurgery

Stereotactic techniques allow the neurosurgeon to precisely localize brain lesions and perform "awake" craniotomies with sedation/analgesia on an outpatient basis.[23,24] These procedures may require the fixation of a frame to the head or radiologically visible markers called fiducials to be fixed to the scalp and forehead with adhesive. Once the frame or markers are attached, a magnetic resonance imaging (MRI) or CT scan is obtained to determine stereotactic coordinates, after which the frame or fiducial markers must not be moved until the procedure is completed. The "key" for removal of the frame must be readily available at all times in the event of an airway emergency (Figure 2-3).

This technique allows biopsy of deep lesions,[25] functional surgery for movement disorders[26], and noninvasive radiation for brain lesions.[27] If the procedure is to be performed with general anesthesia, fiber-optic intubation may be necessary to avoid manipulation of the frame. However, the procedures are usually

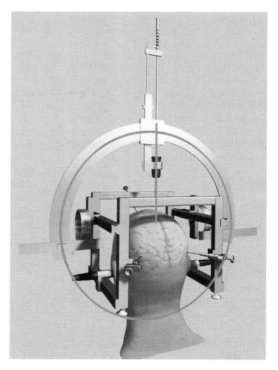

Figure 2-3. Stereotactic frame in position.

performed with local infiltration and sedation/analgesia since the patient must be conversant at all times. Small doses of midazolam and a continuous infusion of propofol together with fentanyl or remifentanil may be used for sedation. During deep brain stimulation, propofol and dopaminergic agonists and antagonists (metoclopramide and droperidol) should be avoided.

Postoperative pain is usually minimal, but nausea and vomiting may be significant, and prophylactic antiemetics should always be administered. Patients are observed until they are able to ambulate and tolerate oral intake and are evaluated by the neurosurgeon prior to discharge. In most cases, patients receive a follow-up visit by a home care nurse later the same day. Postoperative bleeding is the most common complication and usually presents within the first 6 hours or more than 24 hours postoperatively. Patients are discharged with explicit instructions to contact the surgeon and return to the emergency room if specific signs or symptoms develop. For this reason, adequate support at home and access to the hospital for readmission are important selection criteria for performing these surgeries on an ambulatory basis. These procedures are usually performed in hospital-based centers due to the specialized equipment needs and potential complications.

Spinal neurosurgery

Microdiscectomy and percutaneous discectomy are minimally invasive procedures for decompression of the lumbar nerve roots and are performed to relieve radicular irritation due to herniated lumbar discs. Several studies have demonstrated the feasibility of performing these procedures on an outpatient basis.[28,29] A small incision is made over the proposed interspace, the soft tissue is displaced to expose the ligamentum flavum which is removed, the nerve root is retracted, and the disc material is removed.

Preoperatively, neurologic findings should be carefully documented. Patients are frequently on nonsteroidal anti-inflammatory agents or aspirin, and hematologic status may need to be evaluated. Microdiscectomy may be performed under local anesthesia with sedation or regional or general anesthesia. Percutaneous discectomies are usually performed only with sedation/analgesia to allow the patient to inform the surgeon of inadvertent nerve root contact, which is usually extremely painful. Sedation/analgesia with a small dose of midazolam and low-dose propofol infusion, supplemented with an opioid, will result in a comfortable but arousable patient.

Subarachnoid block with tetracaine (10–14 mg) or bupivacaine (8–12 mg) may also be used for this surgery. A group of patients who underwent microdiscectomy with subarachnoid block (isobaric 0.5% bupivacaine) combined with wound infiltration had lower pain scores and analgesic requirements compared to those who had received general anesthesia.[30]

Postoperatively, there is a high incidence of moderate to severe pain (34%), vomiting is in the range of 9.5%, and the unanticipated admission rate is approximately 5.7%.[31] Patients are discharged once standard discharge criteria are met and postoperative examination by the neurosurgeon has been performed. Major vascular injury is a rare complication (1.6 per 10,000) that, if not recognized intraoperatively, will be identified in the postanesthesia care unit. Urinary retention may occur postoperatively, and for this reason all patients are required to void prior to discharge. The role of the surgical procedure in the etiology of this complication is unclear. However, the factors predictive of early postoperative failure to void have been found to be age of more than or equal to 50 years, intraoperative fluid administration of more than or equal to 750 mL, and bladder volume of more than or equal to 270 mL on admission to the postanesthesia care unit.[32]

Ophthalmic procedures

Vitreoretinal surgery

Although the great majority of ophthalmic surgeries are performed on an ambulatory basis, vitreoretinal surgeries have traditionally been considered inpatient procedures. However, there is a recent trend toward ambulatory vitreoretinal surgery. There is a suggestion that outcomes may be improved in ambulatory patients due to greater vigilance in maintenance of special positioning postoperatively by supportive family members as compared to busy hospital nurses.[33] Vitreoretinal surgery is performed for repair of retinal detachment, vitreous hemorrhage, macular epiretinal membrane peeling, posterior segment foreign bodies, and trauma. The surgery may involve scleral buckling, vitrectomy, gas–fluid exchange, and injection of vitreous substitutes. The scleral buckle is an extraocular surgery and consists of suturing a silicone rubber appliance to the sclera to indent the eye and functionally close the retinal tear. Vitrectomy is an intraocular procedure and consists of partial or complete removal of the vitreous and introduction of saline, perfluorocarbon gas, or silicone oil in exchange.

Preoperatively, a thorough evaluation of the cardiac and renal status is essential since patients may have received acetazolamide or mannitol preoperatively to decrease intraocular pressure (IOP). Rapid infusion of mannitol may precipitate congestive heart failure and electrolyte abnormalities and possibly myocardial ischemia. Acetazolamide also inhibits renal carbonic anhydrase, and patients receiving it may be acidotic, hypokalemic, and hyponatremic. Many patients undergoing retinal surgery are diabetic and are at increased risk for aspiration if they have gastroparesis. These patients will also require close monitoring of their blood sugar in order to maintain it within the normal range perioperatively.

Retinal surgery may be performed under regional or general anesthesia. Nitrous oxide is usually avoided since the ophthalmologist may inject hexafluoride (SF_6) or perfluoropropane (C_3F_8) into the posterior chamber and diffusion of nitrous oxide into the gas bubble may cause a dramatic increase in IOP which may compromise retinal blood flow. The gas is absorbed very slowly, and if the patient undergoes subsequent general anesthesia, nitrous oxide should be avoided for several days following air injection (Box 2-5).

Postoperatively, the most common reason cited for admission has been pain and nausea. These symptoms are more severe in the presence of increased IOP (>40 mm Hg) or with scleral buckling[34] and may be minimized by the preemptive administration of antiemetics and the use of regional anesthetic blocks.

Box 2-5. Intravitreal gas absorption	
Air	5 days
SF_6	10 days
C_3F_8	15–30 days

Thoracic procedures

Mediastinoscopy

Mediastinoscopy is performed to diagnose mediastinal masses and to sample lymph nodes in order to stage pulmonary tumors. The procedure involves the introduction of a short endoscope into the anterior mediastinum through a small incision in the suprasternal notch. The proximity of major vascular structures is associated with the potential for massive hemorrhage, and the presence of superior vena cava (SVC) obstruction may give rise to markedly distorted anatomy. Nonetheless, in one large series of 1,015 ambulatory mediastinoscopies, only 10 patients experienced postoperative complications that required hospitalization.[35] These included supraventricular arrhythmias and postoperative myocardial ischemia and were related to pre-existing comorbidities rather than the surgery.

The anesthetic management of patients undergoing this procedure presents several challenges. Preoperatively, patients must be evaluated for significant SVC obstruction by checking the blood pressure in both upper extremities, and the equipment for invasive blood monitoring should be available. If SVC obstruction is present, the blood pressure in the right arm will be significantly lower than in the left. Airway compression may present and is manifested by an inability to lay supine or by wheezing or stridor. A preoperative CT scan or MRI will be necessary to confirm these conditions. These patients may not be suitable for ambulatory discharge.

In the case of a large mass, a large bore intravenous catheter should be inserted in the lower extremity. Patients with lung cancer may have myasthenic syndrome, and neuromuscular blockade should be carefully monitored. Postoperative pain is well controlled with oral analgesics. Hoarseness has been reported following this procedure, and laryngeal nerve damage may require reintubation.[36] Less common (0.01%–0.6%) but serious vascular injuries include damage to the pulmonary artery, SVC, azygos vein, aortic arch, and its branches and require immediate thoracotomy. Tracheal and bronchial injury also require operative repair.[37]

Thoracoscopy

Developments in video-assisted thoracoscopic surgery have revolutionized thoracic surgery. The procedure is used to diagnose and treat pleural or parenchymal lung disease, mediastinal masses, and pericardial disease. Thoracoscopy has been used for treatment of pneumothorax due to apical blebs, Heller

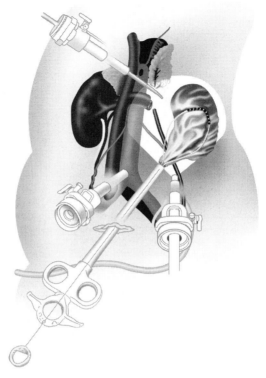

Figure 2-4. Laparoscopic nephrectomy.

myotomy, and upper dorsal sympathectomy. The procedure is associated with fewer cardiopulmonary sequelae than thoracotomy but does require intraoperative one-lung ventilation (Figure 2-4).

A report of patients who underwent the surgery as outpatients indicates that 72.5% were discharged home on the day of surgery and 22.5% the next day (within 23 hours of surgery).[38] Reasons for admission included conversion to open thoracotomy and surgery performed late in the day.

Preoperative pulmonary function tests are an integral part of patient evaluation and predict postoperative pulmonary dysfunction. A forced vital capacity of less than 50%, a forced expiratory volume in one second of less than 50%, a maximal breathing capacity of less than 50%, or a residual volume to total lung capacity ratio greater than 50% are all associated with a high risk of significant postoperative morbidity and mortality.

Regional anesthesia may be used for this procedure and consists of a combination of intercostal nerve blocks, stellate ganglion block, and paravertebral block. Most frequently, however, general anesthesia is used with double-lumen tubes or bronchial blockers to facilitate lung isolation and visualization of the thoracic cavity.

Following closure of the port sites and placement of the chest tube, the collapsed lung is gently reinflated with gradually increasing tidal volumes. The chest tube can be safely removed within 90 minutes of surgery and results in a marked reduction in postoperative pain and analgesic requirements. In most healthy patients, postoperative pain is controlled with nonsteroidal anti-inflammatory drugs and opioid analgesics. Epidural analgesia is used in those patients who have significant cardiac or pulmonary disease. Postoperative complications include hemorrhage, airway obstruction, and air embolism.

Limited thoracotomy

Outpatient open-lung biopsy in non-oxygen-dependent patients has been reported.[39] Lung biopsies are often required to make a definitive diagnosis in patients with interstitial lung diseases. The surgeries are performed with general anesthesia. All patients had a chest radiograph prior to transfer to the day surgery unit and were discharged home several hours later with oral analgesics. Avoidance of rib retractors and a chest tube will minimize postoperative pain and facilitate discharge. The authors stress that patient selection and technical aspects of the surgery are critical to the successful outcome of the surgery. In view of the potential complications and special monitoring needs, mediastinoscopies, thoracoscopies, and limited thoracotomies are not suitable for freestanding ambulatory centers.

Cardiovascular procedures

Cardiac surgery

Video-assisted thoracoscopy has been used to facilitate the interruption of a patent ductus arteriosus.[40] Patients ranged in age from several days to 50 years of age. In the non-neonate group, 18 patients were discharged on the day of surgery, whereas 6 were observed overnight in the day surgery unit and one was admitted because of small size and a history of premature birth. The 50-year-old patient was admitted because of the presence of subcutaneous emphysema related to a bronchial injury following double-lumen endobronchial tube placement.

A recent report of coronary artery bypass grafting in awake patients described 12 patients who underwent median sternotomy and revascularization with thoracic epidural anesthesia.[41] The average procedural time was 98.2 ± 19.8 minutes, and intermediate care stay was 4.9 ± 0.6 hours. Although all patients recovered well, they remained hospitalized for 7.8 ± 0.5 days due to reimbursement regulations. The authors concluded that with further refinement of the procedure, outpatient coronary artery bypass surgery may be feasible! The growth in percutaneous coronary intervention has eclipsed the number of interventions performed by a surgical approach overall, because of the less invasive nature of the revascularization procedure with less procedural mortality and morbidity. These procedures are performed with local anesthesia and mild sedation, and the patients are discharged home after a day's observation and return to work in a week. The introduction of drug-eluting stents has addressed the problem with restenosis, and it is speculated that the role of surgical coronary revascularization will continue to decrease as a proportionate share of total revascularization procedures.

Vascular surgery

Carotid endarterectomy

Carotid endarterectomy is one of the most common vascular surgeries and is now being added to the list of ambulatory surgeries, with patients being discharged following an 8-hour observation period.[42] Thirty-two percent of patients were discharged on the day of surgery and did not experience any adverse sequelae. The surgeons commented that another 34% of patients could have been discharged if their surgery had been scheduled for earlier in the day.

There are two types of patients who undergo carotid surgery: those who have suffered a series of transient ischemic attacks and those who have had strokes. The carotid artery is approached through an incision in the neck, and following administration of heparin, the internal, external, and common carotid arteries are clamped, the vessel is opened to remove the thrombus, and arteriotomy is closed. Heparin effect may be reversed with protamine. In some cases, an indwelling shunt may be used to maintain carotid blood flow during the period of arterial occlusion.

Preoperatively, a careful cardiovascular examination must be conducted. Blood pressure must be measured in both arms, and if there is a difference, it should be measured in the arm with the higher values during and after surgery. A preoperative electrocardiogram is mandatory since at least 1% of patients will have a myocardial infarction postoperatively. It is important to evaluate the effect of hyperextension and lateral rotation of the neck on neurologic symptoms since occlusion of compromised vertebral-basilar flow due to head positioning may result in perioperative cerebral ischemia. Platelet function may be altered in patients who have been on chronic aspirin therapy. Preoperative sedatives should be avoided since they may make it difficult to evaluate neurologic status in the immediate postoperative period.

The combination of superficial and deep cervical plexus block has been used for this surgery. There is some evidence that local anesthesia is associated with a lower incidence of shunting and less hemodynamic instability.[43] The patient's mental status serves as a monitor of the cerebral function during the period of arterial occlusion in these cases. Local anesthetic blockade of the phrenic nerve occurs in all patients undergoing cervical plexus block, and brachial plexus blockade is not an infrequent occurrence.

When general anesthesia is employed, short-acting agents are preferred to allow for evaluation of the neurological status of the patient immediately following surgery. General anesthetics have a cerebral protective effect by decreasing the cerebral metabolic rate and redistributing blood flow to ischemic areas. General anesthesia also blunts the stress response to crossclamping the carotid artery.

Cerebral perfusion monitoring plays an important role when carotid endarterectomy surgery is performed under general anesthesia. Electroencephalography (EEG) is considered to be the standard for monitoring patients undergoing carotid endarterectomy. However, EEG may fail to identify small areas of focal ischemia. Transcranial Doppler is a noninvasive method of monitoring the blood flow in middle cerebral artery and detecting microemboli. Measurement of stump pressure is used to clinically evaluate the adequacy of cerebral perfusion. Cerebral ischemia rarely occurs when the stump pressure is greater than 60 mm Hg. Many of the procedures performed on an ambulatory basis were performed with regional anesthesia, with the patient's mental status serving as a monitor of the cerebral function.

Circulatory instability is common postoperatively and frequently requires pharmacologic therapy. This is related to the loss of normal carotid baroreceptor function which results in hypertension. Loss of chemoreceptor activity also occurs and results in the loss of the normal ventilatory response to hypoxia. Evidence of new neurological findings postoperatively will require emergent cerebral angiography and re-exploration if an intimal flap is suspected.

Gynecologic procedures

Hysterectomy

Hysterectomy is the second most common surgery performed in the United States; approximately 633,000 are performed each year. Vaginal hysterectomy has been associated with fewer complications and shorter hospital stays than abdominal hysterectomy, whereas laparoscopic hysterectomy (which is less painful) has shortened hospitalization further[44,45] and has actually been performed on an ambulatory basis.[46,47] The usual ambulatory procedure is a laparoscopic-assisted vaginal hysterectomy, in which the uterine attachments are freed up laparoscopically and the procedure is completed vaginally. Other variants include total laparoscopic hysterectomy in which the entire surgery is performed through the laparoscope with morcellation and a subtotal laparoscopic hysterectomy which is a supracervical hysterectomy. Many patients have a significant history of uterine bleeding and may be anemic. The procedure is performed with general anesthesia, with patients in the dorsal lithotomy position and often in steep Trendelenberg to displace the abdominal structures.

Complications include acute hemorrhage, perforation of a viscus, and extra-abdominal insufflation such as subcutaneous emphysema, pneumothorax, pneumopericardium, or gas emboli. Carbon dioxide is quickly absorbed, and there is usually no major physiologic compromise.

Urologic procedures

Nephrectomy

Nephrectomies may be performed for benign or malignant conditions and consist of removal of the kidney and a small portion of the ureter or more extensive procedures as in the case of the radical surgery with pelvic lymph node dissection. Advances in laparoscopic surgery have extended to urologic procedures, and urinary diversions, nephrectomy, and nephroureterectomy are performed with this technique. In a series of 51 children who underwent a variety of urologic procedures, 86% of the children were discharged home 7 hours after surgery.[48] The children all received a caudal block (0.25% bupivacaine with 1:200,000 epinephrine), local infiltration of the wound (0.25% bupivacaine), and ketorolac prior to the end of surgery. Another group of 26 children between the ages of 4 months and 11 years underwent laparoscopic nephrectomy with general anesthesia.[49] The mean surgery time was 165 minutes and postoperative analgesic requirements were minimal: six patients received no postoperative morphine but instead were given 0.9 mg/kg of codeine. Three of the children were discharged home 6 hours following their surgery.

Laparoscopic nephrectomies are performed with the patient in the lateral decubitus position, and all pressure points must be protected. In addition, small children must be secured to prevent movement with tilting of the operating table. Considerations for children undergoing laparoscopy are similar to those in adults and have already been described.

Prostatectomy

Transurethral resection of the prostate

Transurethral resection of the prostate (TURP) is performed for benign disease unless the gland is very large. The transurethral resection has been successfully performed as an ambulatory procedure in a freestanding facility.[50] A total of 58 patients had surgery performed with spinal (39 subjects) and general (19 subjects) anesthesia. There were two readmissions, one for tachycardia and one for a fever.

Patients undergoing this surgery are generally elderly with pre-existing medical problems and need careful evaluation and medical optimization preoperatively. Renal function may be impaired due to chronic obstruction, and mental function should be assessed preoperatively in order to allow accurate interpretation of possible perioperative changes due to hyponatremia. Surgery is performed in the lithotomy position, and patients should be positioned carefully and pressure points padded. Regional anesthesia is often preferred because it allows early detection of TURP syndrome by evaluation of mental changes. Considerable bleeding may occur during resection, and large-bore intravenous catheters are necessary for replacement of blood and fluids. Postoperatively, in patients who have had spinal anesthesia, the Foley catheter should be removed only after return of perianal sensation, motor control, and proprioception. Photoselective vaporization of the prostate (PVP) offers a less invasive approach to removing enlarged benign prostate tissue. It combines the effectiveness of TURP, the surgical "gold standard" with the safety, comfort, and ease of a therapeutic alternative. The GreenLight laser system uses a very high-powered "green laser" that absorbs hemoglobin which immediately vaporizes and precisely removes enlarged prostate tissue, reducing any bleeding or the need for large-volume irrigation solutions. Most patients return home a few short hours after the PVP procedure and can return to normal, nonstrenuous activities within days. General anesthesia is used for the procedure because of the discomfort the patient experiences during the laser procedure.

Radical prostatectomy

Prostate cancer is the most commonly diagnosed cancer type in men, affecting about one eighth of the male population of the United States. Radical prostatectomy may be performed by a retropubic or perineal approach. As a result of advances in technology, the procedure may be performed on an ambulatory basis in patients with localized tumors.[51] In a series of 40 patients who underwent retropubic prostatectomy, 80% were discharged on the day of surgery. Patients received extensive preoperative education, and all patients were visited at home by a nurse on the night of surgery. Postoperative pain control is the main reason for hospitalization following prostatectomy, and the authors described a "pelvic block" at the bladder neck and base and along the muscle and fascia, which resulted in sufficient analgesia that no additional postoperative analgesia was required and patients were discharged with oral analgesics.

Radical perineal prostatectomy is less painful and has been performed as an ambulatory procedure with concurrent laparoscopic pelvic lymph node dissection.[52] Ninety-one patients who underwent this surgery were discharged home within 23 hours of the procedure. As with the previous group, these patients received extensive preoperative education and care was standardized by institution of a clinical pathway. All patients were contacted the next day by telephone for follow-up.

General or regional anesthesia may be used, but general anesthesia is preferred if laparoscopic lymph node dissection is planned. Blood transfusion may be necessary with larger prostate glands (more than 30 g). Postoperative peroneal nerve injury has been documented due to high lithotomy position, and patients should be evaluated for this complication after surgery.

Orthopedic procedures

The growth in ambulatory orthopedic surgery has gone hand in hand with the advances in regional analgesic techniques.

Shoulder arthroplasty

Shoulder joint replacement with special implants is performed for severe arthritis or following trauma. Patients presenting for this surgery who have rheumatoid arthritis must be screened for other joint involvement, including occult subluxation of the cervical spines and cricoarytenoid joint involvement, which may manifest as hoarseness. Bony deformities may make positioning difficult and also complicate endotracheal intubation. Surgery is performed in the sitting position, and accurate blood pressure monitoring is crucial. General and regional anesthesia have both been used for the procedure. The surgery has traditionally required hospital admission for postoperative pain control, but continuous perineural infusion with portable infusion pumps has resulted in the procedure being added to the long list of orthopedic surgeries that are performed on an ambulatory basis.[53]

Hip arthroplasty

Hip arthroplasty is a proven treatment for advanced arthritis. Improvements in prostheses and surgical techniques have resulted in shorter hospitalizations and more rapid rehabilitation. Minimally invasive arthroplasty has resulted in decreased blood loss and postoperative pain so that patients have been able to leave the facility within 12 hours of surgery[54] (Figure 2-5). Patients are generally elderly and must be screened preoperatively for comorbidities. Evaluation of cardiac status may be difficult because pain associated with arthritis often limits activity, and pharmacologic stress testing may be necessary in patients suspected of having significant coronary artery disease. Surgery is performed with general or regional anesthesia, with the patient in the lateral decubitus position. Care should be exercised in positioning the patient with supports for the neck, axilla, and upper limbs. Deliberate hypotension will reduce the blood loss during surgery.

Complications include bleeding, nerve damage, and embolization of air, fat, bone, and cement during insertion of the femoral component. Patients are routinely anticoagulated postoperatively to prevent deep venous thrombosis, which

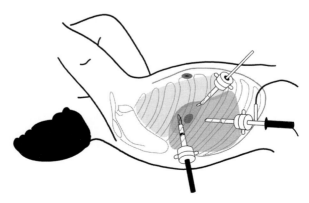

Figure 2-5. Thoracoscopic surgery.

has an impact on the choice of postoperative analgesic technique. In most reports of ambulatory arthroplasty, oral analgesics were used following discharge.

Aesthetic surgery procedures

Abdominoplasty

Abdominoplasty is a common body contouring surgery that may be fairly extensive, consisting of elevation of skin and fat flaps up to the costal margins, umbilical translocation, and musculofascial plication. Patients undergoing abdominoplasty procedures may be healthy or morbidly obese. Obese patients need to be screened for obstructive sleep apnea and other common comorbidities such as hypertension and type II diabetes mellitus. They may require aspiration prophylaxis. Pharmacokinetics is altered in morbidly obese patients, and sedative and opioid medications should be administered with care.

The procedure is usually performed on an inpatient basis; however, a recent publication described a series of 18 ambulatory patients, 16 of whom had their surgery in an office surgery suite under general anesthesia.[55] All patients received premedication with a COX-2 (cyclooxygenase-2) inhibitor and local anesthetic infiltration at the completion of surgery. Postoperatively, patients were prescribed oral opioids and oral diazepam for discomfort. There were no major complications in the ambulatory group; however, careful patient and facility selection was stressed. (See Chapter 11 for further discussion of office-based abdominoplasty).

Summary

The range of ambulatory surgical procedures continues to grow as pressure to reduce health care costs increases from the federal government, businesses, insurance providers, and patients. This review of the more extensive surgeries that are being introduced to the ambulatory arena is presented together with the special features of these procedures in order to guide the anesthesiologist who will be involved in the management of patients undergoing these surgeries as they become commonplace. It is critical for physicians to control the clinical decisions that affect the safety of our patients, and the involvement of the anesthesiologist in all stages of the perioperative care of this expanding patient population is the key to a successful ambulatory outcome.

References

1. Lillemoe KD, Lin JW, Talamini MA, Yeo CF, Snyder DS, Parker SD. Laparoscopic cholecystectomy as a "true" outpatient procedure: initial experience in 130 consecutive patients. *J Gastrointest Surg.* 1999;3:44–49.

2. Lau H, Brooks DC. Predictive factors for unanticipated admissions after laparoscopic cholecystectomy. *Arch Surg.* 2001;136:1150–1153.

3. Fleisher LA, Yee K, Lillemoe KD, et al. Is outpatient laparoscopic cholecystectomy safe and cost effective? A model to study transition of care. *Anesthesiology.* 1999;90:1746–1755.

4. Watkins BM, Montgomery KF, Ahroni JH, Erlitz MD, Abrams RE, Scurlock JE. Adjustable gastric banding in an ambulatory surgery center. *Obes Surg.* 2005;15:1045–1049.

5. Pierin AMG, Alavarce DC, Gusmao JL, Halpern A, Mion D. Blood pressure measurement in obese patients: comparison between upper arm and forearm measurements. *Blood Press Monit.* 2004;9:101–105.

6. Brodsky J, Lemmens H, Brock-Utne J, John G, Saidman LJ, Levitan R. Anesthetic considerations for bariatric surgery: proper positioning is important for laryngoscopy. *Anesth Analg.* 2003;96:1841–1842.

7. Boyce J, Ness T, Castroman P, Gleysteen J. A preliminary study of the optimal anesthesia positioning for the morbidly obese patient. *Obes Surg.* 2003;13:4–9.

8. Ezri T, Hazin V, Warters D, Szmuk P, Weinbroum AA. The endotracheal tube moves more often in obese patients undergoing laparoscopy compared with open abdominal surgery. *Anesth Analg.* 2003;96:278–282.

9. Servin F, Farinotti R, Harberer JP, Desmonts JM. Propofol infusion for maintenance of anesthesia in morbidly obese patients receiving nitrous oxide. *Anesthesiology.* 1993;78:657–665.

10. Song D, Whitten CW, White PF. Remifentanil infusion facilitates early recovery for obese outpatients undergoing laparoscopic cholecystectomy. *Anesth Analg.* 2000;90:1111–1113.

11. Juvin P, Vadam C, Malek L, Herve D, Marmuse JP, Desmonts JM. Postoperative recovery after desflurane, propofol or isoflurane anesthesia among morbidly obese patients: a prospective randomized study. *Anesth Analg.* 2000;91:714–719.

12. Ray S. Result of 310 consecutive patients undergoing laparoscopic Nissen fundoplication as hospital outpatients or at a free-standing surgery center. *Surg Endosc.* 2003;17:378–380.

13. Skattum J, Edwin B, Trondsen E, Mjaland O, Raeder J, Buanes T. Outpatient laparoscopic surgery: feasibility and consequences for education and health care costs. *Surg Endosc.* 2004;18:796–801.

14. Buckenmaier CC, Steele SM, Nielsen KC, Klein SM. Bilateral continuous paravertebral catheters for reduction mammoplasty. *Acta Anaesthesiol Scand.* 2002;46:1042–1045.

15. Karmakar MK. Thoracic paravertebral block. *Anesthesiology.* 2001;95:771–780.

16. Case C, Johantgen M, Steiner C. Outpatient mastectomy: clinical, payer, and geographic influences. *Health Serv Res.* 2001:36:869–884.

17. Ferrante J, Gonzalez E, Pal N, Roetzheim R. The use and outcomes of outpatient mastectomy in Florida. *Am J Surg.* 2000;179:253–260.

18. Margolese RG, Lasry JM. Ambulatory surgery for breast cancer patients. *Ann Surg Oncol.* 2000;7:181–187.

19. Buckenmaier CC, Klein SM, Nielsen KC, Steele SM. Continuous paravertebral catheter and outpatient infusion for breast surgery. *Anesth Analg.* 2003;97:715–717.

20. Steckler RM. Outpatient thyroidectomy: a feasibility study. *Am J Surg.* 1986;152: 417–419.
21. Samson PS, Reyes FR, Saludares WN, Angeles RP, Ricardo A, Tagorda ER. Outpatient thyroidectomy. *Am J Surg.* 1997;173:499–503.
22. Gil IS, Hobart MG, Schweizer D, Bravo EL. Outpatient adrenalectomy. *J Urol.* 2000;163:717–720.
23. Blanshard HJ, Chung F, Manninen PH, Taylor MD, Bernstein M. Awake craniotomy for removal of intracranial tumor: considerations for early discharge. *Anesth Analg.* 2001;92:89–94.
24. Bernstein M. Outpatient craniotomy for brain tumor: a pilot study in 46 patients. *Can J Neurol Sci.* 2001;28:120–124.
25. Bhardwaj R, Bernstein M. Prospective feasibility study of outpatient stereotactic brain lesion biopsy. *Neurosurg.* 2002;51:358–364.
26. Fine J, Duff J, Chen R, Hutchison W, Lozano AM, Lang AE. Long term follow up of unilateral pallidotomy in advanced Parkinson's disease. *N Engl J Med.* 2000;342: 1708–1714.
27. Prasad D, Steiner M, Steiner L. Gamma surgery for vestibular schwannoma. *J Neurosurg.* 2000;92:745–759.
28. Newmann MH. Outpatient conventional laminotomy and disc excision. *Spine.* 1995;20:353–355.
29. Singhal A, Berstein M. Outpatient lumbar microdiscectomy: a prospective study in 122 patients. *Can J Neurol Sci.* 2002;29:249–252.
30. Dagher C, Naccahe N, Narchi P, Hage P, Antakly MC. [Regional anesthesia for lumbar microdiscectomy]. *J Med Liban.* 2002;50:206–210.
31. Shaikh S, Chung F, Imarengiaye C, Yung D, Bernstein M. Pain, nausea, vomiting and ocular complications delay discharge following ambulatory microdiscectomy. *Can J Anaesth.* 2003;50:514–518.
32. Keita H, Diouf E, Tubach F, et al. Predictive factors of early postoperative urinary retention in the postanesthesia care unit. *Amnesty Analg.* 2005;101:592–596.
33. Cannon CS, Gross JG, Abramson I, Mazzei W, Freeman WR. Evaluation of outpatient experience with vitreoretinal surgery. *Br J Ophthalmol.* 1992;76:68–71.
34. Wilson D, Barr CC. Outpatient and abbreviated hospitalization for vitreoretinal surgery. *Ophthalmic Surg.* 1990;21;119–122.
35. Cybulsky IJ, Bennett F. Mediastinoscopy as a routine outpatient procedure. *Ann Thor Surg.* 1994;58:176–178.
36. Foster ED, Munro DD, Dobell ARC. Mediastinoscopy: a review of anatomical relationships and complications. *Ann Thorac Surg.* 1972;13:273–286.
37. Schubach SL, Landreneau RJ. Mediastinoscopic injury to the bronchus: use of in-continuity bronchial flap repair. *Ann Thorac Surg.* 1992;53:1101–1103.
38. Chang AC, Yee J, Orringer MB, Iannettoni MD. Diagnostic thoracoscopic lung biopsy: an outpatient experience. *Ann Thorac Surg.* 2002;74:1942–1947.
39. Blewett CJ, Bennett WF, Miller JD, Urschel JD. Open lung biopsy as an outpatient procedure. *Ann Thorac Surg.* 2001;71:1113–1115.

40. Hines MH, Bensky AS, Hammon JW, Pennington DG. Video-assisted thoracoscopic ligation of patent ductus arteriosus: safe and outpatient. *Ann Thorac Surg.* 1998;66: 853–859.
41. Aybek T, Dogan S, Neidhart G, et al. Coronary artery bypass grafting through complete sternotomy in conscious patients. *Heart Surg Forum.* 2002;5:17–21.
42. Sheehan MK, Greisler HP, Littooy FN, Baker WH. Same-evening discharge after carotid endarterectomy: our initial experience. *J Vasc Surg.* 2004:39;575–577.
43. Watts K, Lin PH, Bush RL, et al. Impact of anesthetic modality on the outcome of carotid endarterectomy. *Am J Surg.* 2004;166;741–747.
44. Olsson JH, Ellstrom M, Hahlin M. A randomized prospective trial comparing laparoscopic and abdominal hysterectomy. *Br J Obstet Gynaecol.* 1996;103:345–350.
45. Raju KS, Auld BJ. Randomized prospective study of laparoscopic vaginal hysterectomy versus abdominal hysterectomy each with bilateral salpingo-oophorectomy. *Br J Obstet Gynaecol.* 1993;101:1068–1071.
46. Galen DI, Jacobson A, Eckstein LN. Outpatient laparoscopi c-assisted vaginal hysterectomy. *J Am Assoc Gynecol Laparosc.* 1994;1:241–245.
47. Thiel J, Gamellin A. Outpatient total laparoscopic hysterectomy. *J Am Assoc Gynecol Laparosc.* 2003;10:481–483.
48. Sprunger JK, Reese CT, Decter RM. Can standard open pediatric urological procedures be performed on an outpatient basis? *J Urol.* 2001;166:1062–1064.
49. Yao D, Poppas DP. A clinical series of laparoscopic nephrectomy, nephroureterectomy and heminephroureterectomy in the pediatric population. *J Urol.* 2000;163: 1531–1535.
50. Gordon NSI. Catheter-free same day surgery transurethral resection of the prostate. *J Urol.* 1998;160:1709–1712.
51. Hajjar JH, Budd HA, Wachtel Z, Howhannesian A. Ambulatory radical retropubic prostatectomy. *Urology.* 1998;51:443–448.
52. Ruiz-Deya G, Davis R, Srivastav SK, M Wise A, Thomas R. Outpatient radical prostatectomy: impact of standard perineal approach on patient outcome. *J Urol.* 2001;166:581–586.
53. Ilfeld BM, Wright TW, Enneking FK, et al. Total shoulder arthroplasty as an outpatient procedure using ambulatory perineural local anesthetic infusion: a pilot feasibility study. *Anesth Analg.* 2005;101:1319–1322.
54. Berger RA, Jacobs JJ, Meneghini M, Valle CD, Paprosky W, Rosenberg AG. Rapid rehabilitation and recovery with minimally invasive total hip arthroplasty. *Clin Ortho Rela Res.* 2004;429:239–247.
55. Mast BA. Safety and efficacy of outpatient full abdominoplasty. *Ann Plast Surg.* 2005;54:256–259.
56. Casati A, Putzu M. Anesthesia in the obese patient: pharmacokinetic considerations. *J Clin Anesth.* 2005;17:134–145.

3. Adult clinical challenges

Donald M. Mathews, MD
Rebecca S. Twersky, MD, MPH

Successful ambulatory surgery begins with proper selection and screening of patients. It then requires intelligent perioperative management of the medical issues that have been identified during the preoperative evaluation. Both of these areas, preoperative evaluation and perioperative management, are constantly evolving, and maintaining a current knowledge base is a challenge for the busy ambulatory anesthesiologist.

Previous chapters have discussed the preoperative evaluation process and the various strategies that can be used. The roles of laboratory screening tests and consultative services have also been considered. This chapter will consider the management of the more common and challenging medical issues identified during the preoperative evaluation of the ambulatory patient. As these management concepts evolve with the generation of new data and new consensus opinion, it is valuable for the ambulatory anesthesiologist to periodically revisit these areas of basic practice. Anesthesiologists should determine whether the ambulatory surgical facility is able to handle the patient's clinical conditions and their associated complications.

Geriatrics

The world's elderly population is quickly growing. In the U.S., there were 3.1 million Americans age 65 and older in 1900, and, today, there are roughly 35.6 million aged persons. By 2030, it is projected there will be about 71.5 million older persons, more than twice their number in 2000. This trend is mirrored in all industrial nations as mortality rates decline and life expectancy rates continue to reach record levels. By the year 2030, 11.9% of world population will be age 65 and older.[1]

People age 85 and older are the fastest growing segment of the entire population, with expected growth from 4 million people today to 20 million by 2050.[2] Not only are our citizens living longer as a result of public health measures, more prescription drugs, and advances in medicine, the nature of illness is changing. Approximately 78% of those over age 65 have at least one chronic condition while almost 63% have two or more. In general, the prevalence of chronic conditions increases with age; presumably persons over 65 with just one chronic condition or two minor chronic conditions would be able to enter and/or remain in the work force. The implications of this "demographic imperative" are dramatic. Increased life expectancy, safer forms of anesthesia, and less-invasive surgical techniques have made it possible for older adults—in their 70s, 80s, and beyond—to have many types of ambulatory surgery. As a result, anesthesiologists—whether in training or in practice—will likely spend a significant proportion of their careers providing care to older patients. Thus, an aging population has implications for our ambulatory anesthesia practices. It is common for patients in their 80s and occasionally in their 90s to be scheduled for cataract extraction, cystocopy, excisional biopsies, and other minor ambulatory procedures. More younger elders are also seeking elective cosmetic surgery.

According to a growing number of studies, overall mental and physical health—not age—is a better predictor of a successful outcome after many elective procedures. At one time, advanced age may have excluded a patient from ambulatory surgery; this is no longer true. Even the very elderly patient (>100 years) should not be excluded from ambulatory surgery solely based on age.[3] Current data show a low rate of postoperative complications and unplanned hospital admissions in this population,[4] although age over 80 is reported to be a risk factor for unplanned admission.[5,6] All patients should be assessed on their medical, physical, and social conditions and the type of surgery and anesthesia being performed. The goal for the geriatric ambulatory patient undergoing elective surgery is to improve and maintain physical functioning and overall quality of life. The provision of high-quality, "gero-sensitive" perioperative care is becoming an even more critical issue in ambulatory anesthesia.

Preoperative evaluation

Preoperative evaluation of the geriatric patient is highly individualized, as different people age at varying rates. Nevertheless, virtually all physiologic systems decline with advancing chronological age, and reduced functional reserve and the ability to compensate for physiologic stress may be manifest in the geriatric patient's response to surgery and anesthesia (Box 3-1). Each disorder must be evaluated for the degree of compensation and its potential impact in the context of the planned procedure. Preoperative functional status can be difficult to accurately assess because elderly patients may have reduced cognitive impairment or general declining state even in the absence of specific associated diseases. Compounded with that are the multiple medications that elderly patients consume, further altering homeostatic mechanisms. Therefore, sufficient preanesthetic assessment and consultation with other treating physicians may be indicated. A multidimensional approach to preoperative evaluation is recommended and should include screening for mental status, depression, and alcohol abuse in addition to functional cardiovascular (CV) capacity and specific medical disease. In addition, the patient should be asked about recent surgeries. For example, following recent retinal detachment surgery, nitrous oxide may diffuse into the gas bubble, expand it, and cause vision loss in the affected eye. If systemic diseases are well controlled and preoperative medical conditions are optimized, there is no increased risk for perioperative complications for geriatric patients undergoing ambulatory surgery. Preoperative approaches to several of these medical problems are discussed in this chapter. For preoperative testing for patients undergoing low-risk surgery associated with low complication rate, the number of preoperative laboratory tests needed has been substantially

Box 3-1. Considerations in the geriatric patient

Multiple comorbidities
Mental health status
Polypharmacy, chronic medications
Cognitive impairment
Sensory deficits (hearing or visual loss)
Limited mobility
Social support situation

reduced or eliminated and is addressed in more detail in Chapter 1. We contend that *routine* screening in elderly patients does not significantly add to information obtained from the patient's history and physical examination. Selective, rather than routine, tests should be ordered only when the history or a finding on physical examination would have indicated the need for the test even if surgery had not been planned. Appropriate preoperative optimization will provide benefit in terms of improving functional status after discharge.

Perioperative care

The normal physiological changes of aging have an effect on perioperative management (Box 3-2). Blood pressure changes may be more exaggerated; older

Box 3-2. Physiologic changes of aging

Cardiovascular
Increased blood pressure
Decreased baroreceptor sensitivity
Increased incidence of arrhythmias, heart block, bradycardia
Increased stroke volume

Pulmonary
Decreased vital capacity, FEV_1 (forced expiratory volume in 1 second), and PaO_2 (partial pressure of oxygen, arterial)
Increased closing capacity and functional residual capacity

Central nervous system
Decreased cerebral blood flow and $CMRO_2$ (cerebral oxygen consumption)
Increased incidence of cerebrovascular disease
Increased incidence of Alzheimer's dementia
Decreased amounts of neuronal substance, neurotransmitters
Impaired thermoregulation

Renal and liver function
Decreased glomerular filtration rate, creatinine clearance less than 1 mL/minute per year >40 years
Decreased hepatic blood flow
Decreased levels of serum proteins

Musculoskeletal
Decreased amounts of muscle mass, lean body mass
Increased amounts of adipose tissue

Miscellaneous
Depressed airway reflexes
Impaired glucose tolerance
Impaired homeostasis of fluid and electrolytes

adults show less of a heart rate response to hypotension and may be at risk for orthostatic hypotension. In addition, patients may be on chronic antihypertensive treatments, which can further compound changes in systemic circulation. For example, diuretic therapy, alpha-adrenergic receptors, and angiotensin-converting enzyme inhibitors can result in intravascular volume depletion and changes in electrolytes. There is also an increased incidence of silent myocardial infarction (MI) and coronary artery disease (CAD); therefore, preoperative electrocardiograms (ECGs) should be available for review.[7] Further investigation is warranted if there is evidence of an old MI, left bundle branch block, left anterior hemiblock, or intraventricular conduction defects that have not been previously noted. Geriatric patients are more at risk for hypoxemia, aspiration, and hypothermia. The physiologic changes of normal aging lead to pharmacological issues with anesthetic agents (Box 3-3). These lead to increased sensitivity to most anesthetic agents. For example, minimum alveolar concentration (MAC) decreases by 6% with each decade of life following age 40.[8] The MAC of sevoflurane (with 65% nitrous oxide) is 2.6% in young patients (average age, 25) and 1.45% in the elderly (average age, 76).[9] Older patients require smaller doses of intravenous (IV) anesthetic agents than younger patients. Propofol requirements decrease by approximately 10% with each decade of life: the effect-site concentration (in µg/mL) needed for similar degrees of electroencephalogram suppression are 2.35, 1.8, and 1.25 in 25-, 50-, and 75-year-olds, respectively.[10] Concurrent administration of IV agents increases anesthetic depth so that dose reductions for propofol are indicated when propofol is given with other drugs. However, even with reduced doses of propofol, hypotension frequently occurs. The nadir for hypotension after loss of consciousness occurs several minutes longer in elderly patients. Less hypotension and bradycardia are seen with sevoflurane inductions than with propofol inductions in the elderly.[11] Regional anesthesia, when appropriate, might be offered as an alternative for the elderly patient, although decreases in neural population, neural conduction velocity, and inter-Schwann cell distance can lead to an increased sensitivity to local anesthetics.[12] In addition, changes in the systematic absorption, distribution, and clearance of local anesthetics lead to an increased sensitivity, decreased dose

---

Box 3-3. Pharmacologic differences in the elderly

Decreased protein binding, resulting in:
    Exaggerated pharmacologic effect
    Rapid rise concentration of drug in brain

Decreased renal and liver function resulting in:
    Reduced drug clearance
    Smaller induction doses of intravenous agents
    Reduced maintenance dose requirements

Decreased neuronal mass, resulting in:
    Decreased minimum alveolar concentration
    Increased sensitivity to drug

requirement, and a change in the onset and duration of action. The practitioner, when administering any anesthetic agents to the elderly, must use appropriately decreased dosing, have heightened vigilance for untoward effect, and anticipate prolonged duration of action.

There may be advantages to higher inhaled oxygen concentrations (80%–100%) even when the SpO_2 (oxygen saturation as measured by pulse oximetry) is 100%. Use of higher intraoperative and postoperative oxygen concentrations after major surgery has led to decreased postoperative tachycardia, possible myocardial ischemia, and perhaps less postoperative cognitive dysfunction (POCD).[13,14] These interventions have not been studied in ambulatory surgery patients.

The emerging research on POCD and neurobehavioral changes in the elderly are derived from inpatient data,[15,16] and more recent evidence suggests that POCD may occur less commonly than previously reported.[17] Nevertheless, because POCD can be both devastating and debilitating, clinicians practicing in the ambulatory setting should be aware of potential factors. The etiology is uncertain but may be related to intraoperative emboli, higher concentrations of inhaled agents, or cerebral hypoxia.[18] It is important to note that the incidence of POCD seems to be similar with spinal, epidural, or general anesthesia (GA).[19] The clinician should identify and manage the remediable causes of postoperative delirium such as pain and hypoxemia in order to try to reduce POCD in the elderly ambulatory surgery patient.[20,21] Because the mechanism of POCD is still uncertain, it is difficult to recommend specific prevention or treatment strategies. Chung et al.[22] reported that cognitive changes occurred in the elderly even after cataract extraction with a retrobulbar block and supplemented sedation. Ventilatory response to hypoxemia and hypercarbia is reduced with residual sedation, and proper recovery period with supplemental oxygen may be helpful to further reduce any POCD.[23] The elderly are often cognitively fragile and need to be treated accordingly. However, there is currently no scientific basis for avoiding or using any specific anesthetic technique.

Postoperative care of the elderly

A longer postoperative period of observation may be needed after GA, although fast-tracking may be feasible after brief GA.[24] Progressive loss of airway reflexes increase with age, and apnea and periodic breathing after administration of narcotics are more common. Because of alterations in pharyngeal function, diminished cough, and a higher incidence of gastroesophageal reflux, elderly patients have an accentuated risk of aspiration, which is compounded by the effects of anesthesia, sedatives, endotracheal intubation, or nasogastric tube placement.[25] Fast-tracking the recovery of patients following MAC should be encouraged provided that there is no need for continued nursing interventions. Restoring a geriatric patient back to their familiar surroundings and environment should be the goal. Nevertheless, a busy ambulatory surgery facility must respect the slow pace of many of the geriatric outpatients, and sufficient time must be provided for their adequate preoperative preparation and postoperative recovery.

Elderly outpatients experience a lower incidence of pain, dizziness, and emetic symptoms than younger patients[26] but have a higher incidence of perioperative CV events and delay in recovery of fine motor skills and cognitive function. Therefore, postoperative management has to balance the need for intervention and treatment of side effects with the advantages of briefer hospitalization. Not only must elderly outpatients be accompanied by an escort at discharge, but also a competent individual should remain with them. Since the elderly are more prone to drowsiness, confusions, falls, urinary retention, and adverse drug reactions, clinicians should provide the patient and his/her caregiver with clear, written postoperative instructions and contact information should problems or questions arise.

The geriatric patient presents challenges for pre- and postoperative teaching. The patient must understand instructions clearly, or assistance must be sought. As part of the preoperative assessment, a plan for administering the patient's regular medications during the perioperative period must be formulated. The advantages of ambulatory surgery for these patients center around the brief hospital stay, avoidance of unnecessary iatrogenic interventions, and an earlier return to their own familiar environment with resumption of their usual daily activities, diet, and medication schedule. Ensuring that the patient is discharged to a responsible home setting will further minimize complications. If necessary, home care support should be arranged.

Cardiovascular disease

CV disease is the most frequently encountered medical problem for most ambulatory anesthesiologists. There is a broad range of CV disease, from patients with mild hypertension to those with end-stage cardiac dysfunction. Ultimately, the goal of the ambulatory anesthesiologist is to determine whether the patient is (a) currently a candidate for ambulatory surgery, (b) a candidate for ambulatory surgery following further medical management, or (c) a patient who should not be cared for in an ambulatory setting. To reach a decision, the anesthesiologist needs to consider the patient's medical history, information from the patient's medical record, and information from or consultation with the patient's physician (internist, family practitioner, or cardiologist). The anesthesiologist also needs to assess the patient's current physical status, their exercise tolerance, and whether their physical status has changed since they were last seen by their medical physician. The components of the evaluation of CV disease are listed in Box 3-4, and the clinical correlation between disease state and physical finding is described in Box 3-5. The decision to proceed also needs to be made in the context of the "size" or expected surgical invasiveness of the planned procedure.

A variety of algorithms and risk assessment scores have been developed to assist with this process. One that has proven very valuable is the American College of Cardiology/American Heart Association (ACC/AHA) Guidelines for the Preoperative Assessment of the Cardiac Patient for Non-Cardiac Surgery.[27] With this approach, the patient is considered according to the level of surgical

Box 3-4. Evaluation of cardiovascular disease

History

Coronary artery disease
Chest pain, dyspnea at rest and with exercise
Stable versus unstable angina
Previous myocardial infarction and associated complications
Coronary artery bypass graft surgery or angioplasty
Coronary stent: bare metal or drug-eluting

Valvular heart disease or congestive heart failure
Dyspnea, angina, cyanosis, edema, nocturia, fatigue
Myocardial infarction, rheumatic fever, congenital heart disease
Recurrent pneumonia or bronchitis

Arrhythmias
Syncope, dizziness, palpitations

Hypertension and vascular disease
Stroke, claudication, renal disease, diabetes

Miscellaneous
Chronic medication
Other diseases affecting cardiovascular function

Physical examination

Level of orientation
Blood pressure, heart rate and rhythm
Cyanosis, capillary filling
Peripheral edema
Hepatomegaly
Jugular venous distension, pulsation
Precordial pulsations, cardiomegaly
Auscultation of heart and lungs
Ventilatory rate and pattern
Body weight, height, temperature
Evidence of peripheral vascular disease

risk (Box 3-6), the level of medical risk (Box 3-7), and the degree of exercise tolerance (Figure 3-1). Previous guidelines considered major, intermediate, and minor clinical predictors. The new guideline considers instead "active clinical conditions" and "clinical risk factors" (Box 3-7), the latter derived from work by Lee et al.[28] Whereas most ambulatory procedures are low-risk procedures, some intermediate-risk procedures (laparoscopic surgery and moderate-sized orthopedic procedures) are being done on an ambulatory basis, and this list is continually evolving. It should be noted that these guidelines were developed primarily for the use of cardiologists to determine which patients should undergo further risk assessment with noninvasive testing of cardiac function. While an anesthesiologist may use these guidelines to determine when surgery may

Box 3-5. Clinical correlation with cardiac examination

Left ventricular dysfunction, myocardial infarction, ischemia
Cardiomegaly, rales, dyspnea, peripheral edema, jugular venous distension, S_4 gallop, apical systolic murmur

Left ventricular regional wall motion abnormalities
Abnormal precordial systolic bulge

Increased left ventricular end diastolic pressure
S_3 gallop

Mitral regurgitation, papillary muscle dysfunction
Apical systolic murmur

Aortic stenosis
Pansystolic murmur with radiation

Mitral stenosis
Diastolic murmur at base

Aortic regurgitation
Diastolic murmur at apex

proceed, some will prefer that a physician who has an ongoing relationship with the patient determine whether the patient is in a stable medical condition. The guidelines present an overall approach to the patient with CV disease; the management of specific medical problems is considered below.

Box 3-6. Cardiovascular risk stratification: surgical risk

High risk
  Emergent major operations, particularly in the elderly
  Aortic and other major vascular surgery
  Peripheral vascular surgery
  Prolonged procedures with large fluid shifts and/or blood loss

Intermediate risk
  Carotid endarterectomy
  Head and neck surgery
  Intraperitoneal and intrathoracic surgery
  Orthopedic surgery
  Prostate surgery

Low risk
  Endoscopic procedures
  Superficial procedures
  Cataract surgery
  Breast surgery

Box 3-7. Cardiovascular risk stratification: medical clinical predictors

Active Cardiac Conditions
> Unstable coronary syndromes
>> Myocardial infarction within 30 days
>> Unstable or severe angina (Canadian class III or IV)
> Decompensated heart failure
>> New York Heart Association Class IV
>> Worsening or new-onset heart failure
> Significant arrhythmias
>> High-grade atrioventricular block
>> Mobitz II atrioventricular block
>> Third-degree atrioventricular block
>> Supraventricular arrhythmia (including atrial fibrillation) with uncontrolled ventricular rate (greater than 100 beats per minute at rest)
>> Symptomatic bradycardia
>> Newly recognized ventricular tachycardia
> Severe valvular disease
>> Severe aortic stenosis (mean pressure gradient greater than 40 mmHg, aortic valve area less than $1.0\,cm^2$, or symptomatic)
>> Symptomatic mitral stenosis (progressive dyspnea on exertion, exertional presyncope, or heart failure)

Clinical Risk Factors
> Ischemic heart disease
>> History of myocardial infarction
>> History of positive treadmill test
>> Use of nitroglycerin
>> Current chest pain thought to be secondary to coronary ischemia
>> ECG with abnormal Q waves
> Congestive heart failure
>> History of heart failure
>> Pulmonary edema
>> Paroxysmal nocturnal dyspnea
>> Peripheral edema
>> Bilateral rales or S_3
>> CXR with pulmonary vascular redistribution
> Cerebral vascular disease
>> History of stroke or transient ischemic attack
> High-risk surgery
>> Abdominal aortic aneurysm or other vascular, thoracic, abdominal, or orthopedic surgery
> Preoperative insulin treatment for diabetes mellitus
> Preoperative creatinine level greater than 2 mg per dL

Adapted from Fleisher et al.[27] Used with permission.

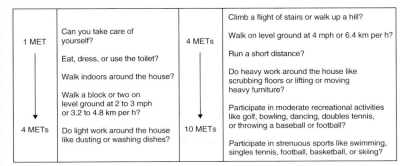

Figure 3-1. Metabolic equivalents (METs) of physical activity. Reproduced from Fleisher et al.[27] Used with permission from the American College of Cardiology Foundation.

The guideline is illustrated in Figure 3-2 and low and intermediate-risk procedures will be considered, as high-risk surgery is not performed on an ambulator basis. In the first step, patients requiring emergency surgery are sent to the operating room. In the second step, clinicians consider whether any of the four active cardiac conditions listed in Box 3-7 (unstable coronary syndromes, decompensated heart failure, significant arrythmias, or severe valvular disease) are present. If so, surgery is postponed. Next, in step 3, the type of surgery is considered: for low-risk procedures (Box 3-6), patients may have surgery without further evaluation. As ambulatory patients are largely undergoing low-risk surgery, this recommendation is very useful to the practicing anesthesiologist. For intermediate-risk procedures, further steps are required.

Next, in step 4, the functional capacity of the patient is considered. If the patient has had a recent favorable exercise test or has a Duke Functional capacity 7 or greater (Figure 3-1), they can proceed to the operating room. For patients with one or more clinical risk factors (Box 3-7), heart rate control with beta-blocker therapy may be considered.

In step 5, those who have a poor or unknown functional capacity are considered. The number of clinical risk factors (Box 3-7: ischemic heart disease, congestive heart failure, cerebral vascular disease, high-risk surgery, diabetes requiring insulin therapy and serum creatinine of greater than $2\,mg/dL$) is determined. Those with none may proceed to the operating room. For those with one or two clinical risk factors, one may proceed to the operating room and consider heart rate control with beta-blocker therapy or consider further functional testing if it will change management of the patient. Those with 3 or more clinical risk factors are a small, high-risk group. For these patients requiring intermediate-risk surgery, it would seem prudent to involve cardiologic consultation to address whether beta-blockade or further non-invasive cardiac testing is appropriate as the guideline finds that there is insufficient data to suggest the best management strategy.

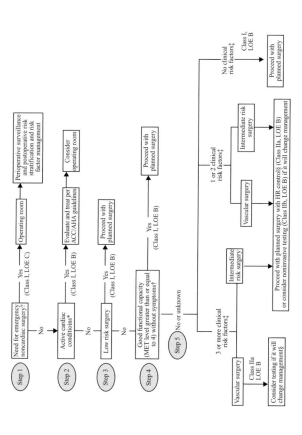

Figure 3-2. American College of Cardiology/American Heart Association algorithm for the evaluation of the cardiac patient for non-cardiac surgery. See Box 3-7 for active cardiac conditions and risk factors. See figure 3-1 for metabolic equivalent (MET) determination. Class I recommendation: procedure/treatment should be performed/administered, class IIa: it is reasonable to perform procedure/administer treatment, class IIb: procedure/treatment may be considered. Level of evidence A: multiple supporting studies, B: several supporting studies, C: few supporting studies, expert opinion. Reprinted from the Journal of the American College of Cardiology, Vol 50, Fleisher et al., ACC/AHA 2007 Guidelines on Perioperative Cardiovascular Evaluation and Care for Noncardiac Surgery, pages 1707–31, 2007. With permission from Elsevier and the American College of Cardiology.

Table 3-1. Antihypertensive drugs

Drug	Perioperative considerations
Diuretics	Hypovolemia, electrolyte abnormalities
Angiotensin-converting enzyme inhibitors (e.g., captopril, enalapril, and fosinopril)	Cough, hypotension upon anesthesia induction, hyperkalemia (especially if taking K^+ supplements)
Angiotensin receptor blockers (e.g., losarten and irbesartan)	Hypotension upon anesthesia induction
Beta-adrenergic blockers (e.g., atenolol, metoprolol, and propoanolol)	Bradycardia, bronchospasm, additive effect of myocardial depression with anesthetics, sudden withdrawal can cause rebound tachycardia, angina, and myocardial infarction
Calcium-channel blockers (e.g., diltiazem. verapamil, and nicardipine)	Atrioventricular block, bradycardia, additive hypotension with anesthesia, decrease MAC, potentiate neuromuscular blocking agents
Alpha-adrenergic blockers (e.g., prazosin and doxazosin)	Additive hypotension with anesthetics, decrease MAC, rebound hypertension on withdrawal
Central alpha-adrenergic agonists (e.g., clonidine and methydopa)	Sedation, decrease MAC, rebound hypertension with withdrawal
Direct vasodilators (e.g., hydralazine)	Tachycardia, postural hypotension
Peripheral adrenergic neuron antagonists (e.g., reserpine)	Bradycardia, orthostatic hypotension, sodium and water retention
Combination products	See both categories above

Hypertension

Hypertension is the most common form of CV disease the anesthesiologist will confront, affecting 25% of all adults and 50% of the elderly in the United States.[29] Perhaps two thirds of these are undiagnosed or under-treated, potentially making management of these patients a daily occurrence. Preoperative evaluation should focus not only on the current blood pressure but also on the presence and severity of end-organ involvement: ischemic heart disease, arrhythmias, cardiomyopathy, and evidence of congestive heart failure (CHF) and cerebrovascular or renal impairment. Classes of antihypertensive medications and the perioperative considerations associated with their use are listed in Table 3-1. With the exception of diuretics, these agents should be continued through the day of surgery. Some advocate the discontinuance of angiotensin system blocking drugs 48–72 hours prior to surgery because of reports of profound and therapy-resistant hypotension following propofol induction, but withholding the agents for more than 10 hours is probably adequate.[30]

Although there is no absolute pressure boundary at which ambulatory surgery should be postponed, most anesthesiologists would be hesitant to proceed with diastolic blood pressure of greater than 110 mm Hg. This is because it has been recognized that the intraoperative problems that occur with the hypertensive patient are magnified in patients who are poorly controlled, leading to difficult perioperative management and increased risk of poor outcome. These problems include contracted overall blood volume causing exaggerated blood pressure decreases with anesthetic induction and "over-reactive" baroreceptors and sympathetic nervous system leading to increased hemodynamic response to surgical stimulation. Blood pressure should be maintained within 20% of baseline to allow for organ autoregulation. Tachycardia should be avoided, especially in those with associated CAD. Anesthetic agents alone may be inadequate to meet these goals, and these patients often require intraoperative vasodilators or beta-blocking agents. The choice of using short- or long-acting vasoactive agents is usually made based on the anticipated need for continued effect in the postoperative period.

Coronary artery disease

The evaluation of severity of CAD as part of preoperative risk stratification was discussed above. Assuming that the AHA/ACC guidelines were followed, those with major clinical predictors were referred for further care, and therefore the most advanced CAD that the ambulatory anesthesiologist will need to consider is the patient with intermediate clinical predictors: stable angina or MI within 4 to 6 weeks. There are several issues in the management of these patients which require the attention of the anesthesiologist.

The first is the change in timing for allowing post-MI elective surgery. Prior doctrine, based on data collected before the era of modern CV care, prohibited elective surgery within 6 months of an MI. Current post-MI care involves evaluation of myocardium at risk through functional assessment, post-MI beta-blockade when appropriate, and cardiac rehabilitation. Those who have undergone this care and are stable 4 to 6 weeks post-MI are eligible for elective surgery. Although these guidelines were first published in 1996, a recent survey shows that most anesthesiologists will still postpone elective surgery for 6 months post-MI.[31]

Patients for whom prudence may be appropriate are those who have undergone percutaneous coronary intervention (PCI), which includes percutaneous balloon angioplasty (PTCA) with or without placement of bare metal or drug-eluting (DES) coronary stents. Issues of atherosclerotic plaque stability and the aggressive anticoagulant regimen given to these patients complicates the timing of elective ambulatory surgery, and are addressed in the ACC/AHA guidelines.[27] Following PTCA, surgery should be postponed for at least 2 to 4 weeks following the procedure,[32] and aspirin therapy continued perioperatively. Following placement of bare metal stents, a 4- to 6-week wait is advisable; thienopyridines (ticlopidine, clopidogrel) are usually stopped one week before surgery and perioperative aspirin therapy continued when possible. Following DES placement, it is recommended to wait one year for elective surgery, maintain perioperative aspirin therapy, and restart thienopyridines as soon as possible postoperatively. For these patients preoperative discussion with the treating cardiologist seems advisable.

Should all patients with CAD risk factors receive perioperative beta-blockers? All of the current data about beta-blocker use have been collected in those undergoing major surgery, defined in one study as surgery requiring 2 or more days of hospitalization. There are currently no data to indicate the appropriate care for those with CAD or risk factors who present for low-risk surgery and are not receiving beta-blockers; the line between risk and benefit of instituting beta-blockade is not entirely clear. Nor is it clear how soon before surgery beta-blocker therapy should be instituted for maximal benefit. Common sense would suggest that patients should be started on these agents if it is in their overall medical benefit, not simply because they are scheduled for low- or medium-risk surgery. Most patients are treated with atenolol (25–100 mg/day) or metoprolol (100–400 mg/day). Patients should receive their usual dose of beta-blockers on the day of surgery.

If a patient receives these agents preoperatively, they should be continued throughout the perioperative period; the consequences of rebound tachycardia can be highly detrimental, leading to ischemia and MI. Oral beta-blockers should be resumed postoperatively. Those who will remain nil per os (NPO) need to receive IV beta-blockers, usually metoprolol 5–10 mg. Other preoperative medications that should be continued through the perioperative period include nitrates, antihypertensive medications, and afterload-reducing agents. Anticoagulants are usually discontinued prior to surgery; however, if the patient has unstable angina or atrial fibrillation, the surgeon and the treating cardiologist should be consulted to plan perioperative anticoagulation. The actual anesthetic technique used is not as important as maintaining a favorable coronary artery oxygen supply/demand relationship: avoid tachycardia, hypoxemia, and peripheral vasoconstriction; maintain adequate hematocrit (>28 mg/dL); and actively warm the patient to avoid hypothermia. Postoperatively, these same goals apply with implementing comprehensive pain therapy to prevent excessive sympathetic stimulation. Postoperative surveillance for ischemia is appropriate. Comparison with a preoperative ECG is often useful to determine the significance of postoperative ECG abnormalities. Aggressive management of postoperative ischemia includes nitrates, beta-blockers, aspirin, and cardiology consultation.

Valvular heart disease

Patients with valvular disease may undergo ambulatory surgery if there is no evidence of CHF or significant impairment in myocardial performance and if compensatory mechanisms for maintaining cardiac output are functioning. Valvular disease can cause dysrhythmias, alterations in pulmonary and peripheral vascular resistance, and changes in preload and myocardial oxygenation. Although the prevalence of rheumatic valvular disease is declining, congenital bicuspid aortic stenosis, mitral valve prolapse (MVP), idiopathic hypertrophic subaortic stenosis, and calcific mitral insufficiency are encountered more frequently.[33]

Table 3-2. Canadian classification of patients with heart disease

Class	Description
0	Asymptomatic
1	Symptoms with strenuous exercise
2	Symptoms with moderate exertion
3	Symptoms with mild exertion
4	Symptoms at any level of physical exertion or symptoms at rest

The preoperative evaluation should assess the severity of the manifestations of the valvular disease. Patients with "significant" valvular disease are considered high-risk and should not be cared for on an ambulatory basis. One method of determining significance is to use the Canadian Classification, also used by the AHA/ACC guidelines (Table 3-2). Those in class 1 and 2 can be cared for with appropriate attention. Those in class 3 should be considered only for minor procedures. Those in class 4 or class 3 who require larger procedures should not be considered for ambulatory care. The patient must be able to lie flat, so "doing it only under local" or regional anesthesia may not be a useful option. CHF, manifesting as dyspnea, orthopnea, and fatigue, should be treated, and myocardial contractility optimized, before ambulatory surgery. Echocardiography is the best noninvasive diagnostic tool for characterizing valvular lesions. Information can be obtained about both the physical and physiological aspects of the lesions such as valve area and flow gradient, respectively. Cardiology consultation may be sought if questions exist about the nature or severity of valvular lesions. Many patients may be taking anticoagulants and the decision to stop anticoagulant therapy or to convert to heparin for the perioperative period should be discussed among the physicians involved in the perioperative management. Box 3-8 lists the cardiac conditions associated with endocarditis. Antibiotic prophylaxis should be followed according to the AHA guidelines (Table 3-3).

Anesthetic management is based on maintaining a cardiac rhythm, blood pressure, and systemic vascular resistance that will minimize the pathophysiology (Box 3-9). Stenotic lesions require strict maintenance of preload, contractility, rate, and rhythm (preferably sinus rhythm) within a narrow range. Aortic stenosis is of particular concern as a decrease in contractility can quickly lead to a downward spiral of decreased cardiac output and decreased coronary perfusion. The anesthesiologist must be prepared to immediately cardiovert a patient with aortic stenosis who develops a dysrhythmia, including atrial fibrillation. All facilities should have functioning defibrillators that are checked regularly. Patients with regurgitant lesions benefit from maintaining lower pulmonary or vascular resistance that maintains forward flow; these patients should be actively warmed, with the goal of maintaining normothermia. Often, combined lesions are present and management should be geared toward the more hemodynamically significant impairment.

Mitral valve prolapse

MVP (Box 3-10) is a fairly common condition, occurring in approximately 4% of the population, with a slightly higher prevalence in women. These patients

Box 3-8. Cardiac conditions associated with the highest risk of adverse outcome from endocarditis for which prophylaxis with dental procedures[+] is recommended

- Prosthetic cardiac valve including bioprosthetic and homograft valves
- Previous Infective Endocarditis
- Certain specific Congenital heart disease (CHD)[*]:
  - Unrepaired or incompletely repaired cyanotic CHD, including palliative shunts and conduits
  - Completely repaired congenital heart defect with prosthetic material or device, whether placed by surgery or by catheter intervention, during the first 6 months after the procedure[†]
  - Repaired CHD with residual defects at the site or adjacent to the site of a prosthetic patch or prosthetic device (which inhibit endothelialization)
- Cardiac transplantation recipients who develop cardiac valvulopathy

[+]Dental procedures involving manipulation of gingival tissue or the periapical region or teeth or perforation of the oral mucosa.

[*]Except for the conditions listed above, antibiotic prophylaxis is no longer recommended for any other form of CHD, ASD, VSD, hypertrophic cardiomyopathy, acquired valvular disease, rheumatic heart disease, bicuspid valve, calcified aortic stenosis, or MVP with or without regurgitation.

[†]Prophylaxis is recommended because endothelialization of prosthetic material occurs within 6 months after the procedure.

Antibiotic prophylaxis is no longer recommended solely to prevent IE in patients who undergo a GI or GU track procedure.

Wilson W, Taubert KA, Gewitz M, et al. Prevention of infective endocarditis: Guidelines from the American Heart Association. A guideline from the American Heart Association Rheumatic Fever, Endocarditis and Kawasaki Disease Committee, Council on Cardiovascular Disease in the Young, and the Council on Clinical Cardiology, Council on Cardiovascular Surgery and Anesthesia, and the Quality of Care and Outcomes Research Interdisciplinary Working Group. JADA 2007;138(6):739–60. © 2007 American Dental Association. Excerpted by JADA with permission of Circulation. Circulation 2007 Apr 19;[Epub ahead of print]. © 2007 American Heart Association. Adapted 2008 with permission of The Journal of the American Dental Association.

Dajani AS, Taubert KA, Wilson W, et al. Prevention of bacterial endocarditis. Recommendations by the American Heart Association. JAMA 1997;277:1794–1801. Used with permission.

Source: Antibiotics and your heart. American Dental Association Web site. Available at http://www.ada.org/public/topics/antibiotics.asp. © 2007 American Dental Association. All rights reserved.

have often undergone an echocardiogram because of the finding of a click or murmur on physical exam or because of symptoms of chest pain, palpitations, anxiety, or embolic phenomena. Patients with prolapse of a structurally abnormal valve have a higher incidence of complications than those with prolapse of

Table 3-3. Antibiotic regimens for infective endocarditis prophylaxis for high risk adult patients undergoing dental procedures[+]

| Situation | Agent | Regimen: Single dose 30 to 60 minutes before dental procedure | |
		Adults	Children
Oral	Amoxicillin	2 g	50 mg/kg
Unable to take oral	Ampicillin	2 g IM or IV	50 mg/kg IM or IV
	OR		
	Cefazolin or ceftriaxone	1 g IM or IV	50 mg/kg IM or IV
Penicillin or ampicillin allergic–oral route	Cephalexin*[#]	2 g	50 mg/kg
	OR		
	Clindamycin	600 mg	20 mg/kg
	OR		
	Azithromycin or clarithromycin	500 mg	15 mg/kg
Penicillin or ampicillin allergic and unable to take oral medication	Cefazolin or ceftriaxone[†]	1 g IM or IV	50 mg/kg IM or IV
	OR		
	Clindamycin	600 mg IM or IV	20 mg/kg IM or IV

[+]Dental procedures involving manipulation of gingival tissue or the periapical region of teeth or perforation of the oral mucosa.
*Or other first- or second-generation oral cephalosporin in equivalent adult dosage.
[†]Cephalosporins should not be used in an individual with a history of anaphylaxsis, angioedema, or urticaria with penicillins or ampicillin.

Wilson W, Taubert KA, Gewitz M, et al. Prevention of infective endocarditis: Guidelines from the American Heart Association. A guideline from the American Heart Association Rheumatic Fever, Endocarditis and Kawasaki Disease Committee, Council on Cardiovascular Disease in the Young, and the Council on Clinical Cardiology, Council on Cardiovascular Surgery and Anesthesia, and the Quality of Care and Outcomes Research Interdisciplinary Working Group. JADA 2007;138(6):739–60. © 2007 American Dental Association. Excerpted by JADA with permission of Circulation. Circulation 2007 Apr 19;[Epub ahead of print]. © 2007 American Heart Association. Adapted 2008 with permission of The Journal of the American Dental Association.

a structurally normal valve. Potential complications include valvular regurgitation, endocarditis, and stroke (Box 3-11). In the absence of significant valvular regurgitation, the perioperative risk is probably not increased. Patients with a structurally abnormal valve and regurgitation need not receive antibiotic prophylaxis for bacterial endocarditis according to updated AHA recommendations (Box 3-8).

Box 3-9. Anesthetic considerations for patients with valvular heart disease

Mitral stenosis
Heart rate: normal to slow
Central blood volume: rapid increases should be avoided
SVR: normal to high
Other: avoid hypoxemia or increase in pulmonary vascular resistance that
  may induce congestive heart failure

Aortic stenosis
Heart rate: normal sinus rhythm
SVR: normal
Central blood volume: keep full

Mitral regurgitation
Heart rate: normal to fast
SVR: normal to low
Other: avoid drug-induced myocardial depression

Aortic regurgitation
Heart rate: normal to high
SVR: normal to low
Other: avoid drug-induced myocardial depression

SVR, systemic vascular resistance.

Box 3-10. Considerations in the patient with mitral valve prolapse

- Documentation of the diagnosis
- Clinical manifestations
  Chest pain
      Dysrhythmia or palpitations
      Valvular insufficiency or ventricular dysfunction
      Neurologic manifestations
      Anxiety
- Keep heart slow and full

Box 3-11. Complications associated with mitral valve prolapse

- Cardiac arrhythmias (junctional rhythm and premature ventricular contractions)
- Atrioventricular heart block
- ST-segment and T-wave changes
- Mitral regurgitation
- Infective endocarditis
- Ruptured chordae tendinae
- Transient ischemic attack
- Sudden death (rare)

Pacemaker

The presence of a functioning pacemaker should not exclude a patient from undergoing ambulatory surgery. In 2005, the American Society of Anesthesiologists (ASA) issued a practice advisory about the management of patients with pacemakers and implantable defibrillators.[34] The patient should be evaluated for the presence of other associated CV disease. Preoperative evaluation should involve determining the reason for the pacemaker, the patient's underlying rhythm, drug therapy, and the exact type of pacemaker (chamber sensed, chamber paced, sensing pattern, and default rhythm). Most pacemakers can be converted to a fixed-rate asynchronous pacemaker to allow the use of electrocautery. This requires obtaining the appropriate magnet for this purpose and the knowledge of how to reprogram a pacemaker if necessary. Bipolar cautery may be used if the pacemaker is not converted to a fixed-rate mode, but this is less advisable. Postoperatively, patients should usually remain in a monitored setting until adequate pacemaker function has been established.

Patients with automatic implantable cardioverter defibrillators are also potential candidates for ambulatory surgery. Improvements in post-MI risk stratification and diagnosis of cardiac electrophysiologic syndromes that can lead to fatal dysrythmias have greatly increased the use of these devices. Ambulatory anesthesiologists will increasingly have to consider the management of these patients in the future. These devices must be disabled before surgery and reset following the procedure. The anesthesiologist must be able to cardiovert the patient during the procedure should this be necessary, and placement of an external pacemaker may be indicated.[35] This coordination usually requires the cooperation and availability of a cardiologist, which may be beyond the capabilities of a freestanding ambulatory practice.

Pulmonary disease

Asthma

Asthma is a common disease in the United States: 11 million people reported having an asthma attack in 2000.[36] Treatment has shifted from providing episodic bronchodilators to long-term chronic treatment of airway inflammation. Research has shown that the class of agents most effective in treating chronic airway inflammation is the inhaled corticosteroid, and they have become the backbone of therapy. Long-acting inhaled beta$_2$-agonists are added for more significant disease. The current definitions of severity of asthma and preferred therapy are presented in Table 3-4. The agents used to treat asthma and their mechanisms of action are presented in Box 3-12.

The assessment of the patient with asthma or chronic obstructive pulmonary disease (COPD) is listed in Box 3-13. The goal of the preoperative evaluation is to determine the severity of the history of reactive airway disease and the state of current therapy. Pulmonary function testing, chest x-ray (CXR), and arterial blood gas determination are usually not required, especially if disease severity can be assessed through history and physical exam. The patient with active

Table 3-4. Asthma classification and preferred therapy

Clinical severity	Symptoms: day	Symptoms: night	PEF or FEV$_1$	Preferred therapy
Severe persistent	Continual	Frequent	≤60%	High-dose inhaled corticosteroids AND long-acting inhaled beta$_2$-agonists
Moderate persistent	Daily	>1 night/week	>60%–<80%	Low-to-medium-dose inhaled corticosteroids and long-acting inhaled beta$_2$-agonists
Mild persistent	>2/week but <1×/day	>2 night/month	≥80%	Low-dose inhaled corticosteroids
Mild intermittent	≤2 days/week	≤2 nights/month	≥80%	No daily medication needed

FEV$_1$, forced expiratory volume in 1 second; PEF, peak expiratory flow.

Box 3-12. Current treatment of asthma

- Inhaled steroids: used to reduce inflammation; bronchiolar relaxation. First-line therapy
- Long-acting beta$_2$ agonists: not for treatment of acute bronchospasm
- Short-acting beta$_2$ agonists: for acute bronchospasm
- Cromolyn and nedocromil: mast cell stabilizers
- Leukotriene modifiers: decrease effect of inflammatory cytokines
- Aminophylline: second-line treatment; least effective; good for nocturnal asthma

Box 3-13. The patient with asthma or chronic obstructive pulmonary disease

- Baseline status (functional status and lung examination)
- Medication use (scheduled and demand medications)
- History of exacerbations: frequency, severity, triggers, intubation
- History of recent exacerbation or respiratory infection
- History of severe bronchospasm may contraindicate ambulatory surgery
- Use of corticosteroids
- Pulmonary function testing not indicated preoperatively in most patients

bronchospasm or a history of continual daily bronchospastic symptoms should not be cared for in an ambulatory setting. There is emerging evidence that patients who are not receiving inhaled corticosteroids preoperatively have increased pulmonary complications postoperatively,[37] and although it is currently not a "standard of care," future preoperative preparation may require this therapy.

All medications should be continued the day of surgery. Many practitioners administer a short-acting beta$_2$-agonists before the patient enters the OR. Regional anesthesia may be preferred since it avoids instrumentation of the airway, although GA is routinely given. Thorough preoxygenation is essential for GA. Propofol is the IV induction agent of choice.[38] For inhalation induction, most practitioners would select sevoflurane. The use of a laryngeal mask airway (LMA) or other non-endotracheal tube device should be used, when possible, to minimize tracheal stimulation. Adequate depth of anesthesia should be provided. Anesthesia can be maintained with propofol or an inhalation agent; most suggest sevoflurane as the agent of choice, but the actual agent delivered is less important once anesthesia has been induced.[39]

Current recommendations about the administration of "stress steroids" for patients who have revived oral corticosteroids should be considered.[40] Those who require 5 mg/day or greater of prednisone or its equivalent (20 mg hydrocortisone = 5 mg prednisone = 4 mg methylprednisolone = 0.75 dexamethasone) or who have been on such therapy in the recent past should be supplemented with exogenous steroids during the perioperative period since their pituitary-adrenal axis may not be able to produce the necessary cortisol in response to surgical stimulation. The duration required for normal pituitary-adrenal function to return following the discontinuation of exogenous steroids is not clear. If there is some doubt, the patient could be referred to an endocrinologist for an adrenocorticotropic hormone stimulation test to assess adrenal function. Patients should take their usual dose the day of surgery and then be given the additional supplemental dose. The dose and duration should be based on the size of the operative procedure: minor procedures (e.g., hernia repair) require only one dose of 25 mg of hydrocortisone.

Acute bronchospasm can be treated, intraoperative, by increasing the anesthetic agent. A short-acting beta$_2$-agonist, such as albuterol, should be administered via nebulizer. Ipratropium bromide may be also given via nebulizer but is not immediate therapy because of a slower onset time. Systemic corticosteroids may be of benefit: 40 to 60 mg of prednisone, methylprednisolone, or prednisolone in a single dose or two divided doses. Severe cases may require an IV beta$_2$-agonist—either epinephrine or terbutaline—although there is no proven advantage of systemic therapy over aerosolized agents. Hospitalization and pulmonary consultation are advisable for significant intra- or postoperative exacerbation.

Chronic obstructive pulmonary disease

The ambulatory patient with COPD, chronic bronchitis, or emphysema can present a great challenge. The pathophysiology of COPD is characterized by an obstruction to air flow with reversible and irreversible components. The degree to which each component is present determines the severity of illness. The reversible component usually consists of bronchospasm, infection, secretion, and atelectasis; treatment consists of bronchodilators, antibiotics, and respiratory therapy prior to outpatient surgery. Preoperative evaluation should involve the same approach as that used for the asthmatic. The patient with COPD may have baseline wheezing and functional limitation, and it can be difficult to determine whether the patient is in medically maximal condition; this will need to be assessed by the patient's own physician. Smokers should be strongly encouraged to abstain prior to surgery. Ideally, the patient will be a nonsmoker for 6 to 8 weeks prior to surgery to have maximal pulmonary benefit: decreased mucus production, return of cilliary function, and improvement in pulmonary compliance.[41] Shorter discontinuation, however, has benefits as recent smoking can cause a hypercoagulable state and interferes with wound healing. In addition, short-term discontinuation favorably shifts the oxygen-hemoglobin binding curve and improves tissue oxygen delivery. Symptoms of nicotine withdrawal can be managed with nicotine transdermal patches.

Intraoperative management considerations are similar to those of the asthmatic. When administering regional anesthesia, practitioners should remember that high spinal levels may not be well tolerated in patients with COPD. Loss of intercostal muscle function and the loss of diaphragmatic function from upper extremity blocks can lead to respiratory distress and even failure.[42] Postoperatively, these patients may be discharged provided that pulmonary function is stable.

Endocrine disorders

Diabetes mellitus

Diabetes mellitus (DM) is the most commonly encountered endocrine disorder in ambulatory surgery, affecting 7% to 8% of the population of the United States.[43] In type 1 diabetes, the insulin-producing islet cells of the pancreas have been destroyed by an autoimmune process. In type 2 diabetes, there is defective insulin secretion and a cellular resistance to the action of insulin. The differences between the types of diabetes are highlighted in Table 3-5. Type 2 DM is increasingly common. It currently accounts for 90% of diabetes and, because of its association with obesity, is expected to develop in one quarter to one third of Americans within the next 25 years![44]

Diabetes leads to multiple medical concerns for the ambulatory anesthesiologist (Box 3-14). The association with CAD is well known and can present with "silent ischemia." Atherosclerotic disease can be present in other arterial beds and lead to central and peripheral vascular disease and cerebrovascular insufficiency. Ventricular stiffness causes decreased compliance and leads to cardiomegaly. Renal involvement can cause renal insufficiency, and autonomic neuropathy results in abnormal blood pressure homeostasis. "Stiff joint syndrome" may be present; of most concern is decreased mobility of the atlantoaxillary joint, leading

Table 3-5. Characteristics of type 1 and type 2 diabetes mellitus

	Type 1	Type 2
Age of onset, typical	Less than 40	Greater than 40
Family history of diabetes	Uncommon	Common
Body habitus	Normal to wasted	Obese
Pathogenesis	Autoimmune mediated	Non-immune-mediated
Associated with metabolic syndrome	No	Yes
Physiologic risk	Prone to ketoacidosis	Prone to hyperosmolar state
Plasma insulin	Low to absent	Normal to high
Insulin therapy	Responsive	Responsive to resistant
Oral hypoglycemic therapy	Unresponsive	Responsive

to difficult endotracheal intubation. The inability to hold together one's palms and fingers with no space between has been called the "prayer sign" and may be a marker for decreased cervical spine mobility. Decreased ability to care for oneself postoperatively due to peripheral neuropathy and retinopathy may require more involved care planning.

Type 2 diabetes is also associated with the metabolic syndrome, which is defined as having three or more of five abnormalities: waist circumference of more than 40 inches (102 cm) for men or more than 35 inches (88 cm) for women, triglyceride level of more than or equal to 150 mg/dL, high-density lipoprotein cholesterol of less than 40 mg/dL in men or less than 50 mg/dL in women, blood pressure of more than or equal to 130/85 mm Hg, and fasting glucose of more than or equal to 110 mg/dL. It is related to insulin resistance, but the two terms are not synonymous.[45]

Box 3-14. Considerations in the diabetic patient

Degree of control
End-organ diseases
 Coronary artery disease
 Stiff ventricle (cardiac diastolic dysfunction)
 Renal insufficiency
 "Stiff joint syndrome," with potential difficult intubation
 Visual impairment (may affect discharge planning)
 Autonomic neuropathy (gastroparesis with nausea and vomiting)
 Peripheral neuropathy

Options for perioperative management
 Administer portion of long-acting insulin
 Administer insulin by sliding scale based on blood sugar
 Administer insulin by infusion
Goal in ambulatory surgery is rapid return to preoperative control
Patient's/family's ability to assess and manage glucose postoperatively

Table 3-6. Insulin preparations

	Onset	Peak	Duration
Rapid-acting (e.g., aspart, lispro, glulisine)	10–30 minutes	30–60 minutes	3–5 hours
Regular	30–60 minutes	1.5–2 hours	5–12 hours
Intermediate-acting (e.g., NPH, lente)	1–2 hours	4–8 hours	10–20 hours
Long-acting (e.g., detemir, glargine, ultralente)	1–4 hours	8–20 hours	16–24 hours

Mixtures: 70/30 = 70% regular/30% NPH; 50/50 = 50% regular/50% NPH. NPH, neutral protamine Hagedorn.

Preoperative evaluation includes evaluation of the type and severity of the diabetes. Most practitioners would avoid caring for "brittle" diabetics in the ambulatory setting. For all diabetics, the patient's type and dose of medical therapy should be determined. Insulin preparations are listed in Table 3-6, and the oral hypoglycemic agents are listed in Table 3-7. Preoperative physical exam should be focused on end-organ disease: for example, symptoms of postural hypotension may be symptoms of autonomic neuropathy and presage difficulty with intraoperative blood pressure control. ECG may be abnormal and so should be obtained preoperatively to determine a baseline. A day-of-surgery glucose determination is advised.[46] Knowledge of the patient's hemoglobin A1C may provide information about the quality of long-term glucose control.

Insulin therapy the day of surgery in the type 1 patient can be managed several ways; the goal is to maintain a level of insulin that prevents the development of ketosis but not so great as to lead to significant hypoglycemia in the setting of reduced caloric input. The practice of administering no insulin until after the surgery can no longer be recommended. Ideally, the diabetic patient, especially the type 1, will be cared for as the first case or early in the day so that they will be NPO for a limited number of hours. The patient may be instructed to hold their a.m. insulin and come to the facility, have their blood glucose checked, and then be given insulin, usually one third to one half their a.m. dose of intermediate or long-acting insulin. Alternatively, patients may take the one third to one half of their usual insulin a.m. dose prior to departure for the ambulatory facility. Blood glucose should be checked preoperatively and postoperatively and the remainder of the a.m. dose can be administered then. The patient can be discharged home with instructions to resume usual insulin therapy with home glucose monitoring. A prescription for an antiemetic agent should be strongly considered. The ability to take fluids should be confirmed before discharge, and discharge instructions should emphasize that the patient needs to return to a medical facility should nausea and vomiting preclude adequate fluid and caloric intake.

Perioperative care of the type 2 patient has traditionally allowed for relatively "loose" glucose control, allowing levels of 200–250 mg/dL. It is probably adequate to discontinue only the day-of-surgery dose of oral hypoglycemic medications. Blood glucose levels should be checked pre- and postoperatively; patients may arrive at the facility with elevated glucose levels. Although it is

Table 3-7. Oral hypoglycemic agents

Type	Mechanism of action	Side effects and considerations
Sulfonylureas—first generation (e.g., chlorpropamide, tolazamide, tolbutamide	Increases insulin secretion via interaction with beta-cell ATP-sensitive K^+ channel	Hypoglycemia (especially in elderly with decreased renal function), effectiveness wanes with time
Sulfonylureas—second generation (glipizide, glyburide	Same as above	As above, also more potent than first generation
Non-sulfonylurea secretogogues (e.g., nateglinide, repaglinide)	Same as above	Rapid onset, taken before meals
Biguanides (e.g., metformin)	Decreases hepatic glucose output, increases peripheral glucose use	Lactic acidosis (especially with renal failure), discontinue prior to surgery and until oral intake resumes, discontinue prior to and for 48 hours after intravenous iodinated contrast dye
Thiazolidinediones (e.g., pioglitazone, rosiglitazone)	Increases insulin sensitivity in adipose, muscle and liver	Rare hepatic failure, fluid retention and weight gain
Alpha-glucosidase inhibitors (e.g., acarbose, miglitol)	Prevents absorption of glucose from small intestines	Abdominal pain, bloating, flatulence
Others (e.g., exenatide, pramlintide)	Incretin mimetic: increases insulin release	Nausea, vomiting, diarrhea
Combinations: metformin with glipizide, glyburide, or rosiglitazone		

not currently clear what the ideal perioperative glucose levels are in these patients, regular insulin should be given if needed.

Recommendations about the ideal "tightness" of perioperative glucose control in the ambulatory surgery patient with either type 1 or type 2 diabetes may change in the future. Traditionally, it was felt that the risk-benefit ratio favored allowing glucose levels to be somewhat elevated, thereby decreasing the chance of unrecognized hypoglycemia. Recent data from the open heart surgery patients demonstrate improved wound healing and better outcomes

Box 3-15. Considerations in the patient with thyroid disease

Hypothyroidism
Symptoms
- Lethargy
- Memory loss
- Constipation
- Cold intolerance
- Hair loss

Physiologic changes
- Weight gain
- Decreased cardiac output
- Decreased intravascular volume
- Decreased ventilatory drive
- Hyponatremia, hypoglycemia
- Pleural, pericardial effusion
- Decreased drug metabolism
- Myxedema coma

Hyperthyroidism
Symptoms
- Tremor
- Heat intolerance
- Tachycardia

Physiologic changes
- Weight loss
- Goiter
- Ophthalmopathy
- Atrial fibrillation

with euglycemic management strategies. Whether these benefits extend to the ambulatory patient is not yet clear.

Administration of metoclopramide preoperatively is not needed unless the patient has symptoms of regurgitation or reflux.[47] If regional anesthesia is chosen, the presence of peripheral neuropathy should be documented preoperatively. Neuropathy may be present and affect intra- and postoperative hemodynamic stability. In addition, postoperative bladder function may be compromised: it is reasonable to require these patients to void prior to discharge.

Thyroid disease

Considerations for the patient with thyroid disease are presented in Box 3-15 and include issues of hypothyroidism, hyperthyroidism, goiter and airway assessment, and the management of thyroid-related medications.

Hypothyroidism

In populations with adequate dietary iodine, the incidence of hypothyroidism is 5 to 10 per 1,000 with perhaps 15 per 1,000 in a sub-clinical state.[48] The incidence increases with age and may be as high as 5% in those over 50 years of age. Patient symptoms include fatigue, cold intolerance, constipation, lethargy, and memory loss. Ideally, patients will be rendered euthyroid prior to ambulatory surgery, and ambulatory surgery in the severely hypothyroid patient should be postponed. Patients with mild disease can undergo ambulatory surgery without significant increased risk.[48] Treatment is with levothyroxine (T4), which has a long half-life (approximately 7 days), so a dose the day of surgery is not usually needed. Caution should be exercised when therapy is begun in patients with significant CAD.

Hyperthyroidism

Hyperthyroidism is most commonly caused by Graves disease, an autoimmune disorder. Signs and symptoms may be overt such as tachycardia, tremor, weight loss, goiter, and ophthalmopathy or more subtle such as frequent atrial premature contractions or new onset of atrial fibrillation. Cardiac effects can also include CHF and ischemic heart disease. Diagnosis is made by a normal or elevated thyroid hormone level with a depressed level of thyroid-stimulating hormone. Treatment is with agents that decrease thyroid hormone production (propothiouracil and methimazole) and beta-blockers to decrease cardiac symptoms.

It usually takes 6 to 8 weeks of therapy to become euthyroid, and ambulatory surgery should be postponed. Thyroid-suppressing drugs and beta-blockers should be continued through the day of surgery. Thyroid storm presents as fever, tachycardia, and delirium and may progress to CV collapse. The chance of thyroid storm is greatly reduced with proper preoperative treatment but may occur in a patient with unrecognized hyperthyroidism and can be misdiagnosed as malignant hyperthermia or pheochromocytoma. Practitioners should be prepared to administer supportive care that includes cooling, hydration, beta-blockers, and thionamides.

Preoperative evaluation

Signs and symptoms of hyper- and hypothyroidism should be elicited. Other endocinopathies should be considered. Thyroid function tests and hemoglobin determination may prove helpful. Particular attention should be paid to the airway, especially in the patient with goiter. Tracheal deviation should be assessed with CXR or computed tomography scan if needed. Dysphonia, dysphagia, respiratory distress, or symptoms of superior vena cava compression warrant further imaging evaluation since goiter can involve mediastinal structures. Practitioners should be prepared to deal with a difficult airway. However, because of the possibility of airway collapse with GA and positive-pressure ventilation, patients with significant mediastinal goiter should probably not be cared for on an ambulatory basis.

Morbid obesity

The United States is in the midst of an obesity epidemic, and an increasing percentage of patients are morbidly obese (body mass index of more than $35\,\mathrm{kg/m^2}$). With proper patient selection, these patients can be cared for on an ambulatory basis.[49] There are a series of comorbidities associated with morbid obesity (MO) which are listed in Box 3-16. These patients have a high incidence of obstructive sleep apnea (OSA) (see below), which may not be diagnosed. Patients who either have sleep apnea or are considered at risk and will require postoperative opioids for pain management should not be cared for on an ambulatory basis. In addition, the patient with resting hypoxemia, daytime somnolence, or Pickwickian syndrome should not be cared for on an ambulatory basis except for the most minor of procedures. A recent survey showed that most anesthesiologists would administer GA on an ambulatory basis to the MO patient without significant comorbidities but would not administer ambulatory GA to the MO patient with significant comorbidities.[31]

Before beginning care, the practitioner should review the facility to ensure that all the specialized equipment needed to care for these oversized people is available. IV access may be difficult and may require ultrasound guidance.

Box 3-16. Considerations in the morbidly obese patient

- Obstructive sleep apnea
- Potential for difficult mask airway or intubation, decreased functional residual capacity
- Potential for increased gastric residual and/or increased intragastric pressure
- Difficult venous access
- Difficult positioning on operating room table
- Altered volume of distribution and drug metabolism
- Potential end-organ manifestations
  - Ventricular failure
  - Pulmonary hypertension
  - Liver dysfunction
  - Thromboembolic disease
- Coexisting disease
  - Diabetes, hypothyroid, Cushing, hyperlipidemia, gastroesophageal reflux disease, renal calculi, chronic back pain
- Surgical risks
  Poor wound healing
- Psychiatric conditions
  Depression, anxiety, low self-esteem

Administration of metoclopromide and H_2 blockers or nonparticulate antacid as recommended could be considered. Regional anesthetic techniques may be used safely, although there is a slightly higher incidence of block failure compared to the nonobese patient.[50] Awake fiber-optic intubation should be planned if exam reveals a potentially difficult airway not amenable to more conventional techniques. Intubation and extubation should be accomplished with the patient in a semi-sitting position, which improves pulmonary mechanics and gas exchange; thorough preoxygenation is essential. Modern, less soluble anesthetics offer distinct advantages in providing faster emergence. Positive end-expiratory pressure should be administered to limit atelectasis. Procedures lasting longer than 4 hours may be associated with muscle breakdown, myoglobinuria, and renal failure in the morbidly obese and should not be planned on an ambulatory basis. Pneumatic thromboelastic stockings should be used and subcutaneous heparin considered to limit thromboembolic events. Postoperative monitoring should be continued until restoration of preoperative oxygen saturation is achieved. Postoperative analgesia should employ multimodal nonopioid techniques.[51]

Obstructive sleep apnea

OSA has emerged as a significant concern for the ambulatory anesthesiologist. No one wants to have a postoperative catastrophe in a patient discharged from an ambulatory facility. Likewise, admitting all patients for postoperative observation may place an undue and unnecessary burden on these patients, their families, and the health care organization. The ASA has recently issued practice guidelines that summarize the current literature and expert opinion about this topic.[52]

The prevalence of OSA is thought to be approximately 2% to 4%. Only a percentage of these patients are formally diagnosed, as diagnosis usually requires a polysonography study. OSA is described as mild, moderate, or severe depending on the number of episodes of apnea or hypoxia. Those without a formal diagnosis may be screened using the criteria such as those listed in Table 3-8. The diagnosis of moderate OSA should be considered in patients who meet criteria in two of the three categories and severe OSA in those with a significantly abnormal finding.[52] The mainstay of therapy for the patient with OSA is to sleep with continuous positive airway pressure (CPAP) or noninvasive positive-pressure ventilation, which can be administered nasally (bi-level positive airway pressure). Patients who have undergone therapeutic surgery such as uvulopalatopharyngoplasty should be considered to be at continued risk unless documented otherwise.

The decision to proceed with ambulatory surgery in the patient with OSA requires consideration of several factors: severity of OSA status, anatomic and physiologic abnormalities, status of coexisting disease, nature of surgery, type of anesthesia, need for postoperative opioids, adequacy of postdischarge observation, and capabilities of the ambulatory facility. The presence of severe OSA, significant physical abnormalities, or significant coexisting disease precludes an ambulatory procedure. Peripheral or superficial procedures that can be performed with local or regional anesthesia are acceptable to a majority of anesthesiologists, whereas upper abdominal, laparoscopic, or airway surgery are

Table 3-8. Identification and assessment of obstructive sleep apnea (OSA)

Predisposing physical characteristics	Body mass index >35 kg/m²
	Neck circumference >17 inches (men), 16 inches (women)
	Craniofacial abnormalities affecting the airway
	Anatomical nasal obstruction
	Tonsils nearly touching or touching in the midline
History of apparent airway obstruction during sleep (two or more)	Snoring (loud enough to be heard through closed door)
	Frequent snoring
	Observed pauses in breathing during sleep
	Awakens from sleep with choking sensation
	Frequent arousals from sleep
Somnolence (one or more)	Frequent somnolence or fatigue despite adequate "sleep"
	Falls asleep easily in a nonstimulating environment despite adequate "sleep"

Positive findings in two categories = moderate OSA, three categories = severe OSA.

not. Other procedures that require GA or postoperative opioids may be decided on a case-by-case basis: some anesthesiologists feel more comfortable sending these patients home if they use a nasal CPAP machine.[53] One proposed approach to making this decision is displayed in Table 3-9. Deep sedation should be avoided; it is preferable to secure the airway and administer GA. The use of perineural infusion catheters with local anesthetics will decrease opioid requirements and may allow an increased number of ambulatory procedures. Ambulatory facilities without the resources to care for these patients in a "worst case" scenario (fiber optics and chest radiography) should consider not caring for these patients.

Following surgery, patients should be observed in a monitored setting until they are no longer at risk for respiratory depression. The postoperative process will take longer in the patient with OSA, and postanesthesia care unit staffing should be prepared. One approach to assessing discharge readiness is to document that the patient is able to maintain their baseline oxygenation when not stimulated and breathing room air. If patients are admitted for observation, continual oxygen saturation monitoring with telemetry is needed.

Table 3-9. Suggested obstructive sleep apnea (OSA) scoring system

Assessment	Degree	Points
A. Severity of OSA	None	0
(subtract 1 point for pre- and postop CPAP or NIPPV)	Mild	1
(add 1 point for $PaCO_2 > 50$)	Moderate	2
	Severe	3
B. Invasiveness of surgery and anesthesia	Superficial, local or nerve block, no sedation	0
	Superficial, moderate sedation or GA	1
	Peripheral with spinal, epidural	1
	Peripheral with GA	2
	Airway surgery with moderate sedation	2
	Major surgery or airway surgery, GA	3
C. Requirement for postoperative opioids	None	0
	Low-dose oral opioids	1
	High-dose oral opioids, intravenous or neuraxial opioids	2

Add results from section A to the greater of B and C. Score of 4 may be at increased risk from OSA, 5 or 6 may be at significantly increased perioperative risk from OSA. CPAP, continuous positive airway pressure; GA, general anesthesia; NIPPV, noninvasive positive pressure ventilation; $PaCO_2$, partial pressure of carbon dioxide, arterial. Adapted from Practice guidelines for the perioperative management of patients with obstructive sleep apnea.[52] Used with permission.

End-stage renal disease

At one time, the patient with end-stage renal disease was not considered eligible for ambulatory surgery. Today, ambulatory surgery, especially minor procedures, is being performed with appropriate caution. The patient with chronic renal failure on dialysis (Box 3-17) may have one or several of the previously described diseases, including CAD, hypertension, CHF, and diabetes. Concerns specific to the dialysis patient include volume and electrolyte status. During the history, signs and symptoms of volume overload and angina should be specifically addressed. Ideally, surgery should be planned for a day following dialysis, when a patient reaches their "ideal" weight. Immediately after dialysis, the patient has relative intravascular volume depletion, whereas after more than 1 day, the patient begins to return to a volume overloaded state. Similarly, electrolyte shifts continue to occur for at least several hours after dialysis. It is also prudent to recheck the serum level of potassium (and glucose, if the patient is

Box 3-17. Considerations in the dialysis patient

- Associated diseases (hypertension, diabetes, coronary disease)
- Electrolyte and acid-base status
- Volume status
- Coagulation status and platelet function
- Timing of dialysis in the preoperative period
- Cognitive impairment common

a diabetic) prior to surgery. Anemia is usually present; a hematocrit of 25% to 28% is normal for the non-erthopoetin-treated patient. Platelet dysfunction may be abnormal if the patient is uremic; the renal failure patient with platelet dysfunction is probably best cared for as an in-patient.

Local or regional anesthesia, when appropriate, may be best for the dialysis patient; GA, if chosen, should be accomplished with agents that minimize CV depression and with agents that do not rely on renal excretion. The altered pharmacokinetics of renal failure should also be remembered, and alternatives to succinylcholine considered if the preoperative serum potassium is elevated. Many agents, such as fentanyl, midazolam, rocuronium, and vecuronium, can be used with the caveat that, while loading doses may not be significantly altered, infusions or repeated doses should be decreased by 30%–50% with an expected prolonged duration of action. An attractive anesthetic consists of propofol, remifentanil, and cisatricurium: none relies on renal excretion.[54] Inhalation anesthetics are also useful since they are excreted predominantly via the lungs. Assuming recent dialysis, uremia-induced gastric dysfunction should not be an issue and the airway can be managed with any airway device including an LMA.

Rheumatoid arthritis

Rheumatoid arthritis (RA) has several important anesthetic implications (Box 3-18). The cervical spine may have limited mobility or instability. Because of the high incidence of asymptomatic instability with severe RA, flexion and

Box 3-18. Considerations in the patient with rheumatoid arthritis

- Potential for difficult airway
- Cervical spine instability or fixation
- Mandibular hypoplasia, particularly in juvenile onset rheumatoid arthritis
- Cricoarytenoid arthritis
- Pulmonary involvement
- Implications of medications
  Aspirin
  Steroids
  Nonsteroidal anti-inflammatory drugs
  Methotrexate

extension radiographs are suggested before ambulatory surgery. The patient with RA may also have cricoarytenoid arthritis, which is frequently asymptomatic and should be anticipated; a smaller endotracheal tube should be considered. Preoperative fiber-optic evaluation may be appropriate in patients with a history of hoarseness or jaw pain. Medication history is also important in this population as chronic aspirin, nonsteroidal anti-inflammatory drugs (NSAIDs), steroids, and methotrexate use are common. If possible, aspirin should be discontinued a week before surgery. NSAID use should not preclude the use of neuraxial techniques. Perioperative steroid coverage should be considered for patients chronically taking these drugs (see discussion in Asthma section).

Alcohol and drug use

Recent or chronic substance use may be a significant problem in patients presenting for ambulatory surgery. A careful history and high index of suspicion are needed, and blood alcohol levels and/or serum toxicology screening may be appropriate. Patients who have signs of acute intoxication should have ambulatory surgery postponed. In the case of chronic use, evaluation of the medical sequelae will help determine the patient's suitability for surgery. IV drug users (Box 3-19) may have difficult venous access and may have undiagnosed HIV infection. IV drug and cocaine users frequently have a low pain threshold and cooperate poorly with minimally painful procedures including IV catheter placement and regional anesthesia.

With acute use, cocaine blocks neuronal uptake of norepinephrine and dopamine, which causes sympathetic nervous system stimulation. Hypertension, cardiac arrhythmias, and ischemia (possibly due to coronary artery vasospasm) may occur in people without prior abnormalities.[55] Seizures, cerebrovascular accident, and hyperthermia may also occur. Patients who have acutely used cocaine should not undergo ambulatory surgery. Chronic cocaine users may have these acute problems as well. In addition, longer duration of use can lead to cardiomyopathy, nasal septal atrophy, and "crack lung" (pulmonary changes

---

Box 3-19. General considerations with intravenous drug and cocaine use

- Difficult intravenous access
- Low pain threshold
- May be poorly cooperative
- HIV transmission risk
- Cardiomyopathy
- Myocardial ischemia
- Pulmonary changes: decreased compliance, chronic granulomatosis
- Nasal septal atrophy
- Altered sympathetic nervous system responses
- Drug withdrawal

Box 3-20. Considerations in alcohol use

Acute
Increased aspiration risk
Metabolic abnormalities
Combativeness
Alcoholic hepatitis

Chronic
Cirrhosis
Coagulopathy
Altered drug volume and kinetics
Pulmonary and extrapulmonary shunting
Acute and chronic gastritis, pancreatitis
Cardiomyopathy, arrhythmia
Delirium tremens, withdrawal seizures, dementia
Bone marrow depression, folate and thiamine deficiency
Unreliable, social problems

such as decreased compliance and chronic granulomatosis from inhaled impurities).

There is an increasing use of amphetamines, methamphetamine (crystal meth), and MDMA (3,4-methylenedioxymethamphetamine, or Ecstasy). The primary pharmacologic action of these agents is through the release of norepinephrine and dopamine, and in the case of Ecstasy, serotonin, from presynaptic autonomic neurons.[56] These agents also inhibit monoamine oxidase, resulting in a sympathomimetic effect similar to cocaine but with a slower onset and longer duration. Use of the agents is associated with stroke, coronary artery occlusion, and MI.

The opioid user may have a history or signs of endocarditis, hepatitis, and chronic pulmonary changes (from suppression of cough reflex and reduced mucociliary clearance). In addition, there is risk of withdrawal; manifestations include tremor, muscle aches, perspiration, rhinorrhea, hot and cold flashes, fever, and gastrointestinal distress. Pain management can be difficult in patients with a history of opioid use; significantly higher amounts of narcotics may be necessary. Alternatives to opioids should be used when feasible, but adequate amounts of pain medication should not be withheld merely from fear of contributing to addiction. Ketamine may be a useful adjunct analgesic in these patients.

Individuals with acute alcohol intoxication (Box 3-20) may have impaired airway reflexes and multiple metabolic abnormalities; these patients are not acceptable for ambulatory surgery. Patients with a history of alcohol use should be questioned carefully about other manifestations, such as liver disease, withdrawal symptoms or history of cardiomyopathy or arrhythmia, and bleeding tendency. Liver disease in the alcoholic patient may range from fatty infiltration to alcoholic hepatitis to cirrhosis; ambulatory surgery should be postponed in patients with acute abnormalities such as alcoholic hepatitis.

Immunosuppression

The ambulatory surgery setting provides a viable option for the immuno-compromised patient who may require procedures that are related to their disease, such as biopsies and line placement, or may require routine procedures unrelated to their disease. Outpatient surgery offers reduced exposure to noso-comial infection and other iatrogenic illness. Preoperative evaluation should be directed toward identifying the systemic effects of both the disease and the treatment that the patient has received.

Cancer patient

The patient with cancer presents several challenges related to both the disease itself and the side effects of therapy; medical considerations are listed in Box 3-21. The patient may be in a debilitated condition with poor nutritional status. Hematologic function should be assessed since myelosuppression is often present; ambulatory surgery should be postponed for significant anemia or low white cell or platelet count. Assessment of coagulation status, electrolyte levels, ECG, and CXR should be considered based on the patient's history, physical exam, chemotherapy regimen, and size of the proposed surgery. Patients are prone to nosocomial infections and require strict aseptic technique.

Cancer treatment can involve both radiation and chemotherapy; both have consequences for the anesthesiologist. Radiation therapy has long-lasting side effects described in Box 3-22. Of greatest concern is radiation pneumonitis and carditis in those who have received radiation therapy of the chest. Airway abnormalities may develop; proper airway evaluation is important and the need for fiber-optic intubation should be considered. The actions of chemotherapeutic agents are directed toward neoplastic cells but can also have significant effects on nonmalignant cells. Cardiac, respiratory, hepatic, renal, and peripheral nervous system function are often altered; effects of several agents on organ function are presented in Table 3-10. Preoperative evaluation should be directed toward these organ systems.

Box 3-21. Considerations for the outpatient with cancer

- Myelosuppression
- Cancer-related ectopic hormone production and associated syndromes
- Coexisting medical problems
- Radiotherapy- and chemotherapy-induced organ dysfunction
- Chemotherapy and anesthesia interactions
- Pain management
- Aseptic technique

Box 3-22. Complications of radiotherapy

Acute
Skin changes, gastrointestinal problems, alopecia, pancytopenia

Intermediate
Bowel obstruction, fistulae

Late
Myocardial fibrosis, radiotherapy-induced coronary artery disease; pericardial effusions; radiation pneumonitis and fibrosis; rib fractures; pleural effusion; hypoxemia; hepatic, renal, central nervous system problems; laryngeal necrosis; and edema

Table 3-10. Major organ toxicity of chemotherapeutic agents

Class	Drug	Major organ toxicity
Alkylating agents	Cyclophosphamide	BMD, pulmonary infiltrates and fibrosis, cardiac toxicity, SIADH
	Busulfan	BMD, pulmonary infiltrates and fibrosis, hepatitis, seizures
	Carboplatin	BMD, peripheral neuropathy, hearing loss, transient cortical blindness
	Cisplatin	Renal damage, ototoxicity, BMD, peripheral neuropathy, electrolyte abnormalities
Antimetabolites	Methotrexate	Oral and GI ulceration, BMD, hepatitic damage, renal toxicity, pulmonary infiltrates and fibrosis, lymphoma
	Flurouracil (5-FU)	Oral and GI ulceration, BMD, neuro defect (cerebellar), arrhythmia, heart failure, seizure
	Gemcitabine	BMD, edema, pulmonary toxicity
	Mercaptopurine	BMD, cholestasis, oral and GI ulceration, pancreatitis
Vinca Alcaloids	Vinblastine	BMD, peripheral neuropathy, stomatitis, muscle pain
	Vincristine	Peripheral neuropathy, BMD, SIADH
Taxanes	Paclitaxel	BMD, peripheral neuropathy, myalgia, cardiac toxicity

(Continued)

Table 3-10. *Continued*

Class	Drug	Major organ toxicity
	Docetaxel	BMD, peripheral neuropathy, fluid retention and pleural effusion, myalgia, hepatic
Antibiotics	Bleomycin	Pneumonitis and pulmonary fibrosis, rash, stomatitis, Raynaud's
	Doxorubicin	BMD, cardiotoxicity (culumative), stomatitis, dermatitis, leukemia
	Idarubicin	BMD, stomatitis, myocardial toxicity
Biologic modifiers	Interferon alfa-2a	BMD, confusion, renal, hepatic arrhythmia, rhabdomyosis
	Interleukin-2	Neuropsychiatric disorder, hypothyroididm, brachial plexopathy
Epipodophylatoxins	Etoposide	BMD, rash, peripheral neuropathy, leukemia
Hormones	Tamoxifen	Thromboembolism, thrombocytopenia, peripheral edema, uterine sarcoma
	Letrozole	Peripheral edema, dyspnea, fatigue
	Flurimid	Hepatic toxicity

BMD, bone marrow depression; GI, gastrointestinal; SIADH, syndrome of inappropriate antidiuretic hormone secretion. Adapted from Drugs of Choice for Cancer.[58] Used with permission.

When planning an anesthetic, familiarity with these treatment-related organ system dysfunctions is important.[57,58] For example, patients who have received high-dose methotrexate therapy are at increased risk for renal failure; monitoring fluid status and urine output is essential. Those who have received anthracycline agents (doxorubicin or daunorubicin) will demonstrate dose-related decreases in cardiac function; they may require careful titration of agents that further depress cardiac function; both isoflurane-N_2O and fentanyl-based anesthetics have been used successfully in these patients.[59] Patients treated with bleomycin or mitomycin C may have developed interstitial fibrosis and pulmonary edema; careful monitoring of fluid status and minimizing inspired FiO_2 (fraction of inspired oxygen) is important. Postoperatively, pain management requires understanding of the patient's preoperative regimen, as the opioid tolerant patient will have a larger-than-average requirement.

In addition, there are concerns about the effects of anesthetics and the OR environment on immunological function that can alter the effectiveness of cancer therapy, at least in theory and in some animal models. Hypothermia should be avoided as it decreases immune function and enhances the chance of nosocomial infection and poor wound healing.[60] The biggest concern with anesthetic agents centers on nitrous oxide, particularly in the patient who is simultaneously receiving methotrexate as they both decrease intracellular folate coenzyme concentrations. The balance between the potentially beneficial cytostatic effects and the metabolically harmful effects of N_2O is still unclear. There is, however, increasing opinion that N_2O should be avoided in these cancer patients.[61]

HIV/AIDS patient

With improvement in therapy, HIV infection has become more of a chronic disease rather than a rapidly fatal illness. It is estimated that approximately 1 million Americans are infected, with more than 20% unaware of their status.[62] Viral load is very high early following infection, decreases in the latent phase, and rises again in the preterminal condition. Assessment of viral load and $CD4^+$ cell count can track disease severity. The disease can affect multiple organ systems (Box 3-23). Classes of therapeutic agents are listed in Box 3-24. Special consideration should be given to patients receiving protease inhibitors, a mainstay of therapy in serious infection. These agents inhibit components of the cytochrome P450 system and inhibit the metabolism of benzodiazepines and potent opioids. Although these agents certainly can be used, the practitioner needs to realize that repeated doses may lead to higher plasma levels and longer duration of action than anticipated.[63] Protease inhibitors also can result in dyslipidemia, which may result in accelerated atherosclerosis and CAD and MI in patients who would otherwise be considered too young to be at significant risk.

Preoperative assessment and testing should be directed to the medical issues listed in Box 3-23. Dilated cardiomyopathy can be seen in 30%–40% of patients with active AIDS, and an echocardiogram may be advisable.[64] A $CD4^+$ count

---

Box 3-23. Considerations for the patient with AIDS

- Opportunistic infections and malignancies
- Cardiomyopathy, myocarditis, coronary artery disease, and myocardial infarction
- Pericardial effusions, pleural effusions
- Pulmonary hypertension
- Diarrhea, esophagitis, dysphagia
- Pancytopenia, coagulopathy
- Cachexia, hypoproteinemia
- Renal and liver involvement
- Central neurologic impairment, encephalopathy, dementia
- Neuropathies: sensory, demylenating polyneuropathy
- Difficult venous access

Box 3-24. Classes of HIV medications
- Nucleoside/nucleotide analogues: headache, nausea, neuropathy, anemia
- Protease inhibitors: inhibit cytochrome P450 system (see text), dyslipidemias
- Reverse transcriptase inhibitors: dizziness, headache, nausea, cytochrome effects
- Fusion inhibitors: insomnia, dizziness, nausea

is useful: a level below 200 counts per microliter denotes a patient at heightened risk for opportunistic infection and may indicate an increased risk for poor outcome following surgery. Coagulation can be affected in advanced disease, and complete blood counts often reflect multiple abnormalities. Electrolyte levels and liver function tests may reveal renal and hepatic involvement. Presence of neuropathy should be elicited and documented.

Patients should continue their antiviral and antiopportunistic infection medications through the morning of surgery. Care should be taken to prevent transmission of disease to health care providers: gloves should be worn, needleless systems should be employed, and blood and body fluid precautions should be rigorously followed. The actual anesthetic technique is probably not critical to the well-being of the patient: effects of anesthetic agents on the immune system found in the laboratory have not been definitively demonstrated *in vivo*. Regional anesthesia is not contraindicated and should be used when appropriate. Previous concerns about spinal anesthesia leading to increased risk of meningitis have proven unfounded.[65] Antiemetic agents should be considered to increase the chance that patients can resume their antiviral medications as soon as possible postoperatively.

Gastroesophageal reflux disease

Gastroesophageal reflux disease (GERD) occurs when the lower esophageal sphincter allows the reflux of acidic gastric contents into the esophagus, causing symptoms (Box 3-25). The incidence is increased in smokers and the obese. The syndrome is often associated with hiatal hernia. Initial treatment is with lifestyle adjustment. If symptoms persist, proton-pump inhibitors (such as omeprazole and esomeprazole) have demonstrated efficacy and have emerged as the mainstay of therapy.[66] H_2 receptor antagonists (such as cimetidine and ranitidine) are also used as first-line therapy or added to proton-pump inhibitors for refractory disease. Prokinetic therapy with metoclopramide is also used. Surgical treatment with fundoplication has emerged as an option for those refractory to medical therapy.

Preoperative evaluation should look for symptoms of supine reflux, including the presence of bronchospastic symptoms, and not merely food-induced symptoms. Medications should be continued through the day of surgery. Preoperative administration of nonparticulate antacid or IV H_2 receptor antagonists

Box 3-25. Symptoms of gastroesophageal reflux disease

Typical
Heartburn, acid regurgitation

Atypical
Dysphagia, noncardiac chest pain, dyspepsia or abdominal pain

Extraesophageal
Hoarseness and/or sore throat, sinusitis, chronic cough, asthma, recurrent aspiration, pulmonary fibrosis

Malignancy
Esophageal adenocarcinoma, head and neck cancer

and/or metoclopramide may be considered. The use of an LMA in patients with controlled disease is controversial; if symptoms are provoked by supine position, most practitioners would secure the airway with an endotracheal tube via an induction that includes cricoid pressure.

Mental health

Psychoactive medications work by altering levels of neurotransmitters in the brain and have the potential to contribute to perioperative morbidity. The major classes of agent, their mechanism of action, and potential perioperative concerns are listed in Table 3-11.[67] Whether these agents should be discontinued prior to surgery is a difficult issue and often requires consultation with the patient's psychiatrist; no blanket statement can be made. The potential benefits of drug discontinuation need to be weighed against the potential risk of exacerbation of the patient's psychiatric illness. In addition, the size of the planned procedure may influence the need to discontinue these medications: minor procedures may be performed safely.

If surgery proceeds without drug discontinuation, the anesthesiologist must be familiar with the potential problems associated with surgical stress and the potential for drug interactions. For example, ephedrine should not be given to those receiving monoamine oxidase inhibitors (MAOIs), as a hyper-catechol-amine state may occur. Also of concern is the development of the serotonin syndrome, which is a progression of symptoms that may be fatal and include clonus, hyperreflexia, mental status changes, and hyperthermia. It is classically described with the combination of MAOIs and selective serotonin uptake inhibitors but has been reported with MAOIs and a variety of serotonergic medications, including phenylpiperidine opioids (meperidine, tramadol, methadone, fentanyl, and dextromethorphan) and $5\text{-}HT_3$ antagonists (ondansetron and granisetron) among others.[68] Morphine and codeine have not been implicated.[69] Care is supportive with the administration of $5\text{-}HT_{2A}$ antagonists such as chlor-promazine in severe cases. Differential diagnosis includes malignant neuroleptic syndrome, malignant hyperthermia, and central cholinergic syndrome.

Table 3-11. Psychiatric medications

Class	Mechanism	Toxicities	Potential interactions
Lithium	Unclear	GI (sinus node dysfunction, bradycardia), central nervous system	Toxicity with drugs that decrease renal function nonsteroidal anti-inflammatory drugs, angiotensin-converting enzyme inhibitors, etc.
MAOIs	Inhibit breakdown of NE and SER by MAO enzyme		Indirect sympathomimetics: pressor effects (can be lethal), meperidine, dextromethorphan: serotonergic syndrome
Tricyclics	Presynaptic inhibition of NE and SER uptake	Conduction deficits, lower seizure threshold	Exaggerated pressor effects with sympathomimetics.
Selective serotonergic reuptake inhibitors	Presynaptic inhibition of SER uptake	GI, agitation, syndrome of inappropriate antidiuretic hormone secretion (rare)	Cytochrome interactions that may lead to serotonergic syndrome: caution with MAOIs, meperidine, and highly protein-bound drugs (lidocaine, midazolam, fentanyl)
Antipsychotics	Block dopamine receptors	Extrapyramidal symptoms, prolonged QT interval	Hypotension with halogenated agents, anticholinergic effects with atropine and scopolamine

GI, gastrointestinal; MAO, monoamine oxidase; MAOI, monoamine oxidase inhibitor; NE, norepinephrine; SER, serotonin. Adapted from Huyse et al.[67] Used with permission.

Latex allergy

Latex allergy has emerged as a significant issue over the past two decades. The latex substance is ubiquitous in society in general and is found in many products used during surgery. It is estimated that 1%–6% of the population and 8%–12% of health care workers have developed a sensitivity to latex.[70] Other groups at risk include the spina bifida patient and others who have undergone multiple genitourinary procedures and those with work-related exposure to latex.

Three clinical entities related to latex are recognized (Box 3-26). The first is a nonallergic skin reaction to latex gloves characterized by sore, chapped hands. This can be treated with changing to nonlatex gloves and routine skin care. A second is an allergic contact dermatitis (type IV) usually caused by additives and accelerants, not latex per se. It is characterized by raised, red lesions that may extend up the arms. The third is the most serious, type I hypersensitivity mediated by antilatex immunoglobulin E antibodies. Reactions include facial swelling, generalized uticaria, respiratory distress, and anaphylaxsis. Treatment involves removal of the latex product, fluids, diphenhydramine, steroids, and epinephrine as needed.

All patients should be questioned for possible latex allergy. Those with possible reactivity should be further questioned about causative agents, symptoms, and sequelae. Some facilities use a formal questionnaire. Most important is to try to separate the patient with contact dermatitis from the type I hypersensitivity patient. Referral for skin testing may be appropriate if a formal diagnosis is desired. The patient with contact dermatitis can be cared for avoiding contact with latex products. The patient with type I hypersensitivity requires more extensive consideration. The powder inside latex gloves aerosolizes the allergen, and the OR must be thoroughly cleaned before the patient enters. Care must be taken to remove all latex-containing products from the OR and all other patient care areas. The practitioner may consider prophylactic treatment with diphenhydramine and steroids, but this is not clearly recommended. One should be prepared to treat a reaction that could include anaphylaxsis. Ideally,

---

Box 3-26. Considerations in latex allergy

Nonallergic contact dermatitis
Chapped, sore hands

Allergic contact dermatitis (type IV)
Chapped sore hands
Raised, red lesions, may extend up arms

Type I hypersensitivity
Uticaria
Facial swelling
Bronchospasm
Hypotension
Anaphylaxis

over time, all latex-containing products will be removed from health care areas and limit the risk of this allergy in the future, for patients and health care workers.

Medical consultation

The anesthesiologist is part of a health care team, and it is sometimes necessary to obtain additional information about a patient prior to ambulatory surgery. The concept of preoperative "medical clearance" is antiquated; only the anesthesiologist has the sufficient knowledge of the operative environment to judge when a patient may undergo ambulatory surgery. However, there are many situations in which information, suggestions, and therapies from medical colleagues are needed to allow the decision to proceed. Table 3-12 contains a partial list of medical situations in which consultation with an internist or cardiologist may

Table 3-12. Consultation with internist or cardiologists with specific questions

Medical issue	Specific question/request
Active cardiac conditions (American Heart Association/American College of Cardiology guidelines)	Can treatment lower risk and allow ambulatory procedure?
Poor or unclear exercise tolerance with one or more clinical risk factors scheduled for greater than low risk surgery.	Need for noninvasive cardiac testing? Need for beta blockers to lower perioperative risk?
Atrial fibrillation or angina on anticoagulant therapy.	Timing of anticoagulant discontinuation? Need for low-molecular-weight heparin?
Known coronary artery disease for intermediate surgical-risk procedure.	Need for beta blockers?
Myocardial infarction within 6 months.	Cardiac status stable? Cardiac function adequate for ambulatory surgery?
Recent percutaneous balloon angioplasty or cardiac stent placement, particularly drug-eluting stents.	Timing of ambulatory surgery? Timing of anticoagulation discontinuation? Need for low-molecular-weight heparin?
Pacemaker	Type and function? How to convert to fixed mode?
Automatic implantable cardioverter defibrillator	Plan for disabling, reenabling?

(Continued)

Table 3-12. *Continued*

Medical issue	Specific question/request
Active bronchospasm	Can therapy be augmented?
Undiagnosed, undertreated significant hypertension.	Begin or augment appropriate therapy.
Undiagnosed, undertreated significant diabetes.	Begin or augment appropriate therapy.
Long-acting psychiatric medications	Risk/benefit of discontinuation?
Bleeding disorder (hemophilia, factor deficiency)	Management strategy
Symptomatic hemoglobinopathy	Management strategy

be appropriate. Note that the request for consultation should contain specific questions or requests.

Summary

The movement toward increased ambulatory surgery will no doubt continue. In the future, the anesthesiologist will be asked to care for patients with increasing medical morbidities and heightened surgical invasiveness. Proper patient selection and medical management are essential for successful outcome. By maintaining an ongoing knowledge of patient management issues, the anesthesiologist can provide state-of-the-art care. To determine whether a patient is suitable for an office-based surgery practice, a freestanding ambulatory surgical facility, or a hospital-based ambulatory unit, the clinician must appreciate the extent of the patient's medical conditions and whether the facility is equipped to handle complications arising from the conditions.

References

1. Kinsella K, Velkoff VA. *An Aging World: 2001*. Washington, DC: U.S. Census Bureau; 2001.
2. Fact Sheet: The American Geriatrics Society (AGS). Available at: http://www. americangeriatrics.org/news/ags_fact_sheet.shtml. Accessed July 5, 2007.
3. Warner MA, Saletel RA, Schroeder DR, Warner DO, Offord KP, Gray DT. Outcomes of anesthesia and surgery in people 100 years of age and older. *J Am Geriatr Soc*. 1998;46:988–993.

4. Aldwinckle RJ, Montgomery JE. Unplanned admission rates and postdischarge complications in patients over the age of 70 following day case surgery. *Anaesthesia.* 2004;59:57–59.

5. Fleisher LA, Pasternak LR, Herbert R, Anderson GF. Inpatient hospital admission and death after outpatient surgery in elderly patients: important of patient and system characteristics and location of care. *Arch Surg.* 2004;139:67–72.

6. Polanczyk CA, Marcantonio E, Goldman L, et al. Impact of age on perioperative complications and length of stay in patients undergoing noncardiac surgery. *Ann Intern Med.* 2001;134:637–643.

7. Kantelip JP, Sage E, Duchene-Marullaz P. Findings on ambulatory electrocardiographic monitoring in subjects older than 80 years. *Am J Cardiol.* 1986;57:398–401.

8. Eger EI. Age, minimum alveolar anesthetic concentration, and minimum alveolar anesthetic concentration-awake. *Anesth Analg.* 2001;93:947–53.

9. Fragen RJ, Dunn KL. The minimum alveolar concentration (MAC) of sevoflurane with and without nitrous oxide in elderly versus young adults. *J Clin Anesth.* 1996;8:352–356.

10. Schnider TW, Minto CF, Shafer SL, et al. The influence of age on propofol pharmacodynamics. *Anesthesiology.* 1999;90:1502–1516.

11. Kirkbride DA, Parker JL, Williams GD, Buggy DJ. Induction of anesthesia in the elderly ambulatory patient: a double-blind comparison of propofol and sevoflurane. *Anesth Analg.* 2001;93:1185–1187.

12. Tsui BC, Wagner A, Finucane B. Regional anaesthesia in the elderly: a clinical guide. *Drugs Aging.* 2004;21:895–910.

13. Marcantonio ER, Goldman L, Orav EJ, Cook EF, Lee TH. The association of intraoperative factors with the development of postoperative delirium. *Am J Med.* 1998;105:380–384.

14. Zakriya KJ, Christmas C, Wenz JF Sr., Franckowiak S, Anderson R, Sieber FE. Preoperative factors associated with postoperative change in confusion assessment method score in hip fracture patients. *Anesth Analg.* 2002;94:1628–1632.

15. Moller JT, Cluitmans P, Rasmussen LS, et al. Long-term postoperative cognitive dysfunction in the elderly ISPOCD1 study. ISPOCD investigators. International Study of Post-Operative Cognitive Dysfunction. *Lancet.* 1998;351:857–861. Erratum in: *Lancet.* 1998;351:1742.

16. Parikh SS, Chung F. Postoperative delirium in the elderly. *Anesth Analg.* 1995;80:1223–1232.

17. Ward B, Imarengiaye C, Peirovy J, Chung F. Cognitive function is minimally impaired after ambulatory surgery. *Can J Anaesth.* 2005;52:1017–1021.

18. Johnson T, Monk T, Rasmussen LS, et al. ISPOCD2 Investigators. Postoperative cognifitive dysfunction in middle-aged patients. *Anesthesiology.* 2002;96:1351–1357.

19. Williams-Russo P, Sharrock NE, Mattis S, Szatowski TIP, Charlson ME. Cognitive effects after epidural vs. general anesthesia in older adults. *JAMA.* 1995;274:44–50.

20. Canet J, Rader J, Rasmussen LS, et al. ISPOCD2 investigators. Cognitive dysfunction after minor surgery in the elderly. *Acta Anaesthesiol Scand.* 2003;47;1204–1210.

21. Vaurio LE, Sands LP, Wang Y, Mullen EA, Leung JM. Postoperative delirium: the importance of pain and pain management. *Anesth Analg.* 2006;102:1267–1273.

22. Chung F, Lavelle PA, McDonald S, Chung A, McDonald NJ. Cognitive impairment after neuroleptanalgesia in cataract surgery. *Anesth Analg.* 1989;68:614–618.

23. Chung FF, Chung A, Meier RH, Lautenschlaeger E, Seyone C. Comparison of perioperative mental function after general anaesthesia and spinal anaesthesia with intravenous sedation. *Can J Anaesth.* 1989;36:382–387.

24. Fredman B, Sheffer O, Zohar E, et al. Fast-track eligibility of geriatric patients undergoing short urologic procedures. *Anesth Analg.* 2002;94:560–564.

25. Cook DJ. Geriatric anesthesia. In: Solomon DH, LoCicero J III, Rosenthal RA, eds. *New Frontiers in Geriatric Research.* New York, NY: American Geriatrics Society; 2004:9–52.

26. Chung F, Mezei G, Tong D. Adverse events in ambulatory surgery. A comparison between elderly and younger patients. *Can J Anaesth.* 1999;46:309.

27. Fleisher LA, Beckman JA, Brown KA, et al. ACC/AHA 2007 guidelines on perioperative cardiovascular evaluation and care for noncardiac surgery: a report of the American College of Cardiology/American Heart Association Task Force on Practice Guidelines (Writing Committee to Revise the 2002 Guidelines on Perioperative Cardiovascular Evaluation for Noncardiac Surgery. *J Am Coll Cardiol.* 2007;50: 159–241.

28. Lee TH, Marcantonio ER, Mangione CM, et al. Derivation and prospective validation of a simple index for prediction of cardiac risk of major noncardiac surgery. *Circulation.* 1999;100:1043–1049.

29. Lackland DT. Systemic hypertension: an endemic, epidemic, and a pandemic. *Semin Nephrol.* 2005;25:194–197.

30. Comfere T, Sprung J, Kumar MM, et al. Angiotensin system inhibitors in a general surgical population. *Anesth Analg.* 2005;100:636–644.

31. Friedman Z, Chung F, Wong DT. Ambulatory surgery adult patient selection criteria—a survey of Canadian anesthesiologists. *Can J Anaesth.* 2004;51:437–443.

32. Kaluza GL, Joseph J, Lee JR, Raizner ME, Raizner AE. Catastrophic outcomes of noncardiac surgery soon after coronary stenting. *J Am Coll Cardiol.* 2000;35: 1288–1294.

33. Forgosh LB, Movahed A. Assessment of cardiac risk in noncardiac surgery. *Clin Cardiol.* 1995;18:556–562.

34. American Society of Anesthesiologists Task Force on Perioperative Management of Patients with Cardiac Rhythm Management Devices. Practice advisory for the perioperative management of patients with cardiac rhythm management devices: pacemakers and implantable cardioverter-defibrillators: a report by the American Society of Anesthesiologists Task Force on Perioperative Management of Patients with Cardiac Rhythm Management Devices. *Anesthesiology.* 2005;103:186–198.

35. Salukhe TV, Dob D, Sutton R. Pacemakers and defibrillators: anaesthetic implications. *Br J Anaesth.* 2004;93:95–104.

36. NAEPP Expert Panel Report: Guidelines for the Diagnosis and Management of Asthma—Update on Selected Topics 2002. Available at: http://www.nhlbi.nih.gov/ guidelines/asthma. Accessed December 30, 2005.

37. Bishop MJ. Preoperative corticosteroids for reactive airway? *Anesthesiology*. 2004; 100:1047–1048.
38. Pizov R, Brown RH, Weiss YS, et al. Wheezing during induction of general anesthesia in patients with and without asthma. A randomized, blinded trial. *Anesthesiology*. 1995;82:1111–1116.
39. Eshima RW, Maurer A, King T, et al. A comparison of airway responses during desflurane and sevoflurane administration via a laryngeal mask airway for maintenance of anesthesia. *Anesth Analg*. 2003;96:701–705.
40. Salem M, Tainsh RE, Bromberg J, Loriaux DL, Chernow B. Perioperative glucocorticoid coverage. A reassessment 42 years after the emergence of a problem. *Ann Surg*. 1994;219:416–425.
41. Warner DO. Helping surgical patients quit smoking: why, when, and how. *Anesth Analg*. 2005;101:481–487.
42. Gentili ME, Deleuze A, Estebe JP, Lebourg M, Ecoffey C. Severe respiratory failure after infraclavicular block with 0.75% ropivacaine: a case report. *J Clin Anesth*. 2002;14:459–461.
43. Flegal KM. Epidemiologic aspects of overweight and obesity in the United States. *Physiol Behav*. 2005;86:599–602.
44. Connery LE, Coursin DB. Assessment and therapy of selected endocrine disorders. *Anesthesiol Clin North Am*. 2004;22:93–123.
45. Hall WD, Watkins LO, Wright JT, et al. African-American Lipid and Cardiovascular Council. The metabolic syndrome: recognition and management. *Dis Manag*. 2006; 9:16–33.
46. Schein OD, Katz J, Bass EB, et al. The value of routine preoperative medical testing before cataract surgery. *N Engl J Med*. 2000;342:168–175.
47. Jellish WS, Kartha V, Fluder E, Slogoff S. Effect of metoclopromide on gastric fluid volumes in diabetic patients who have fasted before elective surgery. *Anesthesiology*. 2005;102:904–909.
48. Farling PA. Thyroid disease. *Br J Anaesth*. 2000;85:15–28.
49. Davies KE, Houghton K, Montgomery JE. Obesity and day-case surgery. *Anaesthesia*. 2001;56:1112–1125.
50. Nielsen KC, Guller U, Steele SM, Klein SM, Greengrass RA, Pietrobon R. Influence of obesity on surgical regional anesthesia in the ambulatory setting: an analysis of 9,038 blocks. *Anesthesiology*. 2005;102:181–187.
51. White PF. The role of non-opioid analgesic techniques in the management of pain after ambulatory surgery. *Anesth Analg*. 2002;94:577–585.
52. Practice guidelines for the perioperative management of patients with obstructive sleep apnea: a report by the American Society of Anesthesiologists Task Force on Perioperative Management of Patients with Obstructive Sleep Apnea. Available at: http://www.asahq.org/publicationsAndServices/sleepapnea103105.pdf. Accessed July 22, 2007.
53. Benumof JL. Obstructive sleep apnea in the adult obese patient: implications for airway management. *Anesthesiol Clin North America*. 2002;20:789–811.
54. Sladen RN. Anesthetic considerations for the patient with renal failure. *Anesthesiol Clin North America*. 2000;18:863–882.

55. Kloner RA, Hale S, Alker K, Rezkella S. The effects of acute and chronic cocaine use on the heart. *Circulation*. 1992;85:407–419.

56. O'Connor AD, Rusyniak DE, Bruno A. Cerebrovascular and cardiovascular complications of alcohol and sympathomimetic abuse. *Med Clin North Am*. 2005:89;1343–1358.

57. Kvolik S, Glavas-Obrovac L, Sakic K, Margaretic D, Karner I. Anaestheic implications of anticancer chemotherapy. *Eur J Anaesth*. 2003;20:859–871.

58. Drugs of choice for cancer. *Treat Guidel Med Lett*. 2003:1;41–52.

59. Thorne AC, Orazem JP, Shah NK, et al. Isoflurane versus fentanyl: hemodynamic effects in cancer patients treated with anthracyclines. *J Cardiothorac Vasc Anesth*. 1993;7:307–311.

60. Sessler DI. Complications and treatment of mild hypothermia. *Anesthesiology*. 2001; 95:531–543.

61. Shaw AD, Morgan M. Nitrous oxide: time to stop laughing? *Anaesthesia*. 1998; 53:213–215.

62. Centers for Disease Control and Prevention. World AIDS Day, December 1, 2003. *MMWR*. 2003;52:1145. www.cdc.gov/mmwr/preview/mmwrhtml/mm5247a1.htm, accessed November 3, 2007.

63. Olkkola KT, Palkama VJ, Neuvonen PJ. Ritonavir's role in reducing fentanyl clearance and prolonging its half-life. *Anesthesiology*. 1999;91:681–685.

64. Barbaro G. Cardiovascular manifestations of HIV infection. *Circulation*. 2002;106: 1420–1425.

65. Ferrero S, Bentivoglio G. Post-operative complications after caesarean section in HIV-infected women. *Arch Gynecol Obstet*. 2003;268:268–273.

66. Fox M, Forgacs I. Gastro-esphageal reflux disease. *Br Med J*. 2006;332:88–93.

67. Huyse FJ, Touw DJ, Strack van Schundel R, de Lange JJ, Slaets JPJ. Psychotropic drugs and the perioperative period: a proposal for a guideline in elective surgery. *Psychosomatics*. 2006;47:8–22.

68. Boyer EW, Shannon M. The serotonin syndrome. *N Engl J Med*. 2005;352: 1112–1120.

69. Gillman PK. Monoamine oxidase inhibitors, opioid analgesics and serotonin toxicity. *Br J Anaesth*. 2005;95:434–441.

70. Reines HD, Seifert PC. Patient safety: latex allergy. *Surg Clin North Am*. 2005: 85;1329–1340.

4. Pediatric clinical challenges

Lucinda L. Everett, MD
Gennadiy Fuzaylov, MD

Pediatric patients present for a wide variety of ambulatory surgical procedures. In general, children are good candidates for ambulatory surgery, but the patient screening and selection process needs to ensure that significant associated conditions are avoided, particularly in the freestanding ambulatory setting. General patient selection concepts and overall risk information for the pediatric patient are presented. Specific clinical challenges presented by pediatric patients are summarized in this chapter, including respiratory issues such as respiratory infection and sleep apnea, gastrointestinal reflux, congenital heart disease, Down syndrome, neuromuscular disorders, and children with hematologic disorders and cancer.

Pediatric ambulatory surgery: basics of preoperative evaluation

Over the past two decades, ambulatory pediatric anesthesia has changed dramatically across the country. The proportion of surgical cases done on an ambulatory basis is frequently estimated to be greater than 70%. Much pediatric surgery is performed in an ambulatory setting since many required procedures are relatively minor and because children represent a population that is largely healthy and free from chronic illness. Also, children (and their parents) generally prefer to recover from surgery in the comfort and security of their home rather than the hospital environment.

In the pediatric ambulatory setting, the anesthesia provider is frequently presented with clinical dilemmas. Patient and procedure selection, as well as availability of appropriate equipment and staff, may be issues in various practice settings. There has been significant evolution in the approach to preoperative evaluation over the past decade. Thorough history and physical examination are the mainstays of preoperative evaluation; the requirements for laboratory testing and other evaluation of coexisting disease depend on the magnitude of the procedure as well as the patient's clinical picture.

The pediatric literature supports testing only in selected situations.[1] For children having anesthesia on an outpatient basis, the final assessment as to appropriateness for ambulatory status should include coexisting diseases, magnitude of the procedure, and home support systems. Willingness to accept a particular patient and procedure may also depend on the specific practice setting; backup in a hospital-integrated ambulatory center makes transfer or unplanned admission much easier than in a freestanding center.

Mechanisms for preoperative evaluation should be designed to identify and potentially exclude high-risk patients, to identify coexisting disease that may have special care requirements, and to identify situations that may require either further evaluation or postponement due to acute illness (especially upper respiratory infection, or URI). Most healthy children do not require a preoperative anesthesia clinic visit prior to the day of surgery as long as surgeons are educated about the appropriate criteria for ambulatory status and patients are instructed to call if they are ill. A screening telephone call from the ambulatory center can be effective in identifying any parental concerns.[2] The remainder of this chapter will discuss common problems that anesthesiologists encounter in pediatric patients in the ambulatory setting.

Risk in pediatric anesthesia

Pediatric anesthesia is extremely safe in experienced hands and with modern anesthetic agents and monitoring.[3] However, the potential for rapid oxygen desaturation with airway obstruction or apnea requires vigilance and the ability to react rapidly and skillfully. Hypoxia can quickly lead to bradycardia and cardiac arrest, particularly in infants.

There are little specific data available about risk in pediatric ambulatory surgery. Patel and Hannallah[4] published data on anesthetic complications in a large series of pediatric outpatients between 1983 and 1986. Preoperative telephone calls were made to obtain screening medical information, give instructions, and check for acute illness. At the time of the study, the most common procedures performed were hernia repair, strabismus surgery, myringotomy, adenoidectomy, and dental restoration; tonsillectomy was not performed on an outpatient basis then. In this study, 10,000 pediatric patients underwent ambulatory surgery and 9,910 were discharged home. The unanticipated admissions (0.9% of patients) were predominantly for protracted nausea and vomiting or for complicated surgery (17%). Postdischarge complications in the 4,998 patients reached for follow-up included the following. No serious adverse outcomes were detailed in this study.

- Vomiting (8.9%)
- Cough (6.5%)
- Sleepiness (5.9%)
- Sore throat (5.1%)
- Fever (4.7%)
- Hoarseness or mild croup (3.4%)

In a large series of patients having myringotomy with tube placement under mask general anesthesia, there was a relatively low incidence of adverse events (9% "minor" events such as upper airway obstruction, prolonged recovery, emesis, and postprocedural agitation; 1.9% "major" events of laryngospasm or stridor). Pre-existing medical conditions or acute illness were associated with a higher risk of adverse events.[5]

Other information may be extrapolated from general studies of pediatric risk. Several studies have shown an increased incidence of complications and mortality in infants less than 1 year of age.[6] In some of these, the increased risk can be attributed to coexisting diseases. Similarly, the pediatric perioperative cardiac arrest (POCA) registry analyzed reported cases of anesthetic-related pediatric cardiac arrest and found that the majority occurred in American Society of Anesthesiologists (ASA) grade 3 to 5 patients.[7] These patients, if their status is properly recognized, would not be candidates for ambulatory surgery.

Analysis of complications in healthy pediatric patients provides useful information about patterns of injury. Closed claims information for pediatric anesthesia showed that pediatric claims were more often related to respiratory events than those in adults and were frequently thought to have been preventable with better monitoring (many of these cases preceded the routine use of pulse oximetery and capnography).[8] Cardiac arrest in healthy patients in the first set of cases reported from the POCA registry was primarily related to anesthetic overdose (halothane) or to airway problems (laryngospasm or underlying airway pathology); the incidence of overdose with volatile anesthetics appears to have decreased since sevoflurane has largely replaced halothane in clinical practice.[9]

Respiratory complications are common in many studies of pediatric adverse events, but with prompt recognition and management, most should not result in serious morbidity. Large series of anesthetic outcomes in children have consistently identified respiratory events as a significant precipitating factor.[10,11] Respiratory adverse events include laryngospasm, bronchospasm, airway obstruction, and decreased systemic oxygen saturation. Improved monitoring has enhanced our ability to detect and treat these problems. Factors that appear to increase the risk of respiratory events include younger age; higher ASA status; ear, nose, and throat surgery;[12] and lack of an anesthetist with significant pediatric experience.[13]

Lower limits of age

Former premature infants are at risk for apnea after general anesthesia or sedation (Box 4-1). The best available evidence about apnea risk comes from an analysis by Coté and colleagues[14] that contains data from 255 former

Box 4-1. Recommendations for the former premature infant

- Risk of apnea is inversely related to postconceptual age and gestational age
- Apnea risk increased by
  - Anemia
  - Ongoing apnea at home
- Admit for observation until 54–56 weeks postconceptual age

premature infants who were administered general anesthesia for inguinal hernia repair. This analysis showed that postoperative apnea in former preterm infants is strongly and inversely related to both gestational age and postconceptual age and that continuing apnea and anemia are also risk factors. No association was found with a number of other historical factors or anesthetic variables, but there were relatively small numbers of infants in each group. This study defined confidence intervals for the risk of apnea at various combinations of gestational and postconceptual age.

For nonanemic infants free of recovery room apnea, the probability of apnea was not less than 1% until postconceptual age 56 weeks for gestational age 32 weeks or postconceptual age 54 weeks with gestational age 35 weeks. Some do question the clinical relevance of apnea detected only by sophisticated monitoring, but most anesthesiologists would require postoperative admission for apnea monitoring in this population. The use of spinal anesthesia in unsedated infants[15] and the administration of caffeine[16] appear to reduce apnea risk but would not be sufficient to allow discharge in this population. The newer anesthetic agents such as sevoflurane have not reduced apnea risk.[17]

Many institutions choose a uniform cutoff age (such as 56 weeks postconceptual age) for ambulatory surgery in former premature infants. There is almost no specific evidence about apnea risk in healthy term infants; these babies are probably acceptable for ambulatory surgery provided that the procedure is not likely to result in significant physiologic changes or postoperative pain requiring opioid medications and that the anesthetic proceeds uneventfully. Most centers either have these patients as early-morning cases with a period of observation (e.g., 4 hours) or choose a minimum age limit (4–6 weeks) for ambulatory surgery in term infants. Parental ability and proximity to medical care are also factors to consider.

Upper respiratory infection

URIs are the primary reason for cancellation of elective surgery in children. One of the most controversial areas in pediatric anesthesia relates to when it is safe to proceed with anesthesia and surgery for patients who present with symptoms of a URI or who have recently recovered from one.[18] Anesthetic complications that commonly occur in children during or shortly after the resolution of

100   L.L. Everett and G. Fuzaylov

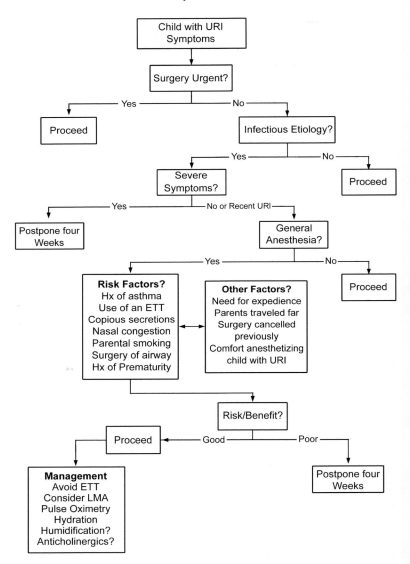

Figure 4-1. Suggested algorithm for the assessment and anesthetic management of the child with an upper respiratory infection. ETT, endotracheal tube; Hx, history; LMA, laryngeal mask airway; URI, upper respiratory infection. Reproduced from Tait and Malviya.[18] Used with permission from Lippincott Williams & Wilkins.

an acute respiratory infection include breath-holding, intraoperative and postoperative oxygen desaturation (to less than 90%), bronchospasm, laryngospasm, atelectasis, and postextubation croup.[19–21]

Risk factors for development of respiratory complications include endotracheal intubation, history of prematurity, surgical procedure involving the airway, reactive airway disease, and nasal congestion.[22] A randomized prospective study demonstrates a significantly lower incidence of bronchospasm in children with URI managed with a laryngeal mask airway rather than an endotracheal tube.[23]

Patients who have signs and symptoms of lower respiratory tract infection (productive cough, crackles, wheezes, or positive chest radiograph finding) or who have a fever greater than 38.5°C should have elective surgical procedures delayed for 4 to 6 weeks after the resolution of symptoms.[24] The algorithm shown in Figure 4-1 is designed to help in the decision-making process of whether to proceed with surgery and anesthesia in children with URIs.

Obstructive sleep apnea

Perioperative risk is felt to increase in proportion to the severity of obstructive sleep apnea (Box 4-2).[25] Children with obstructive sleep apnea may manifest snoring, daytime somnolence, or disruptive behaviors. If uncorrected, chronic sleep apnea with associated hypoxemia can lead to pulmonary hypertension and right heart failure.[26] The term "sleep apnea" is frequently used as a diagnosis in children having tonsillectomy, regardless of whether a precise diagnosis has been made; a more detailed evaluation of the history, physical exam, and (if necessary) sleep studies should be done to delineate the severity of disease and need for continuous positive airway pressure after anesthesia and surgery.

Snoring, body mass index above the 95th percentile for age, and congenital abnormalities of the airway also raise the index of suspicion for sleep apnea. And while we frequently think about sleep apnea in the context of children presenting for adenotonsillectomy, it is important to remember that these patients may also present for other ambulatory surgical procedures and the same history should be sought.

Screening questions in advance of the date of ambulatory surgery should be geared to identify these patients and determine the proper location for surgery as well as any indicated special care in the perioperative period. The ASA

Box 4-2. Obstructive sleep apnea: considerations

- Common in children for tonsillectomy
  - May occur in patients having unrelated procedures
- Risk increases with severity of obstructive sleep apnea
- Consider admission for: age less than 3 years, associated syndromes, need for opioid analgesia
- Patients may be sensitive to opioids

guidelines on sleep apnea state that patients with sleep apnea may undergo procedures under local or regional anesthesia on an outpatient basis; however, the majority of procedures in children require significant sedation or general anesthesia.

The obstructive component does not resolve immediately following tonsillectomy in children with sleep apnea, and respiratory complications are common.[27] Many recommend that tonsillectomy in children under 3 years of age or those with significant sleep apnea or associated diseases be done with overnight postoperative monitoring. For procedures other than tonsillectomy, a clinical determination must be made in each individual case. Severity of sleep apnea, the planned procedure, and the anticipated need for postoperative opioid analgesics should all enter into the decision-making. Sensitivity to opioids is seen in children with sleep apnea.[28,29] Children with significant sleep apnea are best observed overnight with oximetry and respiratory monitoring.

Aspiration risk and gastroesophageal reflux

Gastroesophageal reflux disease is an extremely common diagnosis in children. Manifestations are variable and may range from a sour taste to abdominal or chest pain to outright vomiting. Reflux may also worsen reactive airway disease. The history should certainly address recent, recurrent, or unpredictable vomiting; a history suggestive of delayed gastric emptying would warrant placement of an intravenous catheter and rapid sequence induction of anesthesia. However, the majority of children with reflux, particularly if treated, may safely undergo inhalation induction. The surrogate endpoints of gastric volume and acidity are frequently used to indicate aspiration risk; in a large series of pediatric patients presenting for endoscopy, there was no increase in gastric volume or acidity compared with historical controls.[30]

Aspiration of gastric contents occurs rarely; the reported incidence in the pediatric population is similar to that in adults (1 to 10 cases per 10,000 anesthetics). Aspiration occurs more frequently in emergency cases and "full stomach" situations; these generally should not be seen in the ambulatory setting. Other factors that may increase the risk of aspiration include airway difficulties or coughing during laryngoscopy. If aspiration is suspected on clinical grounds in an outpatient, signs (decreased oxygen saturation, coughing, wheezing, and radiographic abnormality) will generally develop during the first 2 hours if they occur at all. Therefore, an outpatient with suspected aspiration may be safely discharged if there has been no change from baseline clinical status after 2 hours.[31]

Heart murmurs and congenital heart disease

Asymptomatic heart murmurs are common in children; when examining a previously well child for surgery, the anesthesiologist could be the first to hear a heart murmur. Murmurs are either functional or pathologic. Generally, a child who has a murmur but who has a normal S1 and S2, has normal exercise tolerance, is acyanotic, and is growing well can tolerate a general anesthetic without complication. Preoperative assessment of a patient with a heart murmur includes a thorough history and physical examination and an electrocardiogram. If there is any question of a significant structural cardiac abnormality, preoperative echocardiography and evaluation by a pediatric cardiologist should be considered.

Children with known congenital cardiac defects may also present for brief outpatient procedures in an ambulatory setting. The increased prominence of managed care and contracted medical services has had the effect of shifting a sicker and more complicated population of pediatric patients from medical centers and hospitals to ambulatory centers. Therefore, pediatric anesthesiologists and even general practice anesthesiologists may find themselves caring for these children.[32]

This is an excellent example of a situation in which selection criteria for ambulatory surgery may differ between a freestanding ambulatory center and hospital-based ambulatory surgery. Even if the anesthesiologist is comfortable with the physiology of the particular patient's heart disease, the potential need for and availability of a consultant cardiologist and for postoperative admission (including intensive care) should be considered. Children with congenital heart disease should have a cardiac evaluation within 1 year of surgery unless a prior evaluation has dismissed the patient from further follow-up. To develop an effective plan for perioperative care, the anesthesiologist must be knowledgeable about the following.

- Current anatomy and physiology of congenital lesions of the heart
- The precise details of any previous surgery
- Cardiac defects and myocardial function
- Cardiac medications being taken
- The relative stability of the patient's clinical condition

Patients with residual problems such as arrhythmia, heart block, ventricular dysfunction, valvular stenosis or regurgitation, pulmonary vascular stenosis, or pulmonary hypertension are considered to be at increased risk. Patients with congestive heart failure or cyanosis and children with congenital heart disease who are younger than 2 years of age also have an increased frequency of perioperative morbidity.[33]

Children who have had anatomic correction of a congenital heart lesion and have good functional status would be reasonable candidates for minor ambulatory surgery in a freestanding center. The anesthesiologist should have prior access to information regarding the repair and any residual problems; communication with the cardiologist is helpful if there are any questions about the physiology or current status. Patients with simple unrepaired lesions such as a small ventricular septal defect with left to right shunt may be acceptable for an ambulatory center, but unrepaired complex lesions or palliated congenital heart disease (e.g., children with Fontan physiology) are probably best cared for in a hospital setting, even if the procedure is done on an outpatient basis. The American Heart Association guidelines for subacute bacterial endocarditis prophylaxis, which stratify both on patient disease and planned procedure, should be followed[34] (Tables 4-1 and 4-2).

Table 4-1. Cardiac conditions associated with the highest risk of adverse outcome from endocarditis for which prophylaxis with dental procedures[+] is recommended

Prosthetic cardiac valve including bioprosthetic and homograft valves

Previous Infective Endocarditis

Certain specific Congenital heart disease (CHD)*:
    Unrepaired or incompletely repaired cyanotic CHD, including palliative shunts and conduits
    Completely repaired congenital heart defect with prosthetic material or device, whether placed by surgery or by catheter intervention, during the first 6 months after the procedure[†]
    Repaired CHD with residual defects at the site or adjacent to the site of a prosthetic patch or prosthetic device (which inhibit endothelialization)

Cardiac transplantation recipients who develop cardiac valvulopathy

[+]Dental procedures involving manipulation of gingival tissue or the periapical region or teeth or perforation of the oral mucosa.
*Except for the conditions listed above, antibiotic prophylaxis is no longer recommended for any other form of CHD, ASD, VSD, hypertrophic cardiomyopathy, acquired valvular disease, rheumatic heart disease, bicuspid valve, calcified aortic stenosis, or MVP with or without regurgitation.
[†]Prophylaxis is recommended because endothelialization of prosthetic material occurs within 6 months after the procedure.
Antibiotic prophylaxis is no longer recommended solely to prevent IE in patients who undergo a GI or GU track procedure.

Adapted 2008 with permission of The Journal of the American Dental Association.

Table 4-2. Antibiotic regimens for infective endocarditis prophylaxis in high risk pediatric patients undergoing dental procedures[+]

Situation	Agent	Regimen: Single dose 30 to 60 minutes before dental procedure
Oral	Amoxicillin	50 mg/kg
Unable to take oral	Ampicillin OR	50 mg/kg IM or IV
	Cefazolin or ceftriaxone	50 mg/kg IM or IV

(Continued)

Table 4-2. *Continued*

Situation	Agent	Regimen: Single dose 30 to 60 minutes before dental procedure
Penicillin or ampicillin allergic–oral route	Cephalexin*[#] OR	50 mg/kg
	Clindamycin OR	20 mg/kg
	Azithromycin or clarithromycin	15 mg/kg
Penicillin or ampicillin allergic and unable to take oral medication	Cefazolin or ceftriaxone[#] OR	50 mg/kg IM or IV
	Clindamycin	20 mg/kg IM or IV

[+]Dental procedures involving manipulation of gingival tissue or the periapical region or teeth or perforation of the oral mucosa.
*Or other first- or second-generation oral cephalosporin in equivalent pediatric dosage.
[#]Cephalosporins should not be used in an individual with a history of anaphylaxis, angioedema, or urticaria with penicillins or ampicillin.

Adapted 2008 with permission of The Journal of the American Dental Association.

Down syndrome

Patients with Down syndrome (trisomy 21) present a number of anesthetic concerns (Box 4-3). Airway difficulties may occur in patients with Down syndrome; there may be midface hypoplasia with decreased volumes of the oro- and naso-pharynx, relative macroglossia, and persistent mouth-breathing. These patients have a higher incidence of sleep apnea and also a higher incidence of congenital and acquired subglottic stenosis so that age-appropriate endotracheal tubes may be too large.[35] Recovery may be slower after procedures such as tonsillectomy, and these patients should be evaluated carefully as to suitability for a freestanding outpatient setting.

It has been reported that 10% to 30% of Down syndrome patients have some evidence of atlantoaxial instability. Unfortunately, radiographic and clinical findings do not correlate well. One set of recommendations regarding cervical spine evaluation in Down syndrome is to perform a careful history and physical with attention to myelopathic signs and symptoms; screening radiographs (flexion/extension) should be performed for surgery in which significant manipulation of the neck is anticipated (e.g., tonsillectomy).[36] If the plain films are abnormal, further evaluation would include magnetic resonance imaging (MRI). Of course, caution with manipulation of the cervical spine of anesthetized patients is always prudent.

Box 4-3. Anesthetic considerations in down syndrome

- Congenital heart disease
- Airway obstruction
  - Soft tissue
  - Large tongue
  - Potential for obstructive sleep apnea and pulmonary hypertension
- Potential for subglottic stenosis
- Atlantoaxial instability
- Behavioral issues

Cardiac defects, particularly ventricular septal and atrioventricular canal defects, are also common in patients with Down syndrome. Patients should have had an echocardiogram in the neonatal period, and parents are generally aware whether a cardiac abnormality was diagnosed. The information presented in the section on congenital heart defects would apply to these patients.

Neuromuscular disorders

A substantial number of children suffer from a spectrum of neuromuscular diseases that may have anesthetic implications (Box 4-4). Patients with significant impairment related to muscular dystrophy or myopathy would generally not be considered candidates for ambulatory surgery, particularly in a freestanding setting. If the cardiorespiratory status is stable, they may be able to have minor procedures on an ambulatory basis in a hospital setting with somewhat extended postoperative observation. Each patient should be evaluated in terms of overall functional status, risk of cardiovascular compromise, and susceptibility to malignant hyperthermia (MH) or a hyperkalemic response to administration of succinylcholine.

MH is clearly linked to central core disease clinically and genetically; both are caused by mutations of the ryanodine receptor.[37] Other "MH-like" reactions have been reported in patients with myopathy or muscular dystrophy, although the mechanism may not be the same; some concern exists that patients with Duchenne muscular dystrophy may be susceptible to rhabdomyolysis and even cardiac arrest during or after administration of volatile anesthetics without succinylcholine, although the mechanism of this is not entirely clear.[38,39]

Hyperkalemia with cardiac arrest has been reported after succinylcholine in patients with undiagnosed myopathy; this led to the "black box" warning limiting succinylcholine use in children to situations in which urgent control of the airway is required. Patients with a variety of disorders that may lead to upregula-

Box 4-4. Neuromuscular disorders

- Preoperative assessment and patient selection for ambulatory setting
  - Respiratory function
  - Cardiac function
  - Swallowing/airway protection
- Consider possible susceptibility to malignant hyperthermia or to hyperkalemia with succinylcholine
- Metabolic issues in mitochondrial diseases
  - Avoid lactated fluids
  - Give replacement dextrose
  - Be aware of potential for lower anesthetic requirements in some patients

tion of acetylcholine receptors are considered to be potentially at risk of hyperkalemia after the administration of succinylcholine.[40] These states may include upper or lower motor neuron injury, direct muscle injury or inflammation, prolonged immobility, burns, or severe infection.

Duchenne muscular dystrophy is an X-linked recessive disorder characterized by a lack of the sarcolemma protein dystrophin, which leads to muscle cell degeneration. Leg weakness usually develops first; the disease progresses to include respiratory muscle weakness, kyphoscoliosis, and cardiomyopathy. Although many patients with Duchenne muscular dystrophy are confined to wheelchairs by early adolescence, treatment with corticosteroids has shown a beneficial effect on both peripheral and respiratory muscles and delayed the time to functional impairment in these children.[41]

Myotonic dystrophy is an autosomal dominant disorder characterized by persistent contraction of skeletal muscle after stimulation.[42] These children may have respiratory impairment, disordered swallowing and gastrointestinal reflux, cardiomyopathy or conduction abnormalities, and global developmental delay. A careful assessment of the history and functional status should be undertaken prior to considering these patients for outpatient procedures.

Cerebral palsy represents a spectrum of conditions in which some degree of neuromuscular impairment exists related to one of a variety of injuries to the brain either during development or in the peripartum period.[43] These insults include birth hypoxia, prenatal infections, prenatal stroke, or genetic disorders. Developmental status in children with cerebral palsy ranges from normal intellect to severe impairment. These patients may be on medications to control spasticity and may present for surgical procedures related to their disease (orthopedic procedures, antireflux procedures or feeding tubes, or injections of botulinum toxin to treat spasticity). Because of multiple surgical procedures, they should be screened for latex allergy by detailed history. Since there is such a spectrum of disease, it is difficult to make any general statement about suitability for ambulatory anesthesia, but the history and physical should particularly assess the ability to cooperate, control of secretions, reflux, contractures, and respiratory function.

Mitochondrial diseases are a heterogeneous group of diseases caused by structural or functional abnormalities in mitochondria[44], leading to clinical manifestations that may include myopathy, developmental delay, seizures, intestinal dysmotility, and metabolic derangements. These entities have previously been classified either as nonspecific hypotonia or encephalomyopathy or as named syndromes such as Kearns-Sayre syndrome (progressive external ophthalmoplegia) or Leigh's disease (a neurodegenerative disease caused by mutations of mitochondrial DNA or by pyruvate dehydrogenase deficiency).

More recent terminology is based on the attempt to describe the specific clinical manifestations, such as MELAS (mitochondrial encephalomyopathy, lactic acidosis, and stroke-like episodes) syndrome and MERRF (myoclonic epilepsy with ragged red fibers) syndrome. The specific sites of abnormality within the respiratory chain have only recently been delineated.[45] The clinical course of individual patients can be quite variable from mild impairment with stress to severe developmental delay. There is no definitive therapy for mitochondrial disorders, but some patients appear to improve with certain vitamins or supplements and with high carbohydrate diets and adequate hydration.

Patients with mitochondrial disease frequently present for MRI and muscle biopsy in the course of diagnosing the disorder. Preoperative evaluation should include evaluation of neurologic status and aspiration risk as well as cardiac and respiratory status. Cardiomyopathy may develop as may conduction abnormalities. Discussion with the neurologist as well as the parents may yield useful information about the clinical picture and factors that may worsen the child's condition. Although there is a spectrum of disease, these children may deteriorate when fasting and also when administered lactated intravenous solutions, due to inability to metabolize lactate.

Fasting time should be minimized and fluid deficits should be replaced with nonlactated fluid such as normal saline. Maintenance fluids should include dextrose as an energy source. These patients may also be extremely sensitive to anesthetic agents[46] as well as to nondepolarizing relaxants. No one anesthetic regimen has proven superior, but whatever agents are used should be carefully titrated to physiologic signs and consideration given to monitoring level of consciousness where feasible. Some centers have treated these patients as MH-susceptible, but there is no strong link if the disease is known to be mitochondrial in origin; some providers would prefer to use a nontriggering technique (and particularly to avoid succinylcholine) in patients presenting for diagnostic tests to define a myopathy.

Malignant hyperthermia susceptibility

The patient with a personal or family history of MH or a disease with a strong association with MH should be treated as susceptible (Box 4-5). This includes use of a nontriggering anesthetic technique and preparation of the

Box 4-5. Anesthesia machine preparation for malignant hyperthermia-susceptible patients

- Flush anesthesia machine for 20 minutes with high-flow oxygen 10 L/minute
- Disable or remove vaporizers
- Change disposables; consider changing soda lime
- Adequate supply of dantrolene to treat a crisis
- Nontriggering anesthetic technique
- Observe for 2.5 hours before discharge: minimum of 60 minutes in phase I plus 90 minutes in phase II
- Acceptable for outpatient status if no sequelae after nontriggering anesthetic

anesthesia machine with high flows of oxygen 10 L/minute for 20 minutes prior to use. Vaporizers should be disabled or removed to prevent use. Many providers would change the CO_2 absorbent prior to use; this is considered optional by the Malignant Hyperthermia Association of the United States (MHAUS).

Every location where triggering anesthetic agents (volatile anesthetics or succinylcholine) might be used for anesthesia or emergencies, including ambulatory centers and offices, should be equipped to provide initial care for an episode of MH, including an adequate supply of dantrolene. Susceptible patients may be safely treated in an outpatient setting with a nontriggering technique.[47] One recommendation is that MH-susceptible pediatric patients be monitored for 1 hour in the postanesthesia care unit and for an additional 90 minutes in phase II recovery and that they may be safely discharged if no symptoms or temperature elevation have developed.[48] MHAUS recommends a 2.5-hour overall stay (http://www.mhaus.org/index.cfm/fuseaction/OnlineBrochures.Display/BrochurePK/BCD9151D-3048-709E-5A445BC0808B4767.cfm.).

The child with cancer

Childhood leukemias and lymphoma are relatively common, as are solid tumors such as neuroblastoma and nephroblastoma, and intracranial processes such as medulloblastoma, ependymoma, and astrocytoma (Box 4-6). These patients may present for a variety of procedures on an outpatient basis, including vascular access, diagnostic and therapeutic procedures (imaging, bone marrow biopsy, and lumbar puncture with intrathecal chemotherapy), and unrelated surgery. Children who are clinically stable may be good candidates for ambulatory anesthesia. Evaluation should include history of treatment, including surgical procedures, radiation, and/or chemotherapy.

Adriamycin and related drugs may cause cardiomyopathy; generally, children being treated with these drugs will be evaluated periodically with echocardiograms. Bleomycin may produce pulmonary fibrosis. Recent blood counts should be available particularly if the child is still in active chemotherapy cycles.

Box 4-6. Children with cancer: anesthetic concerns

- Sequelae of chemotherapy (e.g., adriamycin cardiotoxicity and bleomycin pulmonary toxicity)
- Bone marrow suppression (neutropenia/infection risk, thrombocytopenia/bleeding risk, and anemia)
- Psychological sequelae of illness and multiple procedures

Attention to infection as well as bleeding risk is prudent. These children often have had multiple procedures and may have particular anxieties or control issues around the induction of anesthesia.

Sickle cell disease

Sickle cell disease occurs as a consequence of a genetic mutation on chromosome 11 and results in an abnormal hemoglobin S.[49] This change causes the characteristic sickle-shaped cells in the deoxygenated state. Classic sickle cell disease occurs in patients who are homozygous for hemoglobin S, but clinical disease may also occur in patients who are heterozygous for hemoglobin S in combination with either hemoglobin C or B-thalassemia. Patients who are heterozygous for hemoglobin S and hemoglobin A (sickle cell trait) are generally asymptomatic except under conditions of extreme hypoxia, altitude, or heat/dehydration. Most patients will have had testing in the neonatal period; however, if the status is not known in a patient from an ethnic group considered at risk for sickle cell disease, laboratory testing or at least a screening hemoglobin should be performed prior to elective surgery.

Patients with sickle cell anemia have chronic hemolysis and intermittent vaso-occlusive crises that are acutely painful and longer term may result in infarction of various organs, particularly bone and kidney. Osteomyelitis is common in sickle cell patients. Acute chest syndrome, a clinical picture of pulmonary consolidation and fever, has a relatively high mortality rate and may be treated with exchange transfusion. Chronic restrictive lung disease may develop, with subsequent right heart failure. Splenic enlargement and subsequent fibrosis is common in sickle cell patients. Stroke may occur by either hemorrhagic or infarctive mechanisms.

Preoperative evaluation of patients with sickle cell disease should include a history of frequency of painful crises and acute chest syndrome, evaluation by history and physical examination of cardiopulmonary function, and recent hematocrit and studies of renal function. Classic teaching on the management of sickle cell disease is to provide adequate oxygenation and hydration intraoperatively, to keep patients warm to avoid vasoconstriction, and to avoid the use of tourniquets which might promote sludging. There are, however, small case series using a tourniquet in sickle cell patients for orthopedic surgery without sequelae. Postoperative management includes effective analgesia (to avoid splinting and hypoventilation), particularly in the case of abdominal surgery.

Overall, sickle cell patients have a higher rate of perioperative complication. The role of preoperative transfusion in preventing perioperative complications from sickle cell disease remains controversial, and the risk of transfusion must be weighed against the potential benefits. Simple transfusion to a hemoglobin of 10 g/dL has been shown to be as effective as exchange transfusion with the endpoint of hemoglobin S to less than 30% and with fewer transfusion-related complications.[50] Patients undergoing minor procedures, if they are otherwise stable clinically, probably do not require preoperative transfusion.[51] Outpatient surgery is a reasonable option in the well-compensated child with sickle cell disease.

Summary

Healthy children are obviously excellent candidates for outpatient anesthesia and surgery. Children with a variety of coexisting medical problems may also be candidates for ambulatory anesthesia, but a careful history and physical examination should be undertaken to exclude those at significant risk for perioperative complications or those who require inpatient services. The magnitude of the procedure, postoperative analgesic requirements, and parental ability and proximity to medical care should also be considered in determining the suitability for outpatient anesthesia in children.

References

1. Meneghini L, Zadra N, Zanette G, et al. The usefulness of routine preoperative laboratory tests for one-day surgery in healthy children. *Paediatr Anaesth.* 1998;8:11–15.
2. Patel RI, Hannallah RS. Preoperative screening for pediatric ambulatory surgery: evaluation of a telephone questionnaire method. *Anesth Analg.* 1992;75:258–261.
3. Murat I, Constant I, Maud'huy H. Perioperative anaesthetic morbidity in children: a database of 24,165 anaesthetics over a 30-month period. *Paediatr Anaesth.* 2004;14: 158–166.
4. Patel RI, Hannallah RS. Anesthetic complications following pediatric ambulatory surgery: a 3-yr study. *Anesthesiology.* 1988;69:1009–1012.
5. Hoffmann KK, Thompson GK, Burke BL, et al. Anesthetic complications of tympanostomy tube placement in children. *Arch Otolaryngol Head Neck Surg.* 2002;128: 1040–1043.
6. Tiret L, Nivoche Y, Hatton F, et al. Complications related to anaesthesia in infants and children. *Br J Anaesth.* 1988;61:263–269.
7. Morray JP, Geiduschek J, Ramamoorthy C, et al. Anesthesia-related cardiac arrest in children: initial findings of the Pediatric Perioperative Cardiac Arrest (POCA) Registry. *Anesthesiology.* 2000;93:6–14.
8. Morray JP, Geiduschek JM, Caplan RA, et al. A comparison of pediatric and adult anesthesia closed malpractice claims. *Anesthesiology.* 1993;78:461–467.

9. Bhananker SM, Ramamoorthy C, Geiduschek JM, et al. Anesthesia-related cardiac arrest in children; update from the Pediatric Perioperative Cardiac Arrest Registry. *Anesth Analg.* 2007;105:344–350.

10. Tiret L, Nivoche Y, Hatton F, et al. Complications related to anaesthesia in infants and children. A prospective survey of 40,240 anaesthetics. *Br J Anaesth.* 1988;61: 263–269.

11. Tay CL, Tan GM, Ng SB. Critical incidents in paediatric anaesthesia: an audit of 10,000 anaesthetics in Singapore. *Paediatr Anaesth.* 2001;11:711–718.

12. Bordet F, Allaouchiche B, Lansiaux S, et al. Risk factors for airway complications during general anaesthesia in paediatric patients. *Paediatr Anaesth.* 2002;12:762–769.

13. Mamie C, Habre W, Delhumeau C, et al. Incidence and risk factors of perioperative respiratory adverse events in children undergoing elective surgery. *Paediatr Anaesth.* 2004;14:218–224.

14. Coté CJ, Zaslavsky A, Downes JJ, et al. Postoperative apnea in former preterm infants after inguinal herniorrhaphy. *Anesthesiology.* 1995;82:809–821.

15. Welborn LG, Rice LJ, Hannallah RS, et al. Postoperative apnea in former preterm infants: prospective comparison of spinal and general anesthesia. *Anesthesiology.* 1990;72:838–842.

16. Henderson-Smart DJ, Steer P. Prophylactic caffeine to prevent postoperative apnea following general anesthesia in preterm infants. *Cochrane Database Syst Rev.* 2001;4: CD000048.

17. Williams JM, Stoddart PA, Williams SAR, et al. Post-operative recovery after inguinal herniotomy in ex-premature infants: comparison between sevoflurane and spinal anaesthesia. *Br J Anaesth.* 2001;86:366–371.

18. Tait AR, Malviya S. Anesthesia for the child with an upper respiratory tract infection: still a dilemma? *Anesth Analg.* 2005;100:59–65.

19. Schreiner MS, O'Hara I, Markakis DA, et al. Do children who experience laryngospasm have an increased risk of upper respiratory tract infection? *Anesthesiology.* 1996;85:475–480.

20. Tait AR, Reynolds PI, Gutstein HB. Factors that influence an anesthesiologist's decision to cancel elective surgery for the child with an upper respiratory tract infection. *J Clin Anesth.* 1995;7:491–499.

21. Levy L, Pandit UA, Randel GI, et al. Upper respiratory tract infections and general anaesthesia in children. Peri-operative complications and oxygen saturation. *Anaesthesia.* 1992;47:678–682.

22. Tait AR, Malviya S, Voepel-Lewis T, et al. Risk factors for perioperative adverse respiratory events in children with upper respiratory tract infections. *Anesthesiology.* 2001;95:299–306.

23. Tait AR, Pandit UA, Voepel-Lewis T, et al. Use of the laryngeal mask airway in children with upper respiratory tract infections: a comparison with endotracheal intubation. *Anesth Analg.* 1998;86:706–711.

24. Jacoby DB, Hirshman CA. General anesthesia in patients with viral respiratory infections: an unsound sleep? *Anesthesiology.* 1991;74:969–972.

25. Gross JB, Bachenberg KL, Benumof JL, et al. Practice Guidelines for the Perioperative Management of Patients with Obstructive Sleep Apnea. American Society of

Anesthesiologists. Available at: http://www.asahq.org/publicationsAndServices/slee-papnea103105.pdf. Accessed July 5, 2007.

26. Blum RH, McGowan FX Jr. Chronic upper airway obstruction and cardiac dysfunction: anatomy, pathophysiology and anesthetic implications. *Paediatr Anaesth.* 2004; 14:75–83.

27. Wilson K, Lakheeram I, Morielli A, et al. Can assessment for obstructive sleep apnea help predict postadenotonsillectomy respiratory complications? *Anesthesiology.* 2002;96:313–322.

28. Strauss SG, Lynn AM, Bratton SL, et al. Ventilatory response to CO_2 in children with obstructive sleep apnea from adenotonsillar hypertrophy. *Anesth Analg.* 1999;89: 328–332.

29. Brown KA, Laferriere A, Moss IR. Recurrent hypoxemia in young children with obstructive sleep apnea is associated with reduced opioid requirement for analgesia. *Anesthesiology.* 2004;100:806–810.

30. Schwartz DA, Connelly NR, Theroux CA, et al. Gastric contents in children presenting for upper endoscopy. *Anesth Analg.* 1998;87:757–760.

31. Warner MA, Warner ME, Warner DO, et al. Perioperative pulmonary aspiration in infants and children. *Anesthesiology.* 1999;90:66–71.

32. Morris CD, Menashe VD. 25-year mortality after surgical repair of congenital heart defect in childhood. A population-based cohort study. *JAMA.* 1991;266:3447–3452.

33. Warner MA, Lunn RJ, O'Leary PW, et al. Outcomes of noncardiac surgical procedures in children and adults with congenital heart disease. *Mayo Clin Proc.* 1998; 73:728–734.

34. Wilson W, Taubert KA, Gewitz M, et al. Prevention of Infective Endocarditis— Guidelines from the American Heart Association. Circulation (online publication); April 19, 2007 found at: http://circ.ahajournals.org/cgi/reprint/CIRCULATIONAHA. 106.183095.

35. Kanamori G, Witter M, Brown J, Williams-Smith L. Otolaryngologic manifestations of Down syndrome. *Otolaryngol Clin North Am.* 2000;33:1285–1292.

36. Brockmeyer D. Down syndrome and craniovertebral instability. Topic review and treatment recommendations. *Pediatr Neurosurg.* 1999;31:71–77.

37. Sei Y, Sambuughin NN, Davis EJ, et al. Malignant hyperthermia in North America: genetic screening of the three hot spots in the type I ryanodine receptor gene. *Anesthesiology.* 2004;101:824–830.

38. Yemen TA, McClain C. Muscular dystrophy, anesthesia and the safety of inhalational agents revisited; again. *Paediatr Anaesth.* 2006;16:105–108.

39. Girshin M, Mukherjee J, Clowney R. The postoperative cardiovascular arrest of a 5-year-old male: an initial presentation of Duchenne's muscular dystrophy. *Paediatr Anaesth.* 2006;16:170–173.

40. Martyn JAJ, Richtsfeld M. Succinylcholine-induced hyperkalemia in acquired pathologic states: etiologic factors and molecular mechanisms. *Anesthesiology.* 2006;104:158–169.

41. Ames WA, Hayes JA, Crawford MW. The role of corticosteroids in Duchenne muscular dystrophy: a review for the anesthetist. *Paediatr Anaesth.* 2005;15: 3–8.

42. White RJ, Bass SP. Myotonic dystrophy and paediatric anaesthesia. *Paediatr Anaesth.* 2003;13:94–102.

43. Wongprasartsuk P, Stevens J. Cerebral palsy and anaesthesia. *Paediatr Anaesth.* 2002; 12:296–303.

44. Shipton EA, Prosser DO. Mitochondrial myopathies and anaesthesia. *Eur J Anaesthesiol.* 2004;21:173–178.

45. DiMauro S, Schon EA. Mitochondrial respiratory-chain diseases. *N Engl J Med.* 2003;348:2656–2668.

46. Morgan PG, Hoppel CL, Sedensky MM. Mitochondrial defects and anesthetic sensitivity. *Anesthesiology.* 2002;96:1268–1270.

47. Yentis SM, Levine MF, Hartley EJ. Should all children with suspected or confirmed malignant hyperthermia susceptibility be admitted after surgery? A 10-year review. *Anesth Analg.* 1992;75:345–350.

48. Pollock N, Langtont E, Stowell K, et al. Safe duration of postoperative monitoring for malignant hyperthermia susceptible patients. *Anaesth Intensive Care.* 2004;32: 502–509.

49. Firth PG, Head CA. Sickle cell disease and anesthesia. *Anesthesiology.* 2004;101: 766–785.

50. Vichinsky EP, Haberkern CM, Neumayr L, et al. A comparison of conservative and aggressive transfusion regimens in the perioperative management of sickle cell disease. *N Engl J Med.* 1995;333:206–213.

51. Griffin TC, Buchanan GR. Elective surgery in children with sickle cell disease without preoperative blood transfusion. *J Pediatr Surg.* 1993;28:681–685.

5. Pediatric perioperative management

Raafat S. Hannallah, MD

Children are excellent candidates for ambulatory (outpatient) surgery. Most children are healthy, and most surgical procedures performed on children are simple and associated with prompt recovery.[1] It is not surprising, therefore, that up to 70% of pediatric surgery in this country is performed on an ambulatory basis. In fact, in many cases, ambulatory surgery is now synonymous with elective surgery. Avoiding hospitalization is particularly advantageous for preschool children who benefit from minimizing separation from parents and for infants who are spared the exposure to a potentially contaminated hospital environment.

Preparation of children for ambulatory surgery

The successful management of pediatric ambulatory patients requires careful attention to proper selection, screening, and preparation well ahead of the day of scheduled surgery. Specific criteria for patient selection and screening have been addressed in Chapter 4. In general, the child should be in good health (American Society of Anesthesiologists [ASA] physical status 1 or 2). Patients who have chronic illness do not need to be excluded from ambulatory surgery, but their medical condition must be optimally controlled before they are acceptable.

Pediatric perioperative environment

The Section on Anesthesiology of the American Academy of Pediatrics introduced specific guidelines for patient care facilities and their medical staff who wish to provide pediatric anesthesia care.[2] The document emphasizes important facility-based issues such as the experience and training of the health care team and the resources committed to the care of infants and children throughout the perioperative period. Competency by the staff in addressing such issues as airway management, fluid administration, temperature regulation, monitoring, vascular catheter insertion, and postoperative pain are as important as the skill and experience of the individual anesthesiologist in determining the type of patient and/or procedure to be performed in any specific outpatient facility.

Preoperative fasting

The need for prolonged fasting (nil per os, or NPO) before elective surgery in healthy pediatric ambulatory patients has been challenged.[3] Studies have shown that children who are allowed to drink clear liquids until 2 hours of anesthesia induction do not manifest an increase in gastric volume or acidity over those who fast overnight.[4,5] Accordingly, most pediatric anesthesiologists have now liberalized NPO requirements for their patients according to the ASA guidelines[6] (Table 5-1).

Solid foods, which include milk, formula, and milk products, are not allowed on the day of surgery. Breast-fed infants, however, can nurse up to 4 hours

Table 5-1. Fasting recommendations

Ingested material	Minimum fasting period (hours)
Clear liquids (*water, fruit juices without pulp, carbonated beverages*)	2
Breast milk	4
Infant formula	6
Nonhuman milk	6
Light meal	6
Heavy (high fat) meal	8

preoperatively.[7] Children may drink clear liquids (up to 10 mL/kg) until 2 hours of the posted surgical time. The main advantage of these liberal guidelines is that children are not thirsty and irritable while waiting for surgery.[8] Other possible benefits include that the patients are less likely to become hypotensive or hypoglycemic during anesthesia.

Preoperative laboratory testing

The incidence of anemia in healthy children is extremely low and does not usually require modification in the anesthetic management.[9] Accordingly, a preoperative hemoglobin or hematocrit level determination is not indicated unless the medical history suggests that significant anemia may be present (e.g., in infants, adolescent females, or in the presence of chronic disease). Routine urinalysis adds little to the preoperative evaluation of a healthy child and is usually omitted. Routine pregnancy testing in young adolescent girls is still controversial.[10]

Psychological preparation

Most ambulatory surgical facilities today have some form of a preoperative information/preparation program for children awaiting surgery. Typically, these programs provide reading material to the family, allow for telephone counseling, and/or organize visits to the facility sometime before the scheduled day of surgery. The program at Children's National Medical Center (CNMC) is described here as an example only since we appreciate that no one way is expected to work everywhere or even for every child in the same institution.

The basic approach to preoperative preparation of children presenting for ambulatory surgery at CNMC is to have the admitting office contact the parents as soon as possible after the procedure is scheduled. A mailing is sent, which includes a coloring book that depicts some basic information about surgery, anesthesia, and being a patient in a hospital. The parents are invited to come to the hospital for a preoperative preparation visit on the Sunday preceding the day of surgery or sooner if they wish. Often these preoperative visits are also mentioned and promoted by the surgeons when they counsel the parents about surgery in the first place.

Volunteer staff under the direction of child life specialists conducts the actual visit. The script is reviewed by many health care professionals, including the anesthesiologist. During the visit, the children are told what to expect on the day of surgery. They are shown the preoperative area where they'll be waiting for surgery, allowed to see and handle special anesthesia equipment such as face mask and breathing circle, and shown the recovery areas where they will re-unite with their parents. At CNMC, a video is shown to reinforce the ideas presented in person. Other facilities may have interactive videos for the child and parents to explore.

Although most people believe that these preparation programs are invaluable in allaying the children's anxiety, there exists little objective evidence that they are indeed useful. Rosen et al.[11] attempted to objectively examine the effect of the preparation program at CNMC on the children's behavior during induction of anesthesia. They found that children who participated in the preoperative preparation program were more likely to be cooperative during induction than those who did not.

Rosen et al. found, however, that only a small percentage of the parents who were invited to come to the tour did in fact participate. Most of the ones who came were extremely motivated parents who admitted to having prepared their children in so many other ways. In addition, parents of very young children and of children who were coming for repeat surgery were less likely to come for the tour. These were the children who, in the study of Rosen et al., were at the highest risk for being upset during induction.

The value of the preoperative visit with the anesthesiologist in allaying the fears of the child and parents cannot be overemphasized, especially for the ambulatory patient who does not have enough time to get familiar with the surgical routine. A full explanation of the anesthetic plan must be offered to the parents *and* the child as appropriate for his age. Although a brief discussion of the risks associated with anesthesia and surgery is appropriate, and often desired by the parents,[12] this should not be presented in a way that adds to the inevitable apprehension of awaiting surgery on one's child.

Pharmacological premedication

An ideal preanesthetic drug should result in preoperative sedation without delaying recovery and discharge from the facility. Oral midazolam can be administered in a dose of 0.5 mg/kg, 20–45 minutes before induction of anesthesia to facilitate separation from the parents and improve the cooperation with anesthesia induction.[13] In some cases, children can be separated from their parents as early as 10 minutes after receiving midazolam. Oral midazolam, in this dose, does not appear to prolong recovery even after ambulatory procedures lasting less than 30 minutes. Oral ketamine in a dose of 6 mg/kg can be a satisfactory alternative to midazolam (Table 5-2). It provides predictable sedation within 15–25 minutes and allows calm separation from parents without significant side effects.

Table 5-2. Premedication/preinduction agents

Drug	Route	Usual dose
Midazolam	Per os	0.5 mg/kg
Midazolam	Nasal	0.2 mg
Midazolam	Rectal	1 mg/kg
Ketamine	Per os	6 mg/kg
Ketamine	Intramuscular	2 mg/kg

Preinduction techniques

Preinduction techniques can be useful for last-minute sedation in children who refuse to separate from their parents or as an alternative to a forced-mask induction in young children who are unable to cooperate with an inhalational induction (Table 5-2). The real practical difference between premedication and preinduction is in the speed of onset. Useful preinduction drugs should have a quick onset time, generally less than 10 minutes. Low-dose intramuscular (IM) ketamine in a dose of 2 mg/kg induces enough sedation to allow acceptance of inhalational induction in children who have been struggling with the mask prior to its administration.[14]

Onset time is less than 3 minutes, and recovery is not prolonged even when the technique is used for short surgical procedures. Because IM injections are undesirable in children, this technique is reserved for very combative patients when other forms of sedation have failed. When low-dose ketamine is followed by an inhalational anesthetic, there is minimal likelihood of delirium or bad dreams during recovery. Although the combination of IM midazolam and ketamine is predictably effective, it is more likely to delay recovery and discharge[15] and should be reserved for extremely combative children.

Both midazolam (0.2 mg/kg) and sufentanil (2 μg/kg) have been used intranasally as preinduction drugs to facilitate separation from the parents and to improve mask acceptance.[16] Although effective, the technique is rather unpleasant and can be associated with serious complications, especially if sufentanil is used. Nasal midazolam is very irritating and induces prolonged crying in almost all the children who receive it. Sufentanil can result in chest wall rigidity and oxygen desaturation.

Parents' presence during induction

Since one of the main reasons for administering routine premedication or having to resort to using a preinduction technique is to facilitate separation of the child from the parents, some anesthesiologists find that they can reduce or even eliminate the need for such agents by allowing the parents to stay with the child during the induction of anesthesia.[17] Some institutions have specially built induction rooms where the parents can accompany their children without having to wear special operating room (OR) attire. Others allow selected parents to wear a cover-all gown or scrubs and walk with the child into the actual OR. In all these situations, the parents are there only for the early part of the induction and are escorted back to the waiting area as soon as the child is asleep.

Although unconventional, this approach is popular in some institutions and is being requested by many parents. Studies have shown that most children are less upset when the parents are present.[17] Parent selection and education are essential for the success of this approach, since anxious parents can make their children even more upset.[18]

Pediatric equipment

Most modern anesthetic machines can be used for patients of all ages. The safe and efficient management of children, however, requires familiarity with certain additional types of equipment and the availability of appropriately smaller sizes of airway and monitoring devices. For practitioners who do not work with children on a regular basis, or when the surgical schedule includes adults and young children in the same anesthetizing location, it is extremely convenient and time-saving to have a special "pediatric cart" that contains all these extras in a single place. Assuming the routine availability of a standard basic adult set-up, the following additional equipment should be considered.

Airway equipment

A complete set of smaller sizes of everything is needed. This includes pediatric face masks (and a selection of food flavors to apply inside the mask), endotracheal tubes, laryngeal mask airways (LMAs), oro- and naso-pharyngeal airways, suction catheters, bite blocks, etc.

Breathing system

The decision to use a pediatric circle system or a Mapleson circuit is largely a matter of preference as long as the anesthesiologist is familiar with the advantages and limitations of each. The circle system is readily available on all anesthesia machines, is a familiar system that is easy to use with mechanical or controlled ventilation, allows the use of economical fresh gas flow (FGF) rates, and helps conserve heat and moisture.

Circle absorber systems, however, are bulky, have a large internal volume that may delay the wash-in and -out of anesthetic agents unless a high FGF is used, and may result in an increase in dead space and resistance to breathing. Mapleson-classified systems (e.g., Jackson Rees modification), on the other hand, are lightweight and easy to move away from the anesthetic machine and allow for quick changes in the inspired anesthetic gas mixtures when the dials on the machine are adjusted.

Table 5-3. Size of pediatric laryngeal mask airways (LMAs)

LMA size	Patient weight (kg)	Cuff volume (mL)
1	<5	2–5
1½	5–10	7
2	10–20	10
2½	20–30	15
3	30–50	20
4	>50	20–30

Airway maintenance

Many of the pediatric ambulatory procedures are superficial, do not require intense muscle relaxation, and especially when general anesthesia is supplemented with a regional block, do not require a depth of anesthesia that can significantly depress ventilation. Patients undergoing these types of procedures (e.g., hernia repair) can be managed quite successfully with face mask airways or LMAs. LMAs are especially useful in brief procedures in which the airway needs to be maintained without interfering with the surgical field (e.g., lachrymal duct probing or ophthalmic examination). They also help free the hands of the anesthesiologist to start intravenous (IV) lines and/or prepare for the following case (Table 5-3).

The use of an endotracheal tube in pediatric ambulatory patients requires careful attention to the selection of a tube size appropriate for the age of the child (Table 5-4), avoiding traumatic instrumentation to minimize the possibility of postintubation croup. There has been a recent trend to use cuffed tracheal tubes routinely in small children.[19] Selection of a tube size that is one size smaller than a noncuffed tube, choosing well-designed cuffs that are low-pressure and short, will produce an adequate seal in the mid-tracheal region and minimize tracheal irritation at the cricoid level (Figure 5-1) or the possibility of accidental endobronchial intubation.[20]

Children who develop postintubation croup must be treated aggressively with cool mist as soon as the symptoms are apparent, which is usually within the first 30 minutes of extubation. If racemic epinephrine inhalation is used, the child must be closely monitored for 2–3 hours afterward to detect possible rebound edema and recurrence of symptoms. Should this happen, repeat treatment is indicated, and overnight admission to a hospital for observation may be required.

Monitoring equipment

Parameters that should be monitored in anesthetized children include heart rate, heart sounds, and breath sounds by means of a precordial or an esophageal stethoscope; blood pressure by means of an appropriate-size cuff that is wide

Table 5-4. Recommended tracheal tube sizes by age

| Age | Internal diameter (mm) | |
---	Noncuffed	Cuffed
Term newborn	3.0	
6 months	3.5	
12 months	4.0	3.5
18–24 months	4.5	4.0
4 years	5.5	5.0
6 years	6.0	5.5
8 years	6.5	6.0
10 years		6.5
12 years		7.0
14 years		7.5
Adult		8.0

Children of the same age vary in size: occasionally a size 0.5 mm ID smaller or larger may be required. Cuffs are generally not used with tube size smaller than 4.0. General formula for children over 2 years:

$$\text{Tube size mm ID} = \frac{\text{Age (years)}}{4} + 4.0$$

| Oral length (cm) | = | 12 | + | Age/2 |
| Nasal length (cm) | = | 15 | + | Age/2 |

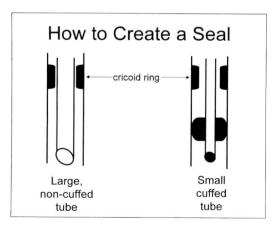

Figure 5-1. Use of a small cuffed tracheal tube provides a seal in the mid-tracheal region and minimizes mucosal irritation in the cricoid area.

enough to cover about two thirds of the length of the upper arm; electro-cardiogram for diagnosis of dysrhythmias; oxygen saturation; and expired CO_2. Temperature-monitoring devices should be available and used when indicated. Monitoring of neuromuscular function is strongly recommended if muscle relaxants are used. Additional monitoring techniques should be available when indicated (e.g., arterial blood gases if malignant hyperthermia is suspected).

Anesthetic agents and techniques

The ideal anesthetic technique for pediatric ambulatory patients is that which provides rapid smooth onset, ease of adjustment and control of anesthetic depth during surgery, prompt emergence, as well as rapid recovery that is free of pain, vomiting, and other unpleasant side effects. Usually, a combination of agents and techniques is used to achieve these goals in children.

Inhalational anesthetics

Inhalational induction is the most popular technique in pediatric anesthesia in this country. When the patient is cooperative and the anesthesiologist enjoys working with children, the onset is usually smooth and rapid. Recovery is quick after short procedures. Unfortunately, up to 10%–15% of all children—especially those who did not receive adequate preoperative sedation—will not cooperate with attempted mask induction.[1]

Some of the reluctance can be overcome with gentle persuasion, distraction, or the use of pleasant food flavors (e.g., bubble gum) to conceal the plastic smell of the anesthetic mask or the pungent odor of the agent. If, in spite of all attempts, the child continues to struggle and refuse the mask, an alternate induction or preinduction technique should be chosen. This is preferable to continuing with a forced-mask induction that can be extremely unpleasant or psychologically traumatic to the child.[1]

Sevoflurane

Sevoflurane is the most commonly used inhalational agent for induction of anesthesia in the U.S. today. It has a pleasant smell and is the least irritating inhalational induction agent available. Because of its low blood/gas solubility coefficient, sevoflurane results in extremely rapid and smooth induction with no airway irritation even when an 8% inspired concentration is used initially. In brief procedures, sevoflurane can be used for both induction and maintenance of anesthesia in children. Although emergence and recovery times are faster when compared to halothane, they are less predictable compared to desflurane.[21]

Sevoflurane undergoes metabolic breakdown in the body, resulting in release of free fluoride ions. The clinical significance of this breakdown appears to be negligible, especially in children undergoing short ambulatory surgical procedures.

Desflurane

Desflurane's low blood/gas partition coefficient (0.42) makes it a very suitable agent for pediatric outpatients. However, desflurane is not indicated for the start of anesthesia induction in children, because it results in a high incidence of airway irritation, coughing, and laryngospasm. Desflurane, however, can be easily introduced following other induction agents, typically sevoflurane. This results in significantly faster emergence and recovery than when halothane or sevoflurane is used.[21] Desflurane maintenance, following sevoflurane induction, is particularly useful in patients undergoing airway procedures such as tonsillectomy and/or adenoidectomy when the timing of the end of surgery cannot be accurately predicted and when rapid awakening and return of airway reflexes is desirable.

Recovery following unsupplemented sevoflurane and desflurane anesthesia has been associated with a higher incidence of excitement than when halothane is used. Attempts to modify the emergence agitation that is frequently seen with these agents have not been completely successful. Attention must be given to ensuring adequate analgesia in these patients. Even in the absence of pain, as is usually seen in children who have a functional regional block or who are undergoing diagnostic radiological procedures, agitation still occurs. More recent experience indicates that a dose of 2–3 μg/kg of fentanyl is effective in reducing this emergence phenomenon without delaying emergence or discharge when desflurane or sevoflurane is used in pediatric ear, nose, and throat patients.[22,23]

Intravenous anesthetics

Because of the unwillingness to subject awake children to the trauma of venipuncture, IV induction of anesthesia is not widely used in pediatric ambulatory surgery (Table 5-5). In situations in which an IV induction is the only option (e.g., an office practice in which an anesthetic machine with vaporizers is not

Table 5-5. Pediatric intravenous induction agents

Drug	Dose (mg/kg)
Thiopental	4–6
Methohexital	1.5–2
Propofol*	2.5–3.5

*To minimize pain on injection, use large antecubital veins or add lidocaine 1–2 mg/mL of propofol prior to its administration.

available), the topical application of the eutectic mixture of the two local anesthetics lidocaine and prilocaine (EMLA) or more recent alternatives such as the Synera topical patch (lidocaine 70 mg and tetracaine 70 mg) can be used to perform painless venipuncture in children.[24,25]

The use of EMLA in ambulatory patients requires careful planning, since approximately 1 hour of contact time under an occlusive dressing is required for full effect. S-Caine Patch, on the other hand, has the distinct advantage of a shorter onset time (20 minutes). In most cases, EMLA should be applied to two potential IV sites to have a backup site available in case the first venipuncture is not successful. Although the use of EMLA does produce skin analgesia, it does not take away the fear of needles in children who have been previously accustomed to expect pain.

Propofol is now the standard IV agent in ambulatory patients. Propofol can be used in a dose of 2.5–3.5 mg/kg for induction of anesthesia in children who accept venipuncture. Pain on injection can be minimized by mixing lidocaine with propofol (1–2 mg lidocaine/1 mL of propofol) immediately prior to its injection. Alternatively, propofol infusion can be started following a brief inhalational induction and establishment of an IV access. Because of their higher volume of distribution and increased clearance, young children require a higher infusion rate initially (250–300 µg/kg per minute) than adults.[26]

When propofol induction is followed by an inhalational agent (e.g., halothane maintenance), recovery is significantly faster than when thiopental induction is followed by halothane.[27] Recovery is fastest if propofol induction is followed by a propofol infusion for the maintenance of anesthesia.[27] In children younger than 3 years of age, propofol infusion has a hemodynamic and recovery profile similar to sevoflurane.[28]

Propofol anesthesia has been consistently shown to be associated with an extremely low incidence of postoperative vomiting even following surgical procedures that normally result in vomiting (e.g., strabismus surgery). Propofol has been extensively used as part of a TIVA (total IV anesthesia) technique for children undergoing endoscopic or radiologic diagnostic procedures outside the OR.[29,30]

Adjunct agents

Muscle relaxants

Muscle relaxants are not routinely needed in ambulatory patients, because of the brief and superficial nature of most types of surgery performed on these patients (Table 5-6). Muscle relaxants may be used to facilitate tracheal intubation or as part of a balanced technique to allow the use of the lightest possible level of anesthesia.

When muscle relaxation is indicated for tracheal intubation only, it is desirable to use the shortest-acting agent available. To avoid the possible confusion about ruling out "masseter spasm" in the small number of patients in whom incomplete relaxation is observed, succinylcholine is currently not indicated for elective use in children.[31]

Table 5-6. Pediatric adjunct agents

Agent	Dose	Route
Muscle relaxants:		
Succinylcholine	2 mg/kg	IV
	5–6 mg/kg	IM
Mivacurium (not currently available in the U.S.)	0.2 mg/kg	IV
Atracurium	0.5 mg/kg	IV
Vecuronium	0.1 mg/kg	IV
Rocuronium	0.6–1 mg/kg	IV
Opioids:		
Fentanyl	0.5–2 μg/kg	IV
Morphine	0.05–0.1 mg/kg	IV
Antiemetics:		
Metoclopramide	0.15 mg/kg	IV
Ondansetron	0.1 mg/kg (maximum 4 mg)	IV
	4 mg for children >20 kg	ODT
Dexamethasone	0.15 mg/kg (maximum 4 mg)	IV
Promethazine	12.5–25 mg	Rectally
Prochlorperazine	2.5–5 mg	Rectally

Doses should be titrated starting with the lower recommended dose. IM, intramuscular; IV, intravenous; ODT, oral disintegrating tablet.

Intermediate-acting relaxants are particularly suitable for use in pediatric ambulatory patients (Table 5-6). Of those, mivacurium seems to be particularly attractive because of its very short duration of action and its spontaneous degradation that often makes pharmacological antagonism unnecessary following a single intubating dose in a surgical procedure that lasts 20 minutes or longer.[32] Avoiding pharmacological antagonism may decrease the incidence of gastrointestinal disturbances, including nausea and vomiting in those patients. Unfortunately, mivacurium is not available at this time. For longer procedures, atracurium, vecuronium, or rocuronium has been extensively used, although pharmacological antagonism is almost always indicated.

Opioids

Short-acting opioids (e.g., fentanyl and/or remifentanil) can be used as part of the main anesthetic or for postoperative analgesia in pediatric ambulatory patients. By decreasing the dose of potent inhalational or IV agents needed, opioids may actually contribute to more rapid awakening. To avoid delaying recovery, the shortest-acting agent that is appropriate for the particular surgical procedure should be selected (Table 5-6).

Antiemetics

Postoperative nausea and vomiting (PONV) can be a significant problem in pediatric outpatients. Tools to predict an increased risk for developing PONV have been developed in adults[33] and more recently in children.[34] The following are four independent risk factors for postoperative vomiting in children.[34]

- During surgery of 30 minutes or longer
- Age 3 years or older
- Strabismus surgery
- History of postoperative vomiting in a previous operation or PONV in relatives (mother, father, or sibling)

By means of this four-item risk score, the incidence of postoperative vomiting can be predicted to be 9%, 10%, 30%, 55%, and 70% when 0, 1, 2, 3, and 4 risk factors, respectively, are present (Figure 5-2). Prophylactic use of antiemetic drugs has become a common approach to minimizing emetic symptoms after outpatient surgery because it is more effective than trying to treat vomiting after it occurs. Patient satisfaction is increased, and discharge home is faster.

Several multicenter trials concluded that IV ondansetron prophylaxis (0.1 mg/kg, maximum 4 mg) was more effective than placebo in preventing postoperative vomiting in children 1–12 years old and 1–24 months old during both the 0- to 2-hour and 0- to 24-hour study periods.[35,36] IV ondansetron was also found effective in treating established postoperative emesis in yet another multicenter trial of 2,720 pediatric outpatients.[37] In the absence of an IV line, or if vomiting occurs after the IV is removed, ondansetron orally disintegrating tablet (4 mg disk for children with greater than 20 kg body weight) can be placed over the tongue for quick absorption without the need for swallowing.[38]

For high-risk patients (e.g., strabismus surgery or adenotonsillectomy), a combination antiemetic regimen, possibly including the intraoperative use of ondansetron (0.1 mg/kg, maximum 4 mg) and dexamethasone (0.15 mg/kg,

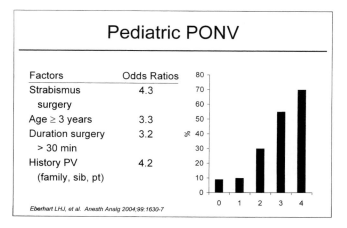

Figure 5-2. Risk factors to predict postoperative nausea and vomiting (PONV) in children. PV, postoperative vomiting. Source: Eberhart et al.[34]

maximum 4 mg), is recommended. For patients with persistent postoperative vomiting, our approach is to stop offering oral fluids and ensure adequate IV hydration.[39] A different class of antiemetic should be administered. Occasionally, rectal promethazine 0.5 mg/kg (Phenergan 12.5–25 mg) or prochlorperazine 0.1 mg/kg (Compazine 2.5–5 mg) is administered in the hospital and/or given to the parents to administer at home.[1]

Perioperative fluid management

Most pediatric ambulatory patients undergo brief surgical procedures that are not associated with significant fluid loss. Fluid management in the perioperative period, therefore, is designed to replace any excessive preoperative deficit and/or anticipated postoperative needs.

Children undergoing very brief surgical procedures (e.g., myringotomies) may not need any parenteral fluid administration as long as they are not excessively starved preoperatively and are expected to be able to ingest and retain oral fluids soon after they are awake.[1] For most other children, intraoperative maintenance fluid administration can be calculated based on the child's body weight according to standard formulae (Table 5-7).[40]

Although hypotonic solutions (e.g., 1/2 or 1/3 normal saline) can be used for that purpose, most anesthesiologists find it more appropriate to use a replacement type solution such as lactated Ringer for that purpose so that the same solution can be used to replace any intraoperative loss (e.g., during tonsillectomy) or continuing postoperative loss that may result from protracted vomiting. If continuing postoperative loss through vomiting or inability to tolerate per os intake is anticipated, it is advisable to start making up that anticipated deficit early on so that the child is well hydrated when ready to go home, thereby avoiding a delay in discharge while "catch-up" fluid administration is instituted.

Adequate parenteral hydration also obviates the need for forcing children to ingest oral fluids before they are allowed to go home. Recent studies confirm that children who are forced to drink before leaving the facility have higher incidence of vomiting and are discharged home later than children who are allowed to drink only when they are thirsty enough to request a drink.[39]

Table 5-7. Maintenance fluid therapy

Child's weight (kg)	Basic hourly rate (mL)
<10	wt × 4
10–20	(wt × 2) + 20
>20	wt + 40

During the first hour of surgery, up to four times the basic hourly rate may be administered as a hydrated solution.

Postoperative analgesia

Adequate postoperative analgesia is a key requirement for successful pediatric ambulatory anesthetic management. Anticipation of the child's requirements, pre-emptive multimodal analgesic therapy, and early scheduled supplementation postoperatively ensure the patient's comfort and may even speed recovery and discharge home.

The selection of the specific analgesic drug or technique is not as vital as the awareness that the individual patient's need can vary tremendously and that treatment must be individualized and titrated to effect. Regional blocks or local infiltration should be used whenever possible to supplement general anesthesia and to limit the need for narcotics during recovery.[1] For some pediatric ambulatory patients, postoperative analgesia can be ensured by continuing to titrate short-acting opioids intravenously during recovery. For most others, postoperative analgesia can be provided by one or a combination of the following methods (Tables 5-8 and 5-9).

Mild analgesics

Acetaminophen (10–15 mg/kg per os) is the most commonly used mild analgesic for pediatric ambulatory patients. For young children, the initial dose is often administered rectally (30–40 mg/kg) prior to awakening from anesthesia. Early administration is best since the onset time can be 60–90 minutes. Supplemental scheduled doses should be given orally every 4–6 hours (not as needed) to maintain adequate blood level and therefore effective analgesia.[41]

Table 5-8. Pediatric analgesic drug dosage

Drug	Route	Dose	Duration of action (hours)
Acetaminophen	Rectally	30–40 mg/kg*	4–6
	PO	10–15 mg/kg	4–6
Ketorolac	IV	0.5 mg/kg (maximum 30 mg)	6–8
	PO	1 mg/kg (maximum 10 mg)	4–6
Ibuprofen	PO	5 mg/kg	6–8
Codeine	PO	0.5–1 mg/kg	4–6
Naproxen	PO	10 mg/kg	6–8
Fentanyl	IV	1–2 µg/kg	0.5–1
Meperidine	IV/IM	0.5–1 mg/kg	2–4
Morphine	IV	0.05–0.1 mg/kg	2–4

Doses should be titrated starting with the lower recommended dose.
*Acetaminophen suppositories are available in sizes of 120, 325, and 650 mg. Usually, the calculated dose is rounded up or down to the nearest whole or half size suppository.
IM, intramuscular; IV, intravenous; PO, per os.

Table 5-9. Regional techniques for pediatric ambulatory surgery

Surgical procedure	Block	Drug/dose
Inguinal hernia hydrocelectomy orchiopexy	Caudal ilioinguinal/ iliohypogastric Instillation	Bupivacaine* 1/4–1/8% 0.75–1.0 mL/kg Bupivacaine* 1/4% 0.3–0.5 mL/kg Bupivacaine* 1/4% 0.5 mL/kg
Umbilical hernia	Infiltration Rectus sheath	Bupivacaine* 1/4% 0.3–0.5 mL/kg Bupivacaine* 1/4% 1.0 mL/kg
Circumcision/hypospadias	Caudal Dorsal nerve Ring block Topical (end of surgery)	Bupivacaine* 1/4% 0.5 mL/kg Bupivacaine* 1/4% 4–6 mL Bupivacaine* 1/4% 4–6 mL Lidocaine jelly or ointment (2%)
Tonsillectomy and adenoidectomy	Infiltration Topical	Bupivacaine 1/4% with Epinephrine 1:200,000 0.5 mL/kg Lidocaine (10%) spray 4 mg/kg
Extremities	Peripheral nerve blocks (e.g., axillary)	Bupivacaine 2.5 mg/kg Lidocaine 5 mg/kg
Airway endoscopy	Topical	Lidocaine 3–5 mg/kg

*Ropivacaine 0.2% can be substituted for bupivacaine in the same volume.

Acetaminophen can be combined with codeine for more effective control of moderately severe pain and/or discomfort.[1] Acetaminophen with codeine elixir contains 120 mg acetaminophen and 12 mg codeine per 5 mL. The usual doses are 5 mL for children 3–6 years old and 10 mL for children 7–12 years old.

Nonsteroidal anti-inflammatory drugs

Nonsteroidal anti-inflammatory drugs (e.g., ketorolac 0.5 mg/kg IV) have proven effective in relieving postoperative pain following minor operations in children.[42] Early administration immediately following induction seems to provide optimal postoperative analgesia. Ketorolac, however, may result in increased surgical bleeding secondary to altered platelet function and is usually avoided in procedures prone to significant postoperative bleeding such as adeno-tonsillectomy.

Regional analgesia

The greatest advantage of regional anesthesia in pediatric ambulatory patients is that local infiltration or regional blocks can be placed intraoperatively after the induction of general anesthesia to help reduce the requirements of other anesthetic agents and promote rapid, pain-free recovery without the need for systemic opioids or other potent analgesics. Many of the surgical procedures performed on these patients are amenable to regional anesthetic supplementation (Table 5-9). The choice of the individual block is determined by the type of operation as well as by the familiarity of the individual anesthesiologist with the available techniques.

Caudal analgesia

This technique can be used to provide analgesia in patients undergoing inguinal, penile, perineal, or lower limb procedures (Figure 5-3). The level of block is determined by several formulae that calculate an appropriate volume of the local anesthetic solution (Table 5-9). A dose of bupivacaine in excess of 2.5 mg/kg is seldom required or justified in pediatric outpatients. The 0.25% and 0.125% solutions of this drug have been shown to be equally effective in providing supplemental intraoperative anesthesia as well as residual postoperative analgesia.[43] The more dilute bupivacaine solution, or alternatively the use of ropivacaine, minimizes the incidence of motor weakness, which is undesirable in ambulatory patients.[43,44]

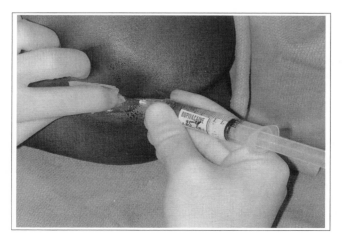

Figure 5-3. Pediatric caudal analgesia.

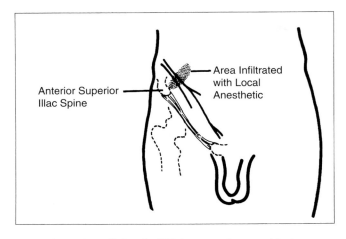

Figure 5-4. Ilioinguinal/iliohypogastric nerve blocks.

Ilioinguinal/Iliohypogastric nerve block

This block is very effective in providing postoperative analgesia following operations performed through an inguinal incision (e.g., hernia repair, hydrocelectomy, or orchiopexy). Since the two nerves enter the inguinal canal through the layers of the anterior abdominal wall muscles, the block can be performed by direct infiltration of these muscles medial to the anterior superior iliac spine using 3–5 mL of 0.25% bupivacaine solution (Figure 5-4).[45] Alternatively, the muscles can be infiltrated through the lateral edge of the inguinal incision[46] or by instillation of bupivacaine directly in the wound to bathe the exposed nerve trunks during dissection.[47]

Penile blocks

Both dorsal nerve block and ring block around the base of the penis can be used to provide analgesia following circumcision or hypospadias surgery (Figure 5-5).[48,49] Epinephrine-free solutions must be used. Alternatively, topical application of local anesthetic cream or ointment to the exposed nerve endings of the skin incision after surgical closure has been found to be effective.[50]

Other blocks

Almost all other regional blocks with which the anesthesiologist is familiar can be adapted for use in children. It is essential, however, that special attention be paid in order not to exceed the safe dose of the local anesthetic solution (Table 5-9). If the calculated maximum safe dose of a standard concentration results in an inadequate volume, a more dilute solution or a different block should be chosen. Examples of these blocks that are frequently used at CNMC include rectus sheath for patients undergoing umbilical hernia repair (Figure 5-6) and axillary and femoral nerve blocks.

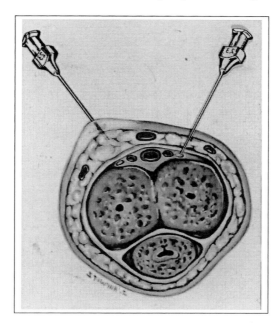

Figure 5-5. Penile blocks.

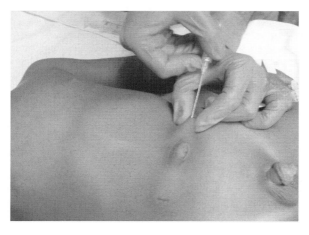

Figure 5-6. Rectus sheath block.

Local infiltration

For operations that are not amenable to a regional technique or for minor peripheral procedures, the surgeon must be encouraged to use local infiltration of the wound area before, during, or at the completion of the operation.

Sedation techniques

Introduction

Sedation and analgesia are frequently required for diagnostic and therapeutic procedures performed on pediatric ambulatory patients. Sedation may be administered by anesthesiologists and nonanesthesiologists in and out of the OR. Sedatives, opioid and nonopioid analgesics, and local anesthetics techniques are frequently used in combination to ensure the comfort and safety of the child. Painful procedures, which are frequently performed outside the OR (e.g., bone marrow aspiration, lumbar puncture, and endoscopy), require the same attention to anxiolysis, analgesia, and sedation as procedures performed in the OR.

Defining the level of sedation

Different levels of sedation/analgesia may be required based on the intensity of the stimulus associated with the procedures. Sedation and immobility are required for nonpainful procedures such as magnetic resonance imaging (MRI) scanning. Sedation with analgesia is required for painful procedures such as lumbar puncture or bone marrow aspiration. Patients undergoing diagnostic gastroduodenoscopies require a level of "sedation" that is equivalent to general anesthesia.[29]

Procedural sedation and analgesia therefore represent a continuum of consciousness to unconsciousness. A clear understanding of the definition of sedation is important in order to recognize when the child has progressed from moderate to deep sedation or general anesthesia and when monitoring and care should be escalated in order to avoid complications.

Although the terminology of sedation is similar in children and adults, the practical applications are different (Figure 5-7). Minimal sedation, or *anxiolysis*, is best exemplified by the use of oral midazolam premedication. The child is sedated if left alone but will not lie still for an extended period or cooperate with an uncomfortable intervention. Moderate sedation/analgesia (*conscious sedation*) is commonly used in adults. In children, however, conscious sedation is often described as an oxymoron. Very few children can become sedated enough to be cooperative and still respond *purposefully* to verbal command or light tactile stimulation.

Children are almost always unconscious when they achieve a level of sedation that allows painful interventions to be performed or even when they lie still

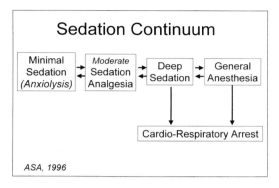

Figure 5-7. Sedation continuum.

for painless radiological examinations. The ability to independently maintain ventilatory function may be impaired. Spontaneous ventilation may be inadequate, and children often require assistance or intervention to maintain a patent airway, especially in the presence of adenotonsillar hypertrophy. Although these observations and required interventions are part of the training anesthesiologists have, the issue has more serious implications when nonanesthesiologists are responsible for providing pediatric sedation.

Although it is not possible to have all pediatric sedation performed by a trained anesthesiologist, there are some models in which all sedation is provided by dedicated sedation teams headed by an anesthesiologist,[51] pediatric intensivist, or emergency medicine physician. A detailed discussion of the merits of these models, however, is not within the scope of this chapter. Patient safety is the utmost priority in these circumstances.

Patient preparation

Requirements for sedation procedures in or outside the OR should be similar to requirements for an anesthetic procedure: a complete history and physical examination, presedation screening phone call, complete drug history and allergy list, appropriate fasting period, etc. Frequently, the anesthesiologist will be the only physician responsible for the child and will need to personally perform these examinations and obtain consent for the sedation.

Standard monitoring and rescue drugs and equipment, including positive-pressure oxygen delivery system and functional suctioning, are mandatory. Pulse oximetry is now universally accepted in all sedating locations. Although capnography is still controversial in some areas, the author finds that a CO_2 tracing obtained from an infant nasal cannula adaptor to be one of the most useful monitors, especially when the child is not completely visible as in the MRI suite (Figure 5-8).

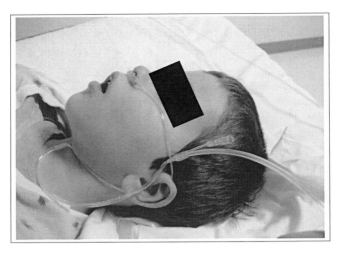

Figure 5-8. Use of capnography during pediatric sedation.

Sedation pharmacology

Most useful sedation drugs require IV titration (Tables 5-10 to 5-12). Although most children dislike and fear injections, IV lines can be started with local skin analgesia or following a brief inhaled induction. At the author's institution, most children presenting for MRI sedation or gastrointestinal endoscopy are started with a brief N_2O/sevoflurane mask induction until an IV line is established and then they are maintained with a propofol infusion. Many of the oncology patients have indwelling central or PICC (peripherally inserted central catheter) lines that can be used from the beginning. It is essential that the sterility

Table 5-10. Oral sedation techniques in children

Drug	Usual dose
Chloral hydrate	25–50 mg/kg (for small infants up to 12 months)
	25–75 mg/kg (for children older than 12 months)
Ketamine	5–10 mg/kg (above 1 year)
Midazolam	0.5–1.0 mg/kg orally
	0.2–0.3 mg/kg intranasally (above 1 year)
Fentanyl (Oralet)	5–15 µg/kg transmucosally (for children weighing more than 15 kg)

Doses should be titrated starting with the lower recommended dose.

Table 5-11. Intramuscular sedation techniques in children

Drug	Usual dose
Ketamine	2–5 mg/kg
Midazolam	0.1 mg/kg
Pentobarbital	4–5 mg/kg

of these lines be strictly maintained and that they be flushed with an appropriate heparin solution before the child is discharged.

The ideal sedating drug should have fast onset and rapid offset with no serious side effects. Propofol is an almost ideal hypnotic agent for many of these procedures. Although it does not provide analgesia, it has a rapid onset and a short duration of action and does not promote postoperative vomiting. It allows the child to wake up, recover, and return to baseline activities and diet sooner than other sedative agents. In the trained hands of an anesthesiologist, it is a safe and familiar drug. Unlike other sedative agents (e.g., midazolam, fentanyl, or morphine), however, there is no reversal agent for propofol. Adverse effects such as airway obstruction and/or apnea must be treated until the drug is redistributed or metabolized.

The use of propofol for procedural sedation by nonanesthesiologists is a subject of intense debate and is not recommended. As stated in the drug label and affirmed by various professional organizations, propofol should be administered only by persons who are trained in the administration of general anesthesia and who are not involved in the surgical/diagnostic procedure.

The combination of midazolam (0.05–0.1 mg/kg) with fentanyl (1–2 μg/kg) is frequently used for procedural sedation in children. In the absence of an IV line, IM injection of midazolam (0.1 mg/kg) and ketamine (2–5 mg/kg) can be used. Discharge criteria and postprocedure follow-up should be similar to other surgical procedures.

Table 5-12. Intravenous sedation techniques in children

Drug	Usual dose
Pentobarbital	2.5 mg/kg; may repeat up to 7.5 mg/kg
Methohexital	0.5 to 1.0 mg/kg; may repeat as needed
Midazolam	0.5–0.1 mg/kg
Propofol	1 to 2 mg/kg; may follow with infusion at 100–250 μg/kg per minute
Ketamine	0.5 to 1.0 mg/kg; may repeat as needed
Fentanyl	0.5 to 2.0 μg/kg

Doses should be titrated starting with the lower recommended dose.

Recovery and discharge

Recovery

Facilities for postoperative care vary among institutions. Many allow parents to be with their children as soon as the operation is completed. Parents can care for and hold, cuddle, and feed the child, and their involvement helps decrease recovery time and reduce the need for a high nurse-to-patient ratio.[52] Several scoring tools to document the return of protective functions have been used in children. Most are based on an adaptation of those used in adult patients. The scoring system currently in use at CNMC is shown in Table 5-13.

Discharge home

Discharge of the child from the hospital should be based on specific criteria approved by the facility. Unlike a scoring system, *all* criteria must be met before the child is allowed to go home. Table 5-14 presents an example of discharge criteria. Every child, regardless of age, must have an escort home. The journey preferably should be by private car or taxicab, and the escort should be provided with written instructions for the home care of the child and be provided with a telephone number to call for further advice or to report complications.

In addition to counseling the parent of each child about postoperative care, most units have designed handouts that specify the care to be provided and the

Table 5-13. Children's National Medical Center postanesthesia care unit scoring tool

Parameter	Score	Description
Motor activity	2	Moves limbs purposefully
	1	Nonpurposeful movements
	0	Not moving
Airway	2	Coughing on command or crying
	1	Maintaining good airway
	0	Airway requires maintenance
Vital signs	2	Stable and appropriate for age
	1	Stable but inappropriate for age
	0	Unstable
Consciousness	2	Awake
	1	Responding to stimuli
	0	Not responding
Pulse oximetry	2	$\geq$95% saturation
	1	90%–94% saturation
	0	<90%

Table 5-14. Discharge criteria (Children's National
Medical Center)

- Stable vital signs
- Absence of respiratory distress
- No or minimal vomiting
- Alert and oriented
- Able to ambulate according to age

---

signs that might herald a complication. For convenience, the handout is usually
limited to postoperative instructions for a specific operative procedure and is
written in the primary language of the parents.

Complications and admissions

Complications

The most commonly reported complications before discharge are sore
throat, headache, muscle pains, nausea and vomiting, and postoperative pain.
Hypothermia is a risk in infants and small children, especially those undergoing
diagnostic procedures without proper insulation. Surgical bleeding must not
be present prior to discharge. Again, this is especially important following
adenotonsillectomies.

Admissions

Complications that result in unplanned admission of the patient to a hospital
are rare. These can be grouped into anesthetic (e.g., protracted vomiting or
severe croup), surgical (e.g., post-tonsillectomy bleeding), and social/adminis-
trative reasons. Surgeons who work in freestanding ambulatory surgery centers
or in an office setting should have arrangements to treat these potential surgical
complications in a hospital environment after regular business hours. In a well-
formulated program in a modern institution, the admission rate is usually less
than 2%. At our institution, the unplanned admission rate for surgical outpatients
has dropped from 0.9% to 0.3%.[53]

Summary

The key to the success of pediatric day surgery lies in careful selection,
screening, and preparation of prospective patients. Selected patients should
be healthy or have a well-controlled medical condition. Screening must be

completed prior to the day of surgery. Liberalized fasting requirements for children may allow clear liquids up to 2 hours before anesthesia induction. Facilities differ in their approach to the use of premedication or allowing the parents to be present during induction.

Monitoring and airway equipment should be appropriate for the child's age and size. Anesthetic techniques should ensure smooth onset, prompt emergence, fast recovery, and safe discharge with good control of postoperative pain and vomiting. Properties of currently used inhalational and IV agents are discussed. A multimodal approach to prevention and treatment of postoperative pain and vomiting is most likely to be effective.

Adequate intraoperative hydration reduces the need for children to ingest fluid before discharge, thereby minimizing dizziness and vomiting. Procedural sedation is frequently required in pediatric ambulatory patients. The requirements for providing safe sedation techniques are outlined. Propofol is the most common agent used by anesthesiologists. Recovery and discharge requirements and complications are discussed.

References

1. Hannallah RS. Outpatient anesthesia. In: Coté CJ, Todres ID, eds. *A Practice of Anesthesia for Infants and Children.* 3rd ed. New York, NY: W.B. Saunders Company; 2001:55–67.
2. American Academy of Pediatrics, Section on Anesthesiology. Guidelines for the pediatric perioperative anesthesia environment. *Pediatrics.* 1999;103:512–515.
3. Coté C. NPO after midnight for children—a reappraisal. *Anesthesiology.* 1990;72: 589–592.
4. Schreiner MS, Triebwasser A, Keon T. Ingestion of liquids compared with preoperative fasting in pediatric outpatients. *Anesthesiology.* 1990;72:593–597.
5. Sethi AK, Chatterji C, Bhargava SK, et al. Safe pre-operative fasting times after milk or clear fluid in children. A preliminary study using real-time ultrasound. *Anaesthesia.* 1999;54:51–59.
6. Practice guidelines for preoperative fasting and the use of pharmacologic agents to reduce the risk of pulmonary aspiration: application to healthy patients undergoing elective procedures. *Anesthesiology.* 1999;90:896–905.
7. Cavell B. Gastric emptying in infants fed human milk or infant formula. *Acta Paediatr Scand.* 1981;70:639–641.
8. Castillo-Zamora C, Castillo-Peralta LA, Nava-Ocampo AA. Randomized trial comparing overnight preoperative fasting period vs oral administration of apple juice at 06:00–06:30 am in pediatric orthopedic surgical patients. *Paediatr Anaesth.* 2005; 15:638–642.
9. Steward DJ. Screening tests before surgery in children—Editorial. *Can J Anaesth.* 1991;38:693–695.
10. Patel RI, DeWitt L, Hannallah RS. Preoperative laboratory testing in children: analysis of current practice. *J Clin Anesth.* 1997;9:569–575.

11. Rosen DA, Rosen KR, Hannallah RS. Anaesthesia induction in children—ability to predict outcome. *Paediatr Anaesth.* 1993;3:365–370.
12. Litman RS, Perkins FM, Dawson SC. Parental knowledge and attitude toward discussing the risk of death from anesthesia. *Anesth Analg.* 1993;77:256–260.
13. Coté CJ, Cohen IT, Suresh S, et al. Comparison of three doses of a commercially prepared oral midazolam syrup in children. *Anesth Analg.* 2002;94:37–43.
14. Hannallah RS, Patel RI. Low dose intramuscular ketamine for anesthesia preinduction in young children undergoing brief outpatient procedures. *Anesthesiology.* 1989;70:598–600.
15. Verghese S, Hannallah R, Patel R, et al. Ketamine/Midazolam combination is not an appropriate preinduction combination in children undergoing brief ambulatory procedures. *Paediatr Anaesth.* 2003;13:228–232.
16. Karl HW, Keifer AT, Rosenberg JL, et al. Comparison of safety and efficacy of intranasal midazolam or sufentanil for preinduction of anesthesia in pediatric patients. *Anesthesiology.* 1992;76:209–215.
17. Hannallah RS. Who benefits when parents are present during anaesthesia induction in their children? *Can J Anaesth.* 1994;41:271–275.
18. Kain ZN, Caldwell-Andrews AA, Maranets I, et al. Predicting which child-parent pair will benefit from parental presence during induction of anesthesia: a decision-making approach. *Anesth Analg.* 2006;102:81–84.
19. Fine GF, Borland LM. The future of the cuffed endotracheal tube. *Paediatr Anaesth.* 2004;14:38–42.
20. Weiss M, Gerber AC, Dullenkopf A. Appropriate placement of intubation depth marks in a new cuffed paediatric tracheal tube. *Br J Anaesth.* 2005;94:80–87.
21. Welborn LG, Hannallah RS, Norden JM, et al. Comparison of emergence and recovery characteristics of sevoflurane, desflurane, and halothane in pediatric ambulatory patients. *Anesth Analg.* 1996;83:917–920.
22. Cohen IT, Finkel JC, Hannallah RS, et al. Effects of fentanyl on the emergence characteristics following desflurane or sevoflurane anesthesia in children. *Anesth Analg.* 2002;94:178–1181.
23. Finkel JF, Hannallah RS, Hummer KA, et al. The effect of intranasal fentanyl on the emergence characteristics after sevoflurane anesthesia in children undergoing surgery for bilateral myringotomy tube placement. *Anesth Analg.* 2001;92:1164–1168.
24. Soliman IE, Broadman LM, Hannallah RS, McGill WA. Comparison of the analgesic effects of EMLA (Eutectic Mixture of Local Anesthetics) to intradermal lidocaine infiltration prior to venous cannulation in unpremedicated children. *Anesthesiology.* 1988;68:804–806.
25. Sethna NF, Verghese ST, Hannallah RS, et al. A randomized controlled trial to evaluate S-Caine™ patch for reducing pain associated with vascular access in children. *Anesthesiology.* 2005;102:403–408.
26. Steur RJ, Perez RS, De Lange JJ. Dosage scheme for propofol in children under 3 years of age. *Paediatr Anaesth.* 2004;14:462–467.
27. Hannallah RS, Britton JT, Schafer PG, et al. Propofol anaesthesia in paediatric ambulatory patients: a comparison with thiopentone and halothane. *Can J Anaesth.* 1994;41:12–18.

28. Cohen IT, Finkel JC, Hannallah RS, Goodale DB. Clinical and biochemical effects of propofol EDTA vs sevoflurane in healthy infants and young children. *Paediatr Anaesth.* 2004:14:135–142.

29. Hammer GB, Litalien C, Wells V, et al. Determination of the median effective concentration (EC50) of propofol during oesophagogastroduodenoscopy in children. *Paediatr Anaesth.* 2001;11:549–553.

30. Khoshoo V, Thoppil D, Landry L, Brown S, Ross G. Propofol versus midazolam plus meperidine for sedation during ambulatory esophagogastroduodenoscopy. *J Pediatr Gastroenterol Nutr.* 2003;37:146–149.

31. Hannallah RS, Kaplan RF. Jaw relaxation following halothane/succinycholine sequence in children. *Anesthesiology.* 1994;81:99–103.

32. Kaplan RF, Garcia M, Hannallah RS. Mivacurium-induced neuromuscular blockade during sevoflurane and halothane anaesthesia in children. *Can J Anaesth.* 1995;42:16–20.

33. Apfel CC, Kortitila K, Abdalla M, et al. A factorial trial of six interventions for the prevention of postoprative nausea and vomiting. *N Engl J Med.* 2004;350:2441–2451.

34. Eberhart LHJ, Geldner G, Kranke P, et al. The development and validation of a risk score to predict the probability of postoperative vomiting in pediatric patients. *Anesth Analg.* 2004;99:1630–1637.

35. Patel RI, Davis PJ, Orr RJ, et al. Single-dose ondansetron prevents postoperative vomiting in pediatric outpatients. *Anesth Analg.* 1997;85:538–545.

36. Khalil SN, Roth AG, Cohen IT, et al. A double-blind comparison of intravenous ondansetron and placebo in prevention of postoperative emesis in 1- to 24-month-old pediatric patients following surgery under general anesthesia. *Anesth Analg.* 2005;101:356–361.

37. Khalil S, Rodarte A, Weldon BC, et al. Intravenous ondansetron in established postoperative emesis in children. *Anesthesiology.* 1996;85:270–276.

38. Cohen IT, Joffe D, Hummer K, et al. Ondansetron oral disintegrating tablets: acceptability and efficacy in children undergoing adenotonsillectomy. *Anesth Analg.* 2005;101:59–63.

39. Schreiner MS, Nicolson SC, Martin T, et al. Should children drink before discharge from day surgery? *Anesthesiology.* 1992;76:528–533.

40. Oh TH. Formula for calculating fluid maintenance requirements. *Anesthesiology.* 1980;53:351.

41. Anderson BJ, Holford NH, Woollard GA, et al. Perioperative pharmacodynamics of acetaminophen analgesia in children. *Anesthesiology.* 1999;90:411–421.

42. Hall SC. Tonsillectomies, ketorolac, and the march of progress. *Can J Anaesth.* 1996;43:544–548.

43. Verghese S, Hannallah R, Rice L, et al. Caudal anesthesia in children: effect of volume vs. concentration of bupivacaine in blocking spermatic cord traction response during orchidopexy. *Anesth Analg.* 2002;95:1219–1223.

44. Da Conceicao MJ, Coelho L, Khalil M. Ropivacaine 0.25% compared with bupivacaine 0.25% by the caudal route. *Paediatr Anaesth.* 1999;9:229–233.

45. Shandling B, Steward DJ. Regional analgesia for postoperative pain in pediatric out-patient surgery. *J Pediatr Surg.* 1980;15:477–480.

46. Hannallah RS, Broadman LM, Belman AB, et al. Comparison of caudal and ilioin-guinal/iliohypogastric nerve blocks for control of post-orchiopexy pain in pediatric ambulatory surgery. *Anesthesiology.* 1987;66:832–834.

47. Casey WF, Rice LJ, Hannallah RS, et al. A comparison between bupivacaine instil-lation versus ilioinguinal/ilio-hypogastric nerve block for postoperative analgesia following inguinal herniorrhaphy in children. *Anesthesiology.* 1990;72:637–639.

48. Soliman MG, Tremblay NA. Nerve block of the penis for postoperative pain relief in children. *Anesth Analg.* 1978;57:495–498.

49. Broadman LM, Hannallah RS, Belman AB, et al. Post-circumcision pain—a prospec-tive evaluation of subcutaneous ring block of the penis. *Anesthesiology.* 1987;67:399–402.

50. Tree-Trakan T, Pirayavaraporn S, Lertakyamanee J. Topical anesthesia for relief of post-circumcision pain. *Anesthesiology.* 1987;67:395–399.

51. Gozal D, Drenger B, Levin PD, et al. A pediatric sedation/anesthesia program with dedicated care by anesthesiologists and nurses for procedures outside the operating room. *J Pediatr.* 2004;145:47–52.

52. Patel RI, Verghese ST, Hannallah RS, et al. Fast-tracking children following ambula-tory surgery. *Anesth Analg.* 2001;92:918–922.

53. Patel RI, Hannallah RS. Anesthetic complications following pediatric ambulatory surgery: a 3-yr study. *Anesthesiology.* 1988;69:1009–1012.

6. Adult preoperative preparation: equipment and monitoring

J. Lance Lichtor, MD

Preoperative instructions for patients

Patient preoperative instructions should include directions on what medications to take prior to the procedure, fasting, what to wear, and what to have available once the procedure is finished. Patients should be told when their surgery is likely to occur and at what time they should arrive at the facility. They should be told what to bring, such as glasses in case they need to read a consent form and a hearing aid so they can understand instructions. Patients should be told not to bring valuables and jewelry, to avoid loss or theft. Rings should be taped on. Whether patients should be required to shower before a procedure depends on patient and facility preference.

Preoperative antiseptic showers have been shown to reduce skin microbial counts, although the evidence to show that they reduce surgical site infection rates is weak. Patients should be told before their surgery what to expect afterward. Due to the effects of the anesthesia, patients may forget what they are told if they are given instructions only after surgery. Patients should be told in advance what criteria they must meet in order to be discharged, approximately when they might be discharged so appropriate plans can be made, what dressings to expect and how they should be managed, and how they should care for the wound.

Box 6-1. Preoperative instructions
- Which medications should be taken before surgery
- Fasting before the procedure
- Appropriate dress
- Times: arrival and time of surgery
- What items to bring
- What items to keep at home
- Shower
- What's going to happen during the procedure
- What the patient should expect after the procedure
- Pain the patient may experience and how it should be handled
- Must have responsible adult escort to take patient home

If drains or tubes will be used, it is best if patients understand how fluids should be measured and disposed and how the drains should be reconnected. The patient should understand what to look for in terms of infection. The patient should understand what pain to expect and how to appropriately manage it. Diet expectations and management should be discussed. Finally, a patient should be told what activities are appropriate and when they can return to their normal activities.

Most patients will benefit from a repeat presentation of their postoperative care needs after surgery as well, optimally in the presence of the individual who will be assisting them after discharge. Brochures can be provided for both specific and general information regarding the surgery and anesthesia. The American Society of Anesthesiologists (ASA) has a number of helpful patient education brochures publicly available on its Web site, http://www.ASAhq.org/patientEducation.htm. See Box 6-1 for a list of preoperative instructions.

Use of current medications

Chronic medications

Most drugs taken to control chronic medical conditions should be taken on the morning of the procedure as usual with a sip of water (Table 6-1). Clonidine and beta-blockers, in particular, should be continued to provide stable perioperative hemodynamics. Some inpatient data suggest that the last dose of angiotensin-converting enzyme and angiotensin II antagonists should be withheld the day of surgery, since perioperative hypotension might be more refractory to vasoconstrictor therapy in patients who continue treatment.[1] Other data reported that the incidence of moderate hypotension was no greater in patients who continued treatment.[2]

Discontinuation of antiplatelet therapy in ambulatory surgery patients depends on the nature of the surgery and proposed anesthesia. Although in the

Table 6-1. Patient medications: which to continue or discontinue on the day of surgery

Continue	Discontinue or withhold
• Antihypertensive agents • Adrenergic beta-antagonists • Calcium channel blockers • Vasodilator agents • Bronchodilator agents • Anticonvulsants • Antidepressive agents, tricyclic • Monoamine oxidase inhibitors (controversial) • Adrenal cortex hormones • Thyroid hormones • Antianxiety agents • Statins (though usually taken in the evening)	• Angiotensin-converting enzyme inhibitors (may take day prior to surgery) • Diuretics • Insulin • Digitalis • Warfarin (if necessary, switch to heparin) • Ticlopidine or clopidogrel: controversial • Aspirin: controversial • Broad-spectrum nonsteroidal anti-inflammatory drugs: controversial • Long- and short-acting sulfonylureas

past many have advocated that aspirin be discontinued before surgery due to bleeding concerns, there is evidence to show, at least in patients undergoing coronary artery bypass graft (CABG), that mortality is decreased if aspirin is continued. Whether high-dose or low-dose aspirin use is important and whether there's a difference in outcome in patients undergoing other types of surgery such as ambulatory surgery require further study. Anesthesiologists and surgeons in each facility should come to an agreement concerning aspirin use prior to surgery.

If patients are taking oral anticoagulants, including antiplatelet agents (e.g., ticlopidine or clopidogrel), or warfarin, the risk of procedure-related bleeding needs to be balanced against the risk of thromboembolism if the drugs are discontinued. For procedures with a low risk of bleeding, the drugs probably do not need to be stopped. For higher risk surgery, the evidence whether to stop oral antiplatelet agents is not decisive but favors stopping.

Small-scale observational studies in nonrandomized series of patients have indicated that preoperative use of combined clopidogrel and aspirin in CABG patients increases the risk of postoperative bleeding. The impact on transfusion requirements and surgical re-exploration rates in the perioperative and immediate postoperative (less than or equal to 48 hours) period is less clear.[3] Warfarin should be stopped 5 days before a procedure, and (if necessary) a heparin infusion should be started. However, this may necessitate hospitalization.

Outpatient perioperative management with low molecular weight heparin, enoxaparin, as bridge therapy for patients on long-term oral anticoagu-lation is a safe and cost-effective alternative. In the case of ticlopidine, clopidogrel, or warfarin, the anesthesiologists, surgeons, and physicians managing the patient's anticoagulation (cardiologists or primary care physicians) should agree about when and if the drugs should be stopped in advance of the surgery.

Instruction concerning discontinuation of oral hypoglycemics varies according to the type of drug. Long-acting sulfonylureas (e.g., chlorpropamide) should be stopped 48 to 72 hours before surgery; short-acting sulfonylureas, other insulin secretagogues, and metformin should be stopped the night before or the day of surgery. Drugs that are extremely long-acting (e.g., thiazolidinediones such as rosiglitazone) can probably be continued through the time of surgery. There are several protocols for managing insulin therapy on the day of surgery.

One recommendation is that patients taking subcutaneous insulin take 2/3 of their bedtime dose of neutral protamine Hagedorn (NPH), Lente, Ultralente, or glargine and then 1/2 of their usual morning dose of insulin.[4] Another recommends the usual night-before dose. Alternatively, patients can hold their morning dose of insulin, their serum glucose can be measured when they arrive in the surgery area, and an appropriate dose of insulin can then be administered; this is widely used in the ambulatory surgery environment to minimize the risk of hypoglycemic symptoms before arrival at the facility. If patients are on an insulin pump, the overnight basal infusion should be reduced by 30% and no bolus from bedtime to the morning of surgery should be given for blood sugar values of less than 200 mg/dL. On the morning of surgery, the insulin delivered through the pump can be switched to the intravenous (IV) line or a subcutaneous injection of glargine insulin can be administered (Figure 6-1).[4,5]

Newer versions of monoamine oxidase (MAO) inhibitors have been found useful in the treatment of neurodegenerative conditions, including Parkinson

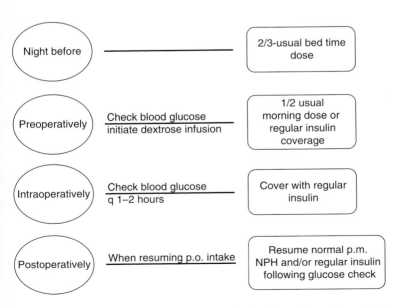

Figure 6-1. Algorithm for managing insulin during the perioperative period.

disease and Alzheimer disease.[6] These isoenzymes of MAO inhibitors (MAOA and MAOB) are generally not associated with cardiovascular effects, and patients who take these drugs do not need to discontinue use prior to surgery. MAO inhibitors are also still used to treat depression, particularly treatment-resistant depression.[7] There are case reports in which MAO inhibitors have been associated with reactions with drugs used during anesthesia. For that reason, many advise that these drugs be discontinued 2 weeks before surgery. Nonetheless, if alternative therapy is not considered or if the drug is not restarted after surgery, patient depression can be exacerbated.

Herbal medicines

More patients are using herbal, vitamin, and over-the counter preparations as alternatives or to supplement a variety of clinical conditions. Several surveys have identified the frequency of herbal medication use to be 22%–32%, common in women 40–60 years of age, and over 70% did not report this information during routine preoperative assessment.[8,9] Because herbal preparations are classified as dietary supplements, they are exempt from safety, efficacy, and regulatory requirements. Different batches of brands of the same herbal compound often contain different amounts of the active ingredient.

The *Physicians' Desk Reference for Herbal Medicines* does provide a comprehensive list, but there are very few peer-reviewed studies evaluating herbals and supplements in the perioperative period. Only a few have been documented to cause problems either through inherent toxicity or through pharmacokinetic and phamacodynamic interactions.[10] The side effects of concern for ambulatory anesthesiologists are primarily cardiovascular problems, bleeding, and prolongation of anesthetic action. The herbals most commonly cited are echinacea, ephedra (ma huang), garlic, ginkgo, ginseng, kava, and St. John's wort. Perioperative concerns and recommendations for discontinuation are noted in Table 6-2.

Fasting guidelines

The ASA approved fasting guidelines in 1999.[11] These general rules allow clear fluids up to 2 hours, light (low-fat) meals up to 6 hours, and heavy (high-fat) meals up to 8 hours before the initiation of anesthesia for adults and children. Coffee is not transparent but is free of particulate matter and is accepted as a clear liquid. Coffee drinkers should follow fasting guidelines but should be encouraged to drink coffee prior to their procedure, since physical signs of withdrawal (e.g., headache) can easily occur.[12] Some surgeons are not aware of these guidelines, so some patients are still being told to fast for longer periods of time; anesthesiologists should work to update these practices. Also, there is evidence that shorter periods of preoperative fasting are accompanied by less

Table 6-2. Clinically important effects, perioperative concerns, and recommendations for perioperative discontinuation of nine commonly used herbal medicines

Herbs (common names)	Important pharmacologic effects	Perioperative concerns	Preoperative discontinuation
Echinacea	Activation of cell-mediated immunity	Allergic reactions	No data
(Purple coneflower root)		Decreased effectiveness of immunosuppressants	
		Potential for immunosuppression with long-term use	
Ephedra (ma huang)	Increased heart rate and blood pressure through direct and indirect sympathomimetic effects	Risk of myocardial ischemia and stroke from tachycardia and hypertension	At least 24 hours before surgery
		Ventricular arrhythmias with halothane	
		Long-term use depletes endogenous catecholamines and may cause intraoperative hemodynamic instability	
		Life-threatening interaction with MAO inhibitors	
Garlic (ajo)	Inhibition of platelet aggregation (may be irreversible)	May increase risk of bleeding, especially when combined with other medications that inhibit platelet aggregation	At least 7 days before surgery
	Increased fibrinolysis		
	Equivocal antihypertensive activity		

(Continued)

Table 6-2. *Continued*

Herbs (common names)	Important pharmacologic effects	Perioperative concerns	Preoperative discontinuation
Ginkgo (duck-foot tree, maidenhair tree, silver apricot)	Inhibition of platelet-activating factor	May increase risk of bleeding, especially when combined with other medications that inhibit platelet aggregation	At least 36 hours before surgery
Ginseng (American ginseng, Asian ginseng, Chinese ginseng, Korean ginseng)	Lowers blood glucose	Hypoglycemia	At least 7 days before surgery
	Inhibition of platelet aggregation (may be irreversible)	May increase risk of bleeding	
	Increased PT/PTT in animals	May decrease anticoagulant effect of warfarin	
	Many other diverse effects		
Kava (awa, intoxicating pepper, kawa)	Sedation	May increase sedative effect of anesthetics	At least 24 hours before surgery
	Anxiolysis	Ability to increase anesthetic requirements with long-term use unstudied	
Saw palmetto (dwarf palm, sabal)	Inhibition of 5-α reductase	May increase risk of bleeding	No data
	Inhibition of cyclooxygenase		

			At least 5 days before surgery
St. John's wort (amber, goat weed, hardhay, hypericum, Klamath weed)	Inhibition of neurotransmitter reuptake	Induction of cytochrome P450 enzymes, affecting cyclosporin, warfarin, steroids, and protease inhibitors and possibly affecting benzodiazepines, calcium channel blockers, and many other drugs	
	MAO inhibition is unlikely	Decreased serum digoxin levels	
		Delayed emergence	
		May increase sedative effect of anesthetics	
Valerian (all heal, garden heliotrope, vandal root)	Sedation	Benzodiazepine-like acute withdrawal	No data
		May increase anesthetic requirements with long-term use	

MAO, monoamine oxidase; PT, prothrombin time; PTT, partial thromboplastin time.
Source: Ang-Lee M et al.[32] © Elsevier. Used with permission.

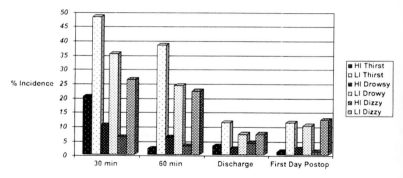

Figure 6-2. Patients had less postoperative thirst (Thirst), were less drowsy (Drowsy), and were less dizzy (Dizzy) if they received 20 mL/kg (HI) versus 2 mL/kg (LI) fluid 30 minutes preoperatively. Measurements were made at 30 minutes (30 M), 60 minutes (60 M), at discharge (DIS), and 24 hours postoperatively (DAY 1). *$p < 0.05$. Source: Yogendran et al.[33] Used with permission.

postoperative nausea and vomiting (PONV), pain, dizziness, drowsiness, and thirst (Figure 6-2). Intraoperative hydration should be used to complete maintenance fluid requirements; however, it is unknown whether rehydration during surgery is equivalent to a shorter fast before surgery in relation to PONV. Table 6-3 provides a summary of fasting guidelines.

Preoperative medications in adults

Broadly speaking, premedication may be used to control anxiety, postoperative pain, nausea, and vomiting to reduce the risk of aspiration during induction of anesthesia and to control infection. Premedication may also help to decrease histamine activity and reduce oral and airway secretions. However, these goals may not all be appropriate for the ambulatory patient. Furthermore, because the outpatient is going home shortly after surgery, the drugs given before anesthesia should not hinder recovery afterward. Most premedicants do not prolong recovery when given in appropriate doses for appropriate indications, although drug effects may be apparent even after discharge. Box 6-2 lists goals for premedication.

Table 6-3. Fasting guidelines before elective operations

Clear liquids (*includes water, apple juice, fruit juices without pulp, black coffee, clear tea, carbonated beverages, flavored gelatin, and clear broth*)	2 hours
Light (low-fat) meals	6 hours
Heavy (high-fat) meals	8 hours

Box 6-2. Possible goals for premedication
- Decrease anxiety
- Control postoperative pain
- Reduce postoperative nausea and vomiting
- Reduce risk of gastric aspiration
- Control infection
- Decrease histamine activity
- Reduce oral and airway secretions

Controlling anxiety

Patients scheduled to undergo surgery can be anxious, and they probably are anxious long before they come to the outpatient area. Anxiety may take different forms. Surprisingly, insomnia is not one. In a study of sleep characteristics of outpatients before elective surgery, no differences in sleep quality between patients before surgery and a community control group was observed.[13] Furthermore, not all ambulatory patients are anxious, and physicians tend to overestimate anxiety that patients are actually experiencing.[14] Anxiety may be procedure-related as well. The most appropriate way to assess patient anxiety is to ask. Visual analog scales are also very easy to use and are an accurate tool to assess and quantify anxiety.[15]

Although historically many classes of drugs (including barbiturates and antihistamines) have been used to reduce anxiety and to induce sedation, benzodiazepines are at present the drugs most commonly used. Midazolam is the drug in this class most commonly used preoperatively, and it can be given intravenously or orally. In adults, it can be used to control preoperative anxiety and also for IV sedation. Even though anxiolytic effects are short-acting, associated fatigue appears to be of longer duration, particularly when midazolam is combined with fentanyl. Adult patients can remain sleepy for up to 8 hours, and this is one reason why patients need an escort even though they may feel well enough to be discharged (Figure 6-3).[16]

Oral diazepam is useful to control anxiety for adult patients, either the day before surgery or the day of surgery before an IV line has been inserted. Indeed, in one study, investigators felt that after 5 mg oral diazepam, it was easier to insert an IV.[17] At proper doses, midazolam places patients at no additional risk for cardiovascular and respiratory depression than does diazepam. Decreased oxygen saturation has also been reported after injection of midazolam, and monitoring of arterial oxygenation as well as administration of supplemental oxygen should be considered and available (if needed) when benzodiazepines are given intravenously. This precaution is important not only when midazolam is given as a premedicant, but also when it is used alone or with other drugs for moderate sedation.

The potential for amnesia after premedication is a benefit and concern. Benzodiazepines can help decrease recall during surgery. They may also play a role in potentiating amnesia where intraoperative use of nitrous oxide is restricted, as may be seen in ambulatory laparoscopic surgeries. Alhough recall during

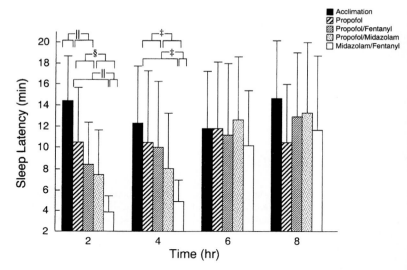

Figure 6-3. Patients can remain sleepy after receiving midazolam and fentanyl even 8 hours after drug administration. The abscissa represents time (in hours) after sedation. The ordinate represents sleep latency (i.e., time to fall asleep). Data are the mean time to fall asleep. An individual is sleepier if less time is required to fall asleep. Subjects receiving the midazolam and fentanyl combination were much sleepier than the same subjects receiving the other types of sedation. Although not seen in the figure, up to 8 hours after sedation, some subjects were still sleepier than before they received drug. Source: Lichtor et al.[16] Used with permission. Sleep latency was longer in the propofol and propofol with fentanyl groups combined than in the midazolam with propofol or midazolam with fentanyl groups combined at 2 h ($\S P < 0.0025$) and at 4 h ($\ddagger P < 0.025$) after injection. The two propofol groups also had shorter sleep latency 2 h after injection compared with the same time during the acclimation session ($\| P = 0.001$). Sleep latency was shorter in the midazolam with fentanyl treatment group compared with the other three treatment groups at 2 h ($\| P = 0.001$) and at 4 h ($\ddagger P < 0.025$).

surgery is a function of many factors, anterograde amnesia increases as benzodiazepine dose increases.[18] But amnesia may be present after a procedure and instructions given postoperatively may be quickly forgotten.

If comfort and support are not sufficient to relieve anxiety, drugs can be used (Table 6-4). For the patient who has been seen at least 24 hours before a scheduled procedure and who expresses a desire for medication to relieve anxiety, oral diazepam (2–5 mg/70 kg body weight) is prescribed for the night before and at 6:00 a.m. on the day of surgery (independent of time of surgery). For patients seen for the first time in the preoperative holding area who seem to need medication, midazolam (0.03 mg/kg) or a small dose of propofol or thiopental (e.g., 10 mg or 25 mg, respectively) is administered intravenously for the average adult.

Table 6-4. Treatment of anxiety

If patient seen >24 hours before procedure:	Oral diazepam 2–5 mg/70 kg night before and at 6 a.m. (even if procedure in afternoon) on day of surgery.
If patient seen for first time on day of surgery:	In preoperative holding area: midazolam 0.03 mg/kg intravenous; or in the operating room before anesthesia induction: propofol 0.7 mg/kg.

When the patient is brought into the operating room (OR), propofol (0.7 mg/kg) can be injected intravenously. Rarely does an average adult need more than 2 mg of midazolam. Elderly patients need even less, often only 0.5 mg. For the challenging mentally handicapped adult, premedication often is necessary to manage them in the holding area and transport them to the OR. Under these circumstances, ketamine (2–4 mg/kg intramuscularly) may also be used in combination with midazolam, administered intramuscularly (0.07–0.1 mg/kg) or orally (0.5–0.75 mg/kg not to exceed 20 mg *per os*) in adult mentally handicapped patients who may not cooperate for IV insertion.

Control of perioperative pain

Preoperative administration of opioids or nonsteroidal anti-inflammatory drugs is also useful for controlling pain in the early postoperative period. Controlled-release oxycodone 10 mg, for example, when given before surgery, was very effective in managing pain after laparoscopic tubal ligation surgery and was even associated with less PONV.[19] Celecoxib, up to 400 mg, is effective in reducing postoperative pain (Table 6-5).[20] Nonsteroidal analgesics may be associated with less nausea compared to narcotics.[21]

Opioids and nonsteroidal anti-inflammatory drugs can also be administered intra-operatively and postoperatively. In a study of patients undergoing adenoidectomy, even a small IV dose of ketoprofen (0.3 mg/kg) given after induction was effective in reducing postoperative pain, although higher doses, up to 3 mg/kg, were more effective in reducing pain and were not associated with an increase in adverse events or intra-operative bleeding.[22] When given postoperatively, these drugs are also effective in reducing pain, although less so than when given preoperatively.[23]

Opioids can also be useful in controlling hypertension during tracheal intubation. Opioid premedication prevents increases in systolic pressure in a dose-dependent fashion. After tracheal intubation, however, systolic, diastolic, and mean arterial blood pressures sometimes decrease below baseline values. The additional consideration that should limit the use of opioids in the ambulatory setting is the increased risk of PONV.

Opioids have other potential uses. Meperidine (but not morphine or fentanyl) is sometimes helpful in controlling shivering in the OR or postanesthesia care

Table 6-5. The efficacy of celecoxib premedication on postoperative pain and recovery times

	Placebo	Celecoxib (200 mg)	Celecoxib (400 mg)
Recovery time (min) from end of surgery to			
Eyes opening (min)	8 ± 5	8 ± 5	6 ± 4
Obeys commands (min)	11 ± 6	13 ± 7	8 ± 4
Orientation (min)	14 ± 8	15 ± 9	12 ± 5
Recovery unit stay			
PACU (min)	69 ± 24	62 ± 27	62 ± 26
DSU (min)	85 ± 39	90 ± 60	81 ± 68
Time to first analgesic (min)	40 ± 39	41 ± 20	34 ± 36
Peak pain scores in PACU (0–10) (n)	5 (2–8)	5 (0–10)	4 (2–6)*
Patients with severe predischarge pain [n (%)]	9 (30)	11 (37)	2 (6)*†
Maximum nausea score (0–10) (n)	2 ± 2	2 ± 2	2 ± 2
Fentanyl in PACU (μg)	120 ± 86	74 ± 67*	56 ± 62*†
Satisfied discharge criteria (min)	141 ± 50	128 ± 26	119 ± 48

Values are mean $\pm$ SD, medians (interquartile range), and percentages (%).

PACU = postanesthesia care unit; DSU = day-surgery unit.

* $P < 0.05$, versus placebo group;

† $P < 0.05$, versus celecoxib 200 mg group.

Patients received either placebo or celecoxib (200 or 400 mg) 30-45 minutes before surgery. Patients who received celecoxib needed less fentanyl postoperatively. After celecoxib 400 mg, severe predischarge pain was less than for patients in the other two groups. Time to first analgesic and nausea was not different between groups. Source: Recart et al.[20] Used with permission.

unit, although treatment is usually instituted at the time of shivering and not in anticipation of the event. Opioids have been used for preoperative sedation. However, the effectiveness of opioids in relieving anxiety is controversial and probably nonexistent, particularly in adults.

Controlling the risk of aspiration

Patients who undergo ambulatory surgery may be at some small risk for aspiration of gastric contents, although this risk is no greater for outpatients than for inpatients. It is important to state that the routine use of medications to "prevent" aspiration is not recommended. All patients should be questioned for a history of positional reflux. Subsets of patients who may be at greater risk for positional reflux and aspiration are pregnant or morbidly obese patients or patients with hiatal hernia.

6. Adult preoperative preparation: equipment and monitoring   157

Preoperative anxiety probably has no effect on gastric acidity for individuals without a history of duodenal ulcer. H_2 receptor antagonists such as cimetidine and ranitidine, omeprazole, sodium citrate, or metoclopramide can be used to reduce acid or gastric volume and thereby control the risk of aspiration. In the case of lansoprazole and omeprazole, two successive doses of the drug, given the night before and day of surgery, are more effective than single doses of either drug the day of surgery in reducing gastric acid secretion.[24] Patients chronically taking large doses of H_2 receptor antagonists may have developed tolerance, and proton pump inhibitors should be given to reduce gastric volume and acidity.[25]

Miscellaneous premedicants

Anticholinergics (e.g., glycopyrrolate, atropine, and scopolamine) are sometimes used to dry oral and airway secretions, especially for upper endoscopy procedures, and when difficult intubation is anticipated. When drying of oral secretions is desired, glycopyrrolate, a quarternary amine compound, is a better choice because it causes less tachycardia than atropine, does not cross the blood-brain barrier, and has no central nervous system effect (Table 6-6).

Nausea and vomiting is still a problem following ambulatory surgery and is addressed in detail in Chapter 12. Nevertheless, high-risk patients should be given prophylactic antiemetics, which are usually given after induction of anesthesia. Histamine receptor blocking agents should be considered as premedication in patients with a history of multiple allergies. H_1 blockers (diphenhydramine 25–50 mg orally or intravenously; hydroxyzine 1.0–1.5 mg/kg intravenously or intramuscularly) and H_2 blocking agents are among those agents used.

Corticosteroids

The administration of small doses of steroids for a short period of time can suppress the hypothalamic pituitary axis for up to 12 months. It is clear that a patient who requires exogenous corticosteroids for health maintenance may not be able to respond to major stressors, like surgery, and thus replacement steroid

Table 6-6. Anticholinergic premedications

Glycopyrrolate	0.2 mg intravenously or intramuscularly; does not cross blood-brain barrier; causes less tachycardia than atropine
Atropine	0.4 mg intravenously or intramuscularly; causes tachycardia; crosses blood-brain barrier; possible central cholinergic syndrome
Scopolamine	0.4 mg intravenously or intramuscularly; has prolonged sedative and amnestic effect; postoperative agitation in older patients; use should be limited to transdermal patch for antiemetic properties

therapy may be necessary to prevent intravascular collapse secondary to adrenal insufficiency.

It appears that patients undergoing minor surgery do not need additional steroid coverage. Chapter 3 discusses the relative potencies of exogenously administered corticosteroids. Regardless, perioperative IV hydrocortisone 100 mg or solucortef 125 mg should be available in the OR and recovery area.

Prophylactic antibiotics

Surgical wounds may be said to be clean, potentially contaminated (e.g., as in procedures entering a bronchus, the gastrointestinal tract, or the oropharyngeal tract), contaminated, or dirty. "Clean" wounds generally involve little contamination by bacteria; in these cases, the most common sources of infection are the patient's skin, the OR environment, and the surgical team and occur where surgery involves the integument or musculoskeletal soft tissues.

"Potentially contaminated" procedures are elective cases involving a hollow viscus. Surgical site infections are higher with higher ASA physical status.[26] Laparoscopic surgery is associated with lower infection rates than open procedures. Although more operations are performed on an outpatient basis, surveillance of surgical site infections for outpatients is not as complete as it is with hospitalized patients and warrants more attention.

Patients undergoing potentially contaminated or contaminated procedures should receive antibiotics. Antibiotics may also be useful in decreasing the incidence of wound infections during certain types of procedures: trauma or burn surgery; surgery in areas having infection, heavy contamination, poor blood supply, or considerable tissue destruction; or lengthy operations.

Antibiotics are also used when active infection exists remote from the operative site. Other candidates for prophylactic administration of antibiotics are patients who are obese, diabetic, old, or malnourished; those whose immune system is suppressed; and those taking steroids. If bone is incised or prosthesis is inserted, antibiotics are also indicated. However, the broad administration of antibiotics must not be taken lightly, as some individuals can become hypersensitive, and use of antibiotics can increase the resistance of indigenous hospital flora to these drugs. Each organization should have a committee (e.g., a policy and therapeutics committee) that is responsible for developing antibiotic policy for that organization.

Prophylactic administration of antibiotics is most effective when the agent is given within 1 hour before the time of incision. The cephalosporins are particularly suited as prophylactic antibiotics because they are effective for a wide range of bacteria. No one cephalosporin, however, has been shown to be more effective than another, and therefore the least expensive option may suffice.

The American Heart Association substantially revised the infective endocarditis (IE) guidelines in 2007 based more on levels of evidence and limiting treatment to those high risk cardiac conditions likely to result in adverse outcome from IE (Table 6-7).[27] These guidelines identify primarily more invasive dental procedures that warrant prophylaxis but emphasize that the risk of IE might be

Table 6-7. Cardiac conditions and endocarditis prophylaxis

Endocarditis prophylaxis recommended

High-risk category

 Prosthetic cardiac valves, including bioprosthetic and homograft valves

 Previous infective endocarditis

 Certain specific congenital heart disease (CHD):

  Unrepaired or incompletely repaired cyanotic CHD, including palliative shunts and conduits

  Completely repaired congenital heart defect with prosthetic material or device, whether placed by surgery or by catheter intervention, during the first 6 months after the procedure†

  Repaired CHD with residual defects at the site or adjacent to the site of a prosthetic patch or prosthetic device (which inhibits endothelialization)

 Cardiac transplantation recipients who develop cardiac valvulopathy

Endocarditis prophylaxis not recommended

Most other congenital cardiac malformations such as ventricular septal defect and atrial septal defect

Acquired valvular dysfunction (e.g., rheumatic heart disease)

Hypertrophic cardiomyopathy

Mitral valve prolapse with or without valvular regurgitation and/or thickened leaflets

Calcified aortic stenosis

Bicuspid valve disease

Physiologic, functional, or innocent heart murmurs

Previous Kawasaki disease without valvular dysfunction

Previous rheumatic fever without valvular dysfunction

Cardiac pacemakers (intravascular and epicardial) and implanted defibrillators

Previous coronary artery bypass graft surgery

even greater from random bacteremia caused by routine daily activities and/or poor oral health. The majority of procedures in previous guidelines have little scientific proof to support routine prophylaxis (Table 6-8). Summary of major changes and current recommendations are noted in Tables 6-9 and 6-10.

Table 6-8. Procedures and endocarditis prophylaxis

**Endocarditis prophylaxis recommended for procedures in high
risk patients**
Dental
  Procedures that involve manipulation of gingival tissue or the periapical
    region of teeth or perforation of the oral mucosa
Respiratory tract
  Tonsillectomy and/or adenoidectomy
  Invasive surgical operations that involve incision and biopsy of respiratory
    mucosa
  Incision and drainage of established infection, abscess, or empyema
Gastrointestinal tract—procedures on infected tissue only
Genitourinary tract—procedures on infected tissue only
Other
  Infected skin, skin structures, or musculoskeletal tissue

Endocarditis prophylaxis not recommended in the following procedures
Dental
  Routine anesthetic injections through noninfected tissue
  Taking dental radiographs
  Placement of removable prosthodontic or orthodontic appliances
  Adjustment of orthodontic appliances
  Placement of orthodontic brackets
  Shedding of deciduous teeth
  Bleeding from trauma to the lips or oral mucosa
Respiratory tract
  Endotracheal intubation
  Bronchoscopy with a rigid or flexible bronchoscope, without incision or
    biopsy
  Tympanostomy tube insertion
Gastrointestinal tract
  Sclerotherapy for esophageal varices
  Esophageal stricture dilation
  Endoscopic retrograde cholangiography with biliary obstruction
  Biliary tract surgery
  Surgical operations that involve intestinal mucosa
  Transesophageal echocardiography
  Endoscopy with or without gastrointestinal biopsy
Genitourinary tract
  Prostatic surgery
  Cystoscopy
  Urethral dilation
  Circumcision
  Vaginal hysterectomy
  Vaginal delivery
  Cesarean section
In uninfected tissue:
  Urethral catheterization
  Uterine dilatation and curettage
  Therapeutic abortion
  Sterilization procedures
  Insertion or other removal of intrauterine devices

(Continued)

Table 6-8. *Continued*

Other
Cardiac catheterization, including balloon angioplasty
Implanted cardiac pacemakers, implanted defibrillators, and coronary stents
Incision or biopsy of surgically scrubbed skin
Ear and Body Piercing
Tattooing

Dajani AS, Taubert KA, Wilson W, et al. Prevention of bacterial endocarditis. Recommendations by the American Heart Association. JAMA 1997;277:1794–1801. Used with permission.
Wilson W, Taubert KA, Gewitz M, et al. Prevention of infective endocarditis: Guidelines from the American Heart Association. A guideline from the American Heart Association Rheumatic Fever, Endocarditis and Kawasaki Disease Committee, Council on Cardiovascular Disease in the Young, and the Council on Clinical Cardiology, Council on Cardiovascular Surgery and Anesthesia, and the Quality of Care and Outcomes Research Interdisciplinary Working Group. JADA 2007;138(6):739–60. © 2007 American Dental Association. Excerpted by JADA with permission of Circulation. Circulation 2007 Apr 19;[Epub ahead of print]. © 2007 American Heart Association. Adapted 2008 with permission of The Journal of the American Dental Association.

Table 6-9. Summary of major changes in updated American Heart Association infective endocarditis (IE) guidelines

- Bacteremia resulting from daily activities is much more likely to cause infective endocarditis (IE) than bacteremia associated with a dental procedure.
- Only an extremely small number of cases of IE might be prevented by antibiotic prophylaxis even if prophylaxis is 100% effective.
- Antibiotic prophylaxis is not recommended based solely on an increased lifetime risk of acquisition of IE.
- Limit recommendations for IE prophylaxis only to those high risk cardiac conditions listed in Table 6-7.
- Antibiotic prophylaxis is no longer recommended for any other form of CHD, except for the high risk cardiac conditions listed in Table 6-7.
- Antibiotic prophylaxis is recommended for all dental procedures that involve manipulation of gingival tissues or periapical region of teeth or perforation of oral mucosa only for patients with underlying cardiac conditions associated with the highest risk of adverse outcome from IE (Table 6-8).
- Antibiotic prophylaxis is recommended for procedures on incision or biopsy of respiratory tract mucosa or for procedures on infected skin, skin structures, or musculoskeletal tissue only for high risk patients (Table 6.8).
- Antibiotic prophylaxis solely to prevent IE is not recommended for GU or GI tract procedures (Table 6-8). High risk patients with established GI or GU infection at the time of procedure may be prophylaxed with an antienterococcal agent.

(Continued)

Table 6-9. *Continued*

- Guidelines reaffirm the procedures noted in the 1997 prophylaxis guidelines for which endocarditis prophylaxis is not recommended and extends this to other common procedures, including ear and body piercing, tattooing, and vaginal delivery and hysterectomy.

Table 6-10. Prophylactic regimens for dental procedures for high risk adult patients

Situation	Agent	Regimen: Single dose 30 to 60 minutes before dental procedure
Oral	Amoxicillin	2 g
Unable to take oral	Ampicillin OR	2 g IM or IV
	Cefazolin or ceftriaxone	1 g IM or IV
Penicillin or ampicillin allergic–oral route	Cephalexin*[#] OR	2 g
	Clindamycin OR	600 mg
	Azithromycin or clarithromycin	500 mg
Penicillin or ampicillin allergic and unable to take oral medication	Cefazolin or ceftriaxone[#] OR	1 g IM or IV
	Clindamycin	600 mg IM or IV

*Or other first- or second-generation oral cephalosporin in equivalent adult dosage.
[#]Cephalosporins should not be used in an individual with a history of anaphylaxis, angioedema, or urticaria with penicillins or ampicillin.

Preanesthetic evaluation on the day of surgery

For some ambulatory surgery patients, their medical history is obtained and physical exam is performed prior to the day of the procedure at a clinic visit. However, although the preoperative clinic evaluation may be performed by either an anesthesiologist or another physician such as an internist, the immediate preanesthetic evaluation is the responsibility of the anesthesiologist who will care for the patient during surgery.

Even if these activities were performed prior to the day of surgery, the findings should be reviewed on the day of surgery and a physical exam that at a minimum should include examination of the airway, heart, and lungs should be performed. Patient education may have been provided the day before surgery, but information related to informed consent should be provided again and consent should be obtained or confirmed. If preoperative laboratory tests are indicated, in the majority of instances, they should have been performed prior to the day of the procedure. Routine preoperative screening tests are not recommended. The ASA developed a practice advisory on preanesthetic evaluation in 2002, as detailed in Chapter 1.[28]

Equipment and monitoring

Despite the fact that the specialty of anesthesia is considered to be a model for patient safety and anesthesia today is considered to be safer than 20 years ago, anesthesia intrinsically is a hazardous undertaking.[29] The potential for complications exists even in the ambulatory surgery setting. Appropriate monitoring may possibly reduce the hazard. The ASA has adopted standards for basic anesthetic monitoring. These standards were last amended in 2005 and which apply in all settings where anesthesia is administered (http://www.asahq.org/publicationsAndServices/standards/02.pdf). A summary of these basic anesthesia monitors is provided in Table 6-11.

Anesthesia monitoring for the ambulatory patient should be no different from the inpatient. One or more individual qualified anesthesia personnel must be in the room at all times that general or regional anesthesia or sedation is undertaken. During that time, patient oxygenation, ventilation, circulation, and temperature must be monitored. Adequate oxygen concen-tration must be measured in the inspired gas mixture and in the patient's blood.

Carbon dioxide concentration must be measured in expired air when an endotracheal tube or laryngeal mask airway (LMA) is used, and monitoring for the presence of exhaled CO_2 is recommended during regional anesthesia and monitored anesthesia care. Circulation must be assessed with blood pressure and heart rate monitoring, electrocardiogram, and a circulatory function monitor such as pulse oximetry. Body temperature should be measured when clinically significant temperature changes may occur.

Table 6-11. Basic anesthesia monitors

- Qualified anesthesia provider in operating room at all times a patient is present
- Inspired gas concentration
- Pulse oximeter
- Qualitative observation of ventilation
- Carbon dioxide particularly if patient's trachea is intubated or if a laryngeal mask airway is used
- Ventilator disconnect monitor if ventilator is used
- Electrocardiogram
- Arterial blood pressure and heart rate at least every 5 minutes
- If general anesthesia, palpation of pulse, auscultation of heart sounds, continuous arterial blood pressure monitoring, ultrasound monitoring of pulse, pulse plethysmography, or pulse oximetry
- Body temperature if temperature change is intended, anticipated, or suspected

Airway devices

Certain airway devices are used more commonly in the ambulatory area. The LMA, or a similar type of airway, provides several advantages that can help patients return to baseline status quickly. Muscle relaxants required for intubation can be avoided. Coughing is less than with tracheal intubation. Anesthetic requirements are reduced. Hoarseness and sore throat are also reduced. Overall, cost savings may result with the use of LMAs.[30] The use of the LMA has been described for laparoscopic procedures, although some are concerned about the potential for aspiration. A list of standard airway devices that should be made available for an ambulatory procedure is presented in Table 6-12.

Table 6-12. Standard airway devices

- Suction catheters
- Oral (#3–5) and nasal (#28–34) airways
- Lidocaine lubricant
- Face masks of varying sizes
- Laryngeal mask airways of varying sizes
- Laryngoscope blades of varying sizes (type user-dependent)
- Endotracheal tubes (6.5–9.0)
- Latex-free and (if desired) latex gloves

Table 6-13. Techniques for difficult airway management

Techniques for Difficult Intubation	Techniques for Difficult Ventilation
Alternative laryngoscope blades	Esophageal tracheal Combitube
Awake intubation	Intratracheal jet stylet
Blind intubation (oral or nasal)	Laryngeal mask airway
Fiberoptic intubation	Oral and nasopharyngeal airways
Intubating stylet or tube changer	Rigid ventilating bronchoscope
Laryngeal mask airway as an	Invasive airway access
intubating conduit	Transtracheal jet ventilation
Light wand	Two-person mask ventilation
Retrograde intubation	
Invasive airway access	

This table displays commonly cited techniques. It is not a comprehensive list. The order of presentation is alphabetical and does not imply preference for a given technique or sequence of use. Combinations of techniques may be employed. The techniques chosen by the practitioner in a particular case will depend upon specific needs, preferences, skills, and clinical constraints.
Source: American Society of Anesthesiologists Task Force on Management of the Difficult Airway.[31] Copyright © 2003, Lippincott Williams and Wilkins, Inc. Used with permission.

In the case of a difficult airway, different airway devices have been used, and every ambulatory surgery facility should have equipment to manage difficult airways consistent with the ASA difficult airway algorithm (Table 6-13 and Figure 6-4). Those airway devices may include the Bullard laryngoscope, other types of laryngoscope blades, video laryngoscope, Combitube, bougie, exchangers, cuffed oropharyngeal airway, LMA as an intubating conduit, light wand, a fiber-optic bronchoscope, intratracheal jet stylet, or invasive surgical airway access. In addition, tracheal intubation can be attempted when a patient is awake. The most recent ASA difficult airway algorithm was published in 2003.[31]

Summary

Since the ambulatory patient will go home the same day and since the effects of anesthesia may interfere with memory after surgery, postoperative instructions should be given before surgery. Safety requires that a reassessment of the patient's status be performed immediately before surgery. Preoperative medications should address anxiety and pain control, but the medications given should not prolong recovery.

Although ambulatory surgery may not be as complex as inpatient surgery, the risks of the anesthesia still exist. Monitoring must follow the same standards. LMAs are used more commonly in the ambulatory setting, but the need for difficult airway management should be anticipated and equipment should be readily available.

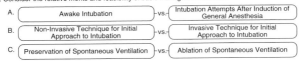

DIFFICULT AIRWAY ALGORITHM

1. Assess the likelihood and clinical impact of basic management problems:
   - A. Difficult Ventilation
   - B. Difficult Intubation
   - C. Difficulty with Patient Cooperation of Consent
   - D. Difficult Tracheostomy

2. Actively pursue opportunities to deliver supplemental oxygen throughout the process of difficult airway management

3. Consider the relative merits and feasibility of basic management choices:

A. Awake Intubation —vs.— Intubation Attempts After Induction of General Anesthesia

B. Non-Invasive Technique for Initial Approach to Intubation —vs.— Invasive Technique for Initial Approach to Intubation

C. Preservation of Spontaneous Ventilation —vs.— Ablation of Spontaneous Ventilation

4. Develop primary and alternative strategies:

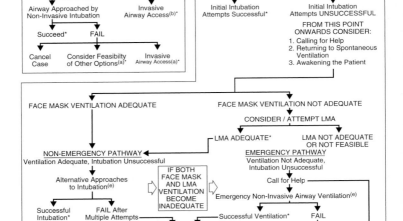

* **Confirm ventilation, tracheal intubation, or LMA placement with exhaled CO_2**

a. Other options include (but are not limited to): surgery utilizing face mask or LMA anesthesia, local anesthesia infiltration or regional nerve blockade. Pursuit of these options usually implies that mask ventilation will not be problematic. Therefore, these options may be of limited value if this step in the algorithm has been reached via the Emergency Pathway.

b. Invasive airway access includes surgical or percutaneous tracheostomy of cricothyrotomy.

c. Alternative non-invasive approaches to difficult intubation include (but are not limited to): use of different laryngoscope blades, LMA as an intubation conduit (with or without fiberoptic guidance), fiberoptic intubation, intubating stylet or tube changer, light wand, retrograde intubation, and blind oral or nasal intubation.

d. Consider re-preparation of the patient for awake intubation or canceling surgery.

e. Options for emergency non-invasive airway ventilation include (but are not limited to): rigid bronchoscope, esophageal-tracheal combitube ventilation, or transtracheal jet ventilation.

Figure 6-4. American Society of Anesthesiologists difficult airway algorithm. Source: American Society of Anesthesiologists Task Force on Management of the Difficult Airway.[31] Copyright © 2003, Lippincott Williams and Wilkins, Inc. Used with permission.

References

1. Bertrand M, Godet G, Meersschaert K, Brun L, Salcedo E, Coriat P. Should the angiotensin II antagonists be discontinued before surgery? *Anesth Analg.* 2001;92:26–30.
2. Comfere T, Sprung J, Kumar MM, et al. Angiotensin system inhibitors in a general surgical population. *Anesth Analg.* 2005;100:636–644.
3. Cannon CP, Mehta SR, Aranki SF. Balancing the benefit and risk of oral antiplatelet agents in coronary artery bypass surgery. *Ann Thorac Surg.* 2005;80:768–779.
4. Glister BC, Vigersky RA. Perioperative management of type 1 diabetes mellitus. *Endocrinol Metab Clin North Am.* 2003;32:411–436.
5. Marks JB. Perioperative management of diabetes. *Am Fam Physician.* 2003;67: 93–100.
6. Youdim MB, Edmondson D, Tipton KF. The therapeutic potential of monoamine oxidase inhibitors. *Nat Rev Neurosci.* 2006;7:295–309.
7. Amsterdam JD, Shults J. MAOI efficacy and safety in advanced stage treatment-resistant depression–a retrospective study. *J Affect Disord.* 2005;89:183–188.
8. Tsen LC, Sega S, Pothier M, et al. Alternative medicine use in presurgical patients. *Anesthesiology.* 2000;93:148–151. Erratum in: *Anesthesiology.* 2000;93:1371.
9. Crowe S, Fitzpatrick G, Jamaluddin MF. Use of herbal medications in ambulatory surgical patients. *Anaesthesia.* 2002;47:203–204.
10. Ang-Lee MK, Moss J, Yuan CS. Herbal medicine and perioperative care. *JAMA.* 2002;286:208–216.
11. [No authors listed]. Practice guidelines for preoperative fasting and the use of pharmacologic agents to reduce the risk of pulmonary aspiration: application to healthy patients undergoing elective procedures: a report by the American Society of Anesthesiologist Task Force on Preoperative Fasting. *Anesthesiology.* 1999;90:896–905.
12. Evans SM, Griffiths RR. Caffeine withdrawal: a parametric analysis of caffeine dosing conditions. *J Pharmacol Exp Ther.* 1999;289:285–294.
13. Kain ZN, Caldwell-Andrews AA. Sleeping characteristics of adults undergoing outpatient elective surgery: a cohort study. *J Clin Anesth.* 2003;15:505–509.
14. Shafer A, Fish MP, Gregg KM, Seavello J, Kosek P. Preoperative anxiety and fear: a comparison of assessments by patients and anesthesia and surgery residents. *Anesth Analg.* 1996;83:1285–1291.
15. Kindler CH, Harms C, Amsler F, Ihde-Scholl T, Scheidegger D. The visual analog scale allows effective measurement of preoperative anxiety and detection of patients' anesthetic concerns. *Anesth Analg.* 2000;90:706–712.
16. Lichtor JL, Alessi R, Lane BS. Sleep tendency as a measure of recovery after drugs used for ambulatory surgery. *Anesthesiology.* 2002;96:878–883.
17. Wittenberg MI, Lark TL, Butler CL, et al. Effects of oral diazepam on intravenous access in same day surgery patients. *J Clin Anesth.* 1998;10:13–16.
18. Bulach R, Myles PS, Russnak M. Double-blinded randomized controlled trial to determine extent of amnesia with midazolam given immediately before general anesthesia. *Br J Anaesth.* 2005;94:300–305.

19. Reuben SS, Steinberg RB, Maciolek H, Joshi W. Preoperative administration of controlled-release oxycodone for the management of pain after ambulatory laparoscopic tubal ligation surgery. *J Clin Anesth*. 2002;14:223–227.

20. Recart A, Issioui T, White PF, et al. The efficacy of celecoxib premedication on postoperative pain and recovery times after ambulatory surgery: a dose-ranging study. *Anesth Analg*. 2003;96;1631–1635.

21. Wennstrom B, Reinsfelt B. Rectally administered diclofenac (Voltaren) reduces vomiting compared with opioid (morphine) after strabismus surgery in children. *Acta Anaesthesiol Scand*. 2002;46:430–434.

22. Kokki H, Nikanne E, Tuovinen K. Intravenous intraoperative ketoprofen in small children during adenoidectomy: a dose-finding study. *Br J Anaesth*. 1998;81:870–874.

23. Bajaj P, Ballary CC, Dongre NA, Baliga VP, Desai AA. Role of parecoxib in preemptive analgesia: comparison of the efficacy and safety of pre- and postoperative parecoxib in patients undergoing general surgery. *J Indian Med Assoc*. 2004;102:272,274,276–278.

24. Nishina K, Mikawa K, Maekawa N, Takao Y, Shiga M, Obara H. A comparison of lansoprazole, omeprazole, and ranitidine for reducing preoperative gastric secretion in adult patients undergoing elective surgery. *Anesth Analg*. 1996;82:832–836.

25. Hirota K, Kushikata T. Preanaesthetic H2 antagonists for acid aspiration pneumonia prophylaxis. Is there evidence of tolerance? *Br J Anaesth*. 2003;90:576–579.

26. [No authors listed]. National Nosocomial Infections Surveillance (NNIS) System Report, Data Summary from January 1992–June 2001, issued August 2001. *Am J Infect Control*. 2001;29:404–421.

27. Wilson W, Taubert KA, Gewitz M, et al. Prevention of Infective Endocarditis: Guidelines from the American Heart Association. Circulation (online publication); April 19, 2007 found at http://circ.ahajournals.org/cgi/reprint/CIRCULATIONAHA.106.183095.

28. Practice advisory for preanesthesia evaluation: a report by the American Society of Anesthesiologists Task Force on Preanesthesia Evaluation. *Anesthesiology*. 2002;96:485–496.

29. Cooper JB, Gaba D. No myth: anesthesia is a model for addressing patient safety. *Anesthesiology*. 2002;97:1335–1337.

30. Macario A, Chang PC, Stempel DB, Brock-Utne JR. A cost analysis of the laryngeal mask airway for elective surgery in outpatients. *Anesthesiology*. 1995;83:250–257.

31. American Society of Anesthesiologists Task Force on Management of the Difficult Airway. Practice guidelines for management of the difficult airway: an updated report by the American Society of Anesthesiologists Task Force on Management of the Difficult Airway. *Anesthesiology*. 2003;98:1269–1277.

32. Ang-Lee M, Yuan C, Moss J. Complementary and alternative therapies. In: Miller RD, ed. *Miller's Anesthesia*. 6th ed. Philadelphia, PA: Elsevier; 2005:607.

33. Yogendran S, Asokumar B, Cheng DC, Chung F. A prospective randomized double-blinded study of the effect of intravenous fluid therapy on adverse outcomes on outpatient surgery. *Anesth Analg*. 1995;80:682–686.

7. Sedation techniques

Tong J. Gan, MB, BS, FRCA
Beverly K. Philip, MD

Minimally invasive surgery and interventional medical specialties are replacing conventional surgery, and increasingly these procedures can appropriately be done under sedation rather than general anesthesia (GA). In part, this is due to advances in minimally invasive surgical techniques that do not require full GA. In addition, patients choose sedation techniques, wanting to recover as quickly as possible and avoid the potential side effects of GA.

Older patients with concomitant diseases may be better served with sedation techniques that cause minimal interference with their homeostasis.[1] Anesthesia care has advanced as well, with the availability of newer shorter-acting drugs and better techniques to use them. Nonetheless, sedation techniques do have complications and hazards specifically their own. This chapter will explore the definitions of sedation and address some of the safety controversies associated with its administration. Perioperative management issues related to sedation will be discussed, as well as specific sedation drugs and techniques.

The goals for a sedation technique are to provide sedation, analgesia, and (as requested) amnesia. This requires a balance between patient comfort and patient safety, while preventing cardiovascular or respiratory compromise or delayed recovery. Sedation may also expedite procedures that require that the patient not move. Sedation facilitates acceptance of local anesthesia or regional anesthesia (RA) by blunting sensations such as pressure, movement, traction, and awareness of the environment. The primary analgesia, however, is based on the administration of local anesthesia or RA, by either surgeon or anesthesiologist.[1]

Definitions

The term "conscious sedation" has been used to describe intravenous (IV) supplementation of local anesthesia and RA with minimal depression of consciousness. This term has been replaced, and today we describe sedation as a continuum, from altered mood to loss of consciousness. The American Society of Anesthesiologists (ASA) has formally defined different levels of sedation and anesthesia in "Continuum of Depth of Sedation: Definition of General Anesthesia and Levels of Sedation/Analgesia" (http://www.asahq.org/publicationsAndServices/standards/20.pdf, 2004; see also Table 7-1).

Table 7-1. American Society of Anesthesiologists continuum of depth of sedation: definition of general anesthesia and levels of sedation/analgesia

	Minimal sedation (anxiolysis)	Moderate sedation/ analgesia ("conscious sedation")	Deep sedation/ analgesia	General anesthesia
Responsiveness	Normal response to verbal stimulation	Purposeful** response to verbal or tactile stimulation	Purposeful** response following repeated or painful stimulation	Unarousable even with painful stimulus
Airway	Unaffected	No intervention required	Intervention may be required	Intervention often required

(Continued)

Table 7-1. *Continued*

	Minimal sedation (anxiolysis)	Moderate sedation/ analgesia ("conscious sedation")	Deep sedation/ analgesia	General anesthesia
Spontaneous ventilation	Unaffected	Adequate	May be inadequate	Frequently inadequate
Cardiovascular function	Unaffected	Usually maintained	Usually maintained	May be impaired

Minimal sedation (anxiolysis) is a drug-induced state during which patients respond normally to verbal commands. Although cognitive function and coordination may be impaired, ventilatory and cardiovascular functions are unaffected.

Moderate sedation/analgesia ("conscious sedation") is a drug-induced depression of consciousness during which patients respond purposefully** to verbal commands, either alone or accompanied by light tactile stimulation. No interventions are required to maintain a patent airway, and spontaneous ventilation is adequate. Cardiovascular function is usually maintained.

Deep sedation/analgesia is a drug-induced depression of consciousness during which patients cannot be easily aroused but respond purposefully** following repeated or painful stimulation. The ability to independently maintain ventilatory function may be impaired. Patients may require assistance in maintaining a patent airway, and spontaneous ventilation may be inadequate. Cardiovascular function is usually maintained.

General anesthesia is a drug-induced loss of consciousness during which patients are not arousable, even by painful stimulation. The ability to independently maintain ventilatory function is often impaired. Patients often require assistance in maintaining a patent airway, and positive-pressure ventilation may be required because of depressed spontaneous ventilation or drug-induced depression of neuromuscular function. Cardiovascular function may be impaired.

Because sedation is a continuum, it is not always possible to predict how an individual patient will respond. Hence, practitioners intending to produce a given level of sedation should be able to rescue*** patients whose level of sedation becomes deeper than initially intended. Individuals administering moderate sedation/analgesia ("conscious sedation") should be able to rescue*** patients who enter a state of deep sedation/analgesia, whereas those administering deep sedation/analgesia should be able to rescue*** patients who enter a state of general anesthesia.

* Monitored anesthesia care does not describe the continuum of depth of sedation, rather it describes "a specific anesthesia service in which an anesthesiologist has been requested to participate in the care of a patient undergoing a diagnostic or therapeutic procedure."

** Reflex withdrawal from a painful stimulus is NOT considered a purposeful response.

*** Rescue of a patient from a deeper level of sedation than intended is an intervention by a practitioner proficient in airway management and advanced life support. The qualified practitioner corrects adverse physiologic consequences of the deeper-than-intended level of sedation (such as hypoventilation, hypoxia, and hypotension) and returns the patient to the originally intended level of sedation.

Source: http://www.asahq.org/publicationsAndServices/standards/20.pdf, 2004. Used with permission.

The central criterion is the patient's level of responsiveness. Importantly, responsiveness to a verbal or physical stimulus must be *purposeful*, and specifically this is not simply reflex withdrawal from a painful stimulus. The assessment of level of responsiveness is supplemented by assessments of the increasing effects of sedation on airway patency, ventilation, and the cardiovascular system.

GA has an additional specific ASA definition. "If the patient loses consciousness and the ability to respond purposefully, the anesthesia care is a general anesthetic, irrespective of whether airway instrumentation is required" (ASA Position on Monitored Anesthesia Care at http://www.ASAhq.org/publicationsAndServices/standards/23.pdf, 2005).

Safety

Although sedation is often offered as "safer than general anesthesia," this may not be altogether correct. There are numerous reports in the literature and the media of adverse cardiovascular and respiratory events associated with sedation techniques. Some are associated with individuals lacking sufficient equipment or training, but the potential for adverse events exists even in more skilled hands. Bailey et al.[2] studied the effect of 0.05 mg/kg midazolam alone, 2 μg/kg fentanyl alone, and the combination in normal volunteers.

Midazolam alone did not produce hypoxia (less than 90% saturation) or apnea. Fentanyl alone produced hypoxia in 50% of individuals, but the combination of the two drugs produced hypoxia in 92% and apnea or obstruction in 50% of these normal volunteers. Studies of patients undergoing aesthetic surgery showed that even clinically appropriate sedation can result in significant increases in arterial CO_2 and decreases in arterial O_2[3] as well as tissue desaturation.[4]

According to the U.S. Food and Drug Administration, midazolam has been implicated in at least 80 deaths during gastrointestinal (GI) endoscopy, and these deaths occurred mainly in the absence of monitoring or an anesthesiologist.[5] Respiratory events were responsible for 78% of the incidents; in 57% of the cases, patients had received a sedative and an opioid. This again highlights the added risk potential when drug combinations are given. Kallar[6] reported no deaths or serious complications in a series of 8,000 cases over 9 years, cared for by anesthesia personnel. Patients expected to be most at risk for complications are the elderly, the obese, and those with significant concomitant illnesses.

Surveys that assessed adverse events comparing sedation with other techniques have corroborated the cautions suggested above. In 1984, Natof[7] conducted a survey in 40 freestanding ambulatory surgery centers, encompassing 87,492 patients (Table 7-2). He reported that the highest incidence of complications occurred in patients who received local anesthesia with sedation, 1:106, compared to 1:120 with GA. Patients who had local anesthesia alone had a lower incidence, 1:268.

A survey of dental office practices found that the risk of death due to GA (1:324,000) was similar to IV sedation (1:314,000).[8] A survey of endoscopists reported 52 deaths in a 2-year period, an incidence of 0.5%.[9] It has been shown that traditional vital signs are insufficient to assess the physiologic effects of sedation.[5,10] In these studies, there was no relationship between changes in heart rate or blood pressure and changes in oxygen saturation. Also, there was no

Table 7-2. Complications and anesthetic technique

Technique	Number of patients	Number of complications	Incidence
Local only	10,169	38	1/268
Local and sedation	10,229	96	1/106
General	61,299	513	1/120
Regional	1,936	7	1/277

Source: Natof H.[7] Used with permission.

relationship between clinical observations of the patients by the anesthesiologist and the SpO_2 (oxygen saturation as measured by pulse oximetry) values.

More recent data from the ASA Closed Claims Project also question the safety advantage with monitored anesthesia care (MAC) compared to GA. The ASA Closed Claims Project recently reported malpractice data for MAC and compared to GA and RA, covering 1,952 claims from 1990–2002.[11] Six percent of claims were associated with MAC, 78% with GA, and 16% with RA. The interesting comparisons relate to GA.

The severity of injury for MAC was similar to that for GA, with a similar proportion of claims for deaths (33% versus 27%) and permanent brain damage (8% versus 10%). The standard of care was judged by reviewers to be substandard in a similar percentage of MAC and GA claims (41% versus 36%), and the proportion of claims resulting in payments (51% versus 52%) and the median amount of the payments were also similar ($159,000 versus $140,000).

There were, however, differences. Compared with the other anesthetics, MAC claims involved more patients older than 70 years and more patients of ASA 3 and 4 ($p < 0.025$).[11] Inadequate oxygen/ventilation was the specific mechanism of injury more often in MAC claims than GA (18% versus 2%). In the MAC claims associated with oversedation, 72% received a combination of drugs (propofol plus others or benzodiazepine plus opioid). In these oversedation claims, 84% resulted in death or brain damage, 78% were judged to involve substandard care, and the median payment was $254,000. Forty-four percent were deemed preventable by better monitoring, including oximetry and capnography, improved vigilance, and audible alarms.

Patient and procedure selection

The success of the sedation technique depends on factors related to the patient, the surgeon, and the procedure. Sedation is ideal for patients who fear GA, who refuse it, or who are at higher risk because of underlying medical conditions. Sedation must be used with caution, however, for impaired, unwilling, or anxious patients or for those who are fearful of pain or of being aware during the procedure. When the procedure can be performed under sedation or GA and when there are no medical indications for preferring one approach over the other, the patient should be given the choice. This, with the safety considerations discussed above, form the basis for valid informed consent.

A patient with significant hypertension, coronary artery disease, or obesity may be more difficult to manage with sedation, since the result may be a situation less under control than that seen with GA. Tachycardia or hypertension can occur only secondary to anxiety, inadequate analgesia, cardiovascular or hormonal response to noxious stimuli, and exogenous epinephrine in the local anesthetic solution. Oxygen desaturation has been reported in unsedated patients having only local anesthesia for oral surgery, possibly caused by breath-holding due to fear or pain.[1] Also, the surgeon must be comfortable with working on a patient who is awake and must be capable of working in a gentle but expeditious manner. The ambulatory procedures that are amenable to management with sedation are numerous and represent the breadth of diagnostic and therapeutic specialties. These include the following:

- Orthopedics
- Aesthetic surgery
- Gynecology
- Urology otolaryngology
- Ophthalmology
- General surgery
- Oral and dental surgery

Many diagnostic cardiologic, GI, and radiologic procedures can also be performed with these techniques. Frequently performed procedures involving sedation include the following:

- Arthroscopy
- Upper extremity surgery
- Dilatation and curettage
- In vitro fertilization
- Rhytidectomy
- Rhinoplasty
- Blepharoplasty
- Superficial skin procedures
- Breast and other biopsies
- Cataract removal and lens insertion
- Cystoscopy
- Insertion of lines and shunts
- Dental extractions and repairs
- Herniography
- Bronchoscopy
- GI endoscopy

Preparation

Preoperative and postoperative medical and administrative requirements for patients receiving sedation techniques should be the same as those for GA or RA. History, physical examination, airway assessment, and appropriate laboratory tests should be performed. Fasting guidelines should be enforced, and an escort at discharge must be available. The extent of preparation and care for sedation techniques should be identical to that for GA.

Psychological preparation of the patient is particularly important. Patients undergoing ambulatory surgery may even be more concerned about their anesthesia than surgery, since surgery is usually minor. Patients also may fear the wait to get into the operating room, loss of control, loss of consciousness, injury, or even death. Though considered trivial, the anesthesia mask and the IV needle may worry some patients. A realistic and informative personal interview in which expectations can be defined is more useful in allaying anxiety than premedication. The ambulatory surgery facility should offer a pleasant physical surrounding and ambiance with a helpful and supportive staff.

During the procedure, it is very important for the anesthesiologist to maintain verbal contact with the patient, provide reassurance, warn of events, and assess nonverbal patient response. The anesthesiologist can influence patient perception, cooperation, and satisfaction.[5]

Monitoring

Central nervous system, cardiovascular, and respiratory monitoring are necessary to ensure patient safety during sedation. Monitoring refines the administration of anesthesia by providing information to assess the effectiveness of drugs and to detect adverse effects. The ASA has "Standards for Basic Anesthesia Monitoring" with specific provisions for sedation (monitored anesthesia) care (Box 7-1).

Vital signs, presence of end tidal CO_2, O_2 saturation, drugs administered, dosages, and interventions performed should be recorded. A precordial stethoscope may be useful for monitoring cardiac and respiratory status. Supplemental oxygen should be considered routinely, although with caution if laser or cautery will be used around the face. Capnography can be performed by placing an adaptor or large-bore IV catheter in the nasal prong and connecting it to the gas sampling tube.[12] Nasal prongs that incorporate a capnographic connection are also commercially available. The ASA "Practice Guidelines for Sedation by Nonanesthesiologists" recommend that "monitoring of exhaled CO_2 should be considered for all patients receiving deep sedation and for patients whose ventilation cannot be directly observed during moderate sedation."

Cardiovascular monitoring may detect changes in heart rate or blood pressure secondary to cardiovascular depression, inadequate sedation, or arrhythmia. Cardiovascular monitoring also serves as an indirect index of hypercarbia or hypoxia. It is important to remember that desaturation cannot be detected visually until oxygenation is dangerously impaired, and use of a pulse oximeter is mandatory. Appropriate monitoring of cardiovascular stability, respiration, and oxygenation should continue into the postoperative period. The personnel who are designated to monitor patients during sedation should be qualified and dedicated for this task, should be present throughout the procedure, and should not also be performing the surgical or diagnostic intervention. See the following sources.

- ASA "Practice Guidelines for Sedation and Analgesia by Nonanesthesiologists," available at http://www.asahq.org/publicationsAndServices/practiceparam.htm#sedation, 2001.

Box 7-1. American Society of Anesthesiologists standards for basic anesthetic monitoring in monitored anesthesia care

Standard I
Qualified anesthesia personnel shall be present in the room throughout the
conduct of all general anesthetics, regional anesthetics, and monitored anesthesia care.

Standard II
During all anesthetics, the patient's oxygenation, ventilation, circulation, and
temperature shall be continuously evaluated.

Oxygenation
Blood oxygenation: During all anesthetics, a quantitative method of assessing
oxygenation, such as pulse oximetry, shall be employed. Adequate illumination and exposure of the patient is necessary to assess color.

Ventilation
During regional anesthesia and monitored anesthesia care, the adequacy of
ventilation shall be evaluated by continual observation of qualitative clinical
signs and/or monitoring for the presence of exhaled CO_2.

Circulation
Every patient receiving anesthesia shall have the electrocardiogram continuously displayed from the beginning of anesthesia until preparing to leave the
anesthetizing location. Every patient receiving anesthesia shall have arterial
blood pressure and heart rate determined and evaluated at least every 5
minutes.

Temperature
Every patient receiving anesthesia shall have temperature monitored when
clinically significant changes are intended, anticipated, or suspected.

Adapted from American Society of Anesthesiologists.[58] Used with permission.

- ASA "Statement on Safe Use of Propofol," available at http://www.
  ASAhq.org/publicationsAndServices/standards/37.pdf, 2004.

Recovery and discharge

The ASA has established "Standards for Postanesthesia Care" that also apply
to patients who receive MAC. All patients who have received sedation should
be recovered in a postanesthesia care unit (PACU) or comparable facility
attended by personnel competent to assess recovery.

Discharge criteria to be met are equivalent to those for GA and include stable
vital signs; orientation; mobilization; and absence of significant pain, nausea, or
bleeding. A responsible escort must be present, and verbal or written discharge
instruction should be given. Information should be provided regarding activity
level and emergency help. Patients should be cautioned not to drive, consume

alcohol, operate machinery, or make important decisions for 12 to 24 hours (see Chapter 13 for specific discharge instructions).

Standards of care

Standards of care and guidelines for sedation techniques have been established by various professional organizations such as the American Dental Association, American Academy of Pediatrics, and ASA, as well as the following facility accrediting organizations:
- Joint Commission (http://www.jointcommission.org/)
- Accreditation Association for Ambulatory Health Care (http://www.aaahc.org)
- American Association for the Accreditation of Ambulatory Surgical Facilities (http://www.aaaasf.org)

Additional guidelines can be found in the booklet "Guidelines for Optimal Ambulatory Surgical Care and Office-based Surgery," published by the American College of Surgeons (http://www.facs.org). These organizations can be contacted directly to obtain their standards.

The role of the anesthesiologist in delivering MAC as originally defined by the ASA (1986) was to provide a service to the patient, to control nonsurgical aspects of medical care, (including monitoring of vital signs), and to remain available to administer anesthetics or deliver other medical care.

ASA has refined and expanded these definitions. MAC includes all aspects of anesthesia care: a preprocedure visit, intraprocedure care, and postprocedure management. Indications for MAC include the nature of the procedure, the patient's clinical condition, and/or the potential need to convert to a general or regional anesthetic. Specific services to be provided may include the following:
- Diagnosis and treatment of clinical problems that occur during the procedure
- Support of vital functions
- Administration of sedatives, analgesics, hypnotics, anesthetic agents, or other medications as necessary for patient safety
- Psychological support and physical comfort
- Provision of other medical services as needed to complete the procedure safely (ASA "Position on Monitored Anesthesia Care")

The same level of care is required for MAC as for GA or RA, and all ASA standards apply. Some of the recommendations for care of patients who receive sedation by nonanesthesiologists can be found in Box 7-2.

Box 7-2. Guidelines for sedation by nonanesthesiologists during diagnostic and therapeutic procedures

Trained professional personnel
- minimum of two: operator and monitor
- trained in airway management
- trained in safe use of drugs for sedation
- protocols to obtain additional support services for emergencies

(Continued)

Box 7-2. *Continued*

Equipment
  - self-inflating positive-pressure oxygen delivery system
  - suction
  - emergency/resuscitation kit
  - pulse oximeter
  - regularly scheduled maintenance

Monitoring of vital functions
  - level (depth) of sedation
    — moderate sedation: performed frequently
    — deep sedation: performed continuously
  - heart rate
  - respiratory rate
  - skin color
  - head position and airway patency
  - oxygen saturation by pulse oximetry

Documentation
  - baseline health evaluation
  - consent for procedure
  - vital functions and medication during procedure
  - postprocedural care in recovery facility
  - discharge plan

Adapted from Holzman et al. in Philip and Minzter.[12] Used with permission.

Current controversies

There is large experience with levels of moderate sedation being provided safely by nonanesthesiologists. However, increasingly, procedures are being done with drugs that can produce deep sedation and even GA. Gastroenterologists have championed "NAPS" (nurse-administered propofol sedation), which is a 2-week training program for registered nurses, now taught nurse-to-nurse.[13] In one series of 9,152 primarily ASA 1 and 2 patients, most complications occurred in 1,836 upper GI endoscopies.

Three patients had "prolonged apnea" with "hypoxemia": two were given mask ventilation and one recovered spontaneously after 30 seconds. Three patients had laryngospasm, and seven had colonic perforations (three due to "forceful sigmoid disruption"). Another series of 2,000 patients excluded ASA 3, aspiration-risk, and difficult-airway patients.[14] In this series, 11 desaturated to less than 90% despite 4 L/minute O_2 and were treated with increased O_2; four desaturated to less than 85% and were "assumed apneic" and treated with mask ventilation. These authors note that experience did not prevent apnea: two of the four desaturations less than 85% occurred in the first 1,000 patients, and two in the second. Two of 2,000 sedations were converted intentionally to GA due to restlessness. Even more illuminating as to the depth of sedation actually achieved was the observation that patients were "often unable to assist with position changes" during colonoscopy.

A cohort study from the Clinical Outcomes Research Initiative database was used to determine the frequency of cardiopulmonary events with gastroenterologist-administered propofol compared with MAC at 69 endoscopy sites in the U.S. For colonoscopy, MAC was associated with a decreased adjusted relative risk of 0.5 (95% confidence interval [CI]: 0.36–0.72). For esophagogastroduodenoscopy, ASA I and II patients who received MAC had a significantly lower relative risk of 0.29 (95% CI: 0.14–0.64).[15] However, these and other series of gastroenterology patients who were given nurse- and gastroenterologist-administered propofol had no major long-term morbidity and no deaths were reported.

Emergency medicine physicians are another group promoting the practice of deep sedation. Here, the series are smaller (20–54 patients) and doses of propofol are higher (e.g., 0.21 mg/kg per minute, 1 mg/kg + 0.5 mg/kg boluses, 1.5 mg/kg).[16] Respiratory depression, hypoxia, and assisted ventilation are consistently reported. Notably, these patients are usually not fasted. Other practitioners such as dentists are also considering giving deep sedation in their practice.[17]

In response to the increasing use of propofol as a preferred sedation agent by nonanesthesiologists, the ASA developed the "Statement on Safe Use of Propofol." Similar concerns apply when other IV induction agents such as thiopental, methohexital, or etomidate are used for sedation. This statement addresses the education, training, and skills needed by the physician who is responsible for the sedation and the education, training, and skills needed by the practitioner who monitors the patient. This document also addresses the potential for reaching unintended deeper levels of sedation/anesthesia than planned and how to rescue patients who do go deeper:

> "Because sedation is a continuum, it is not always possible to predict how an individual patient will respond. Due to the potential for rapid, profound changes in sedative/anesthetic depth and the lack of antagonist medications, agents such as propofol require special attention. Even if moderate sedation is intended, patients receiving propofol should receive care consistent with that required for *deep sedation.*
>
> . . . (N)on-anesthesia personnel who administer propofol should be qualified to *rescue** patients whose level of sedation becomes deeper than initially intended and who enter, if briefly, a state of general anesthesia.
>
> *Rescue of a patient from a deeper level of sedation than intended is an intervention by a practitioner proficient in airway management and advanced life support. The qualified practitioner corrects adverse physiologic consequences of the deeper-than-intended level of sedation (such as hypoventilation, hypoxia, and hypotension) and returns the patient to the originally intended level. It is not appropriate to continue the procedure at an unintended level of sedation."

Optimal sedation: choosing drugs

Physicians strive to provide an optimal level of sedation for the individual patient and the particular procedure. The ability to achieve the desired level of sedation is based on the characteristics of the various sedative drugs. However, the wide variability in the temporal and dose-related response to various sedation agents dictates careful administration and monitoring of sedation in individual patients.

The characteristics of an ideal agent for moderate sedation have not been established by consensus opinion but are accepted to include rapid onset of action, quick recovery of cognitive and physical faculties following the procedure, and a predictable pharmacokinetic and pharmacodynamic profile. A greater understanding of sedation agents will help physicians choose the correct drug, dose, and combination to provide the best possible sedation for their patients.

Pharmacology of sedation drugs

The goal of optimal sedation can be achieved with a combination of sedative drugs and opioid analgesics. A number of sedative drugs, both IV and inhalational, have been used to achieve the sedative state. "Context-sensitive" half-life time, the time to a 50% decrease of an effective site concentration after infusion is stopped, is often used in the literature to describe the clinical duration of a drug and is preferred to t½ beta elimination time. The IV sedatives include propofol, the benzodiazepines, ketamine, barbiturates, etomidate, and dexmedetomidine. Inhalational agents that have been used include sevoflurane and nitrous oxide. Common opioids analgesics include fentanyl, remifentanil, and alfentanil.

Propofol

There is wide consensus that propofol, a sedative hypnotic, has now become the most popular choice for achieving the sedative state. Its rapid onset, distribution, and clearance, with its antiemetic effects, are ideally suited for ambulatory sedation and anesthesia.[18] Propofol is a 2,6-diisopropylphenol with sedative-hypnotic properties. Because of its poor solubility in water, the drug is formulated as an emulsion of 1% propofol, 1.2% egg lecithin, 2.25% glycerol, and 10% soybean oil.

Propofol is highly lipophilic and is structurally unrelated to other sedative agents. The blood concentration-time profile of propofol after an IV bolus injection has a half-life of 2–4 minutes in the initial rapid distribution phase, 30–45 minutes in the metabolic phase, and a longer half-life of 3–63 hours in the final elimination phase. Propofol is extensively metabolized by the liver prior to its elimination by the kidney. Propofol has a short context-sensitive half-time with its recovery profile little affected by the duration of infusion. (Please refer to context-sensitive half-time figures for various induction agents in Chapter 9.)

Propofol is believed to have its primary action in the central nervous system through gamma-aminobutyric acid (GABA) channel binding and potentiating chloride channel conductance. Its sedative effects may also be potentiated through cations on the alpha-2 adrenoreceptor and the N-methyl-D-aspartate

(NMDA) systems. Propofol is a potent vasodilator. During induction, propofol decreases the systolic and diastolic blood pressures by approximately 20%–30% with minimal change in heart rate. The hypotensive effects are especially prominent in hypovolemic, commonly seen in the perioperative period. Reduced dose should be used in elderly patients and debilitated patients and when other drugs are used in conjunction.

Propofol is a potent central respiratory depressant. Apnea occurs commonly, especially when the bolus dose is large and when administered rapidly. Personnel experienced in handling airway emergency should be present when propofol is used. Pain on injection with propofol occurs very commonly. The incidence has been quoted to be between 28% to 90% of patients, even with the low doses of propofol when used for MAC.

The etiology of this pain remains uncertain but two mechanisms have been proposed. First, the phenol may cause immediate pain from a local irritant effect on the vein. This is mitigated when propofol in the aqueous phase is diluted by adding it to fat emulsion. Second, delayed pain (after 10–20 seconds) from an indirect action on the endothelium releasing kininogens may trigger painful stimuli in the nerve endings between the intima and the media of the vessel wall.[19] Newer formulations of propofol (e.g., Propofol-Lipuro [B. Braun], which contains mixed median and long-chain triglyceride and 1% propofol) have been reported to cause less pain on injection.[20]

By virtue of its pharmacokinetic profile, the drug lends itself to continuous infusion for maintenance of anesthesia. The interest of propofol infusion for sedation started at the early stages of clinical use of the drug. Mackenzie et al.[10] demonstrated that, when combined with local anesthesia, a continuous infusion of propofol at subhypnotic doses (3–4 mg/kg per hour) was safe, efficient, and accompanied by a rapid awakening with a low incidence of postoperative side effects. Propofol has also been demonstrated to possess antiemetic properties. The plasma concentration of propofol for 50% reduction in nausea scores (Cp50 for antiemesis) is approximately 0.35 μg/mL, which may be achieved by a low-dose infusion of 10–15 μg/kg per minute.[18]

For IV sedation, an initial bolus of 0.5 mg/kg or an infusion dose of 80–100 μg/kg per minute should be given for 3–5 minutes. Maintenance of bolus increments of 10 to 20 mg, or an infusion rate of 25–75 μg/kg per minute (1.5–4.5 mg/kg per hour), is recommended (Table 7-3).[21–24] The plasma concentrations of propofol associated with an adequate sedation are in the range of 1 to 2 μg/mL.

Midazolam

Midazolam belongs to the family of benzodiazepines. Other drugs in this class sometimes used for perioperative sedation include diazepam and lorazepam, although their effects are longer lasting. Benzodiazepines work via the GABA receptor, although the interaction with the receptor may be different from that of barbiturates. Diazepam and lorazepam are insoluble in water. Outside the U.S., diazepam is also available in an emulsion formulation (Diazemuls), which can be administered intravenously.

Table 7-3. Adult sedative and analgesic drug doses administered as boluses or infusion technique[21–24]

Drugs	Bolus dosage	Infusion rate
Midazolam	25–50 μg/kg 1–2 mg (when used with propofol)	
Propofol	0.25–1 mg/kg	10–75 μg/kg per minute
Methohexital	0.25–1 mg/kg	10–75 μg/kg per minute
Dexmedetomidine		0.2–0.7 μg/kg per hour
Ketamine	0.3–0.6 mg/kg	300–600 μg/kg per hour
Fentanyl	25–50 μg	Not recommended
Alfentanil	5–10 μg/kg	0.25–1 μg/kg per minute
Remifentanil	0.1–0.3 μg/kg	0.025–0.1 μg/kg per minute

Doses should be titrated starting with the lower recommended dose.

Midazolam produces sedation, amnesia, and anxiolysis. Its redistribution and elimination half-lives are much shorter than those of diazepam, and its metabolites have no significant pharmacologic activity. Midazolam possesses amnestic properties, with its amnestic dose being one tenth of the hypnotic dose.

Inter-patient variability is marked with midazolam, and it is important to appreciate that some patients may be very sensitive to its pharmacologic effects. Indeed, when midazolam was initially introduced in the market, there were a number of deaths reported from unrecognized airway obstruction, apnea, and hypoxia, predominantly occurring in elderly patients and those who were debilitated with cardiovascular and respiratory diseases.

Midazolam depresses the slope of the carbon dioxide response curve and attenuates the ventilatory response to hypoxia. Hence, careful titration of the drug and monitoring of its effect are important for the safe use of the drug. In elderly and debilitated patients, elimination is slower and the dose should be appropriately reduced. Midazolam is administered as small IV boluses of between 0.02 and 0.1 mg/kg. In adults, the typical doses are 1–2 mg, given to obtain the desired effects.

IV midazolam (0.04 mg/kg) is shown to reduce performance on motor tests in the PACU but not to delay emergence or discharge readiness in adult patients in a hospital outpatient setting. Midazolam is frequently used as a component of sedation/analgesia by both anesthesia as well as nonanesthesia providers. The combination of midazolam and opioid is widely used and provides greater tolerance and patient satisfaction than midazolam alone.

In elderly and obese patients and those with hepatic impairment, midazolam has a reduced clearance and prolonged half-life compared with those in patients without these characteristics. Important pharmacokinetic characteristics that influence the duration of sedation with midazolam include its relatively long elimination half-life (1.8–6.4 hours) and its distribution to adipose tissue. With repeated dosing, the adipose sites become saturated and the drug redistributes to the blood. Its context-sensitive half-time increases following a prolonged infusion, resulting in delayed recovery.

Flumazenil

Flumazenil is a benzodiazepine antagonist. It is an imidazobenzodiazepine structurally related to midazolam and was approved in 1991. It is a competitive antagonist, with a high receptor affinity and low intrinsic activity. Flumazenil undergoes rapid metabolism in the liver and has a half-life of approximately 60 minutes. This is shorter than the half-life of midazolam and hence may cause resedation as the flumazenil's effects dissipate. Flumazenil is typically administered incrementally in doses of 0.2–1 mg.[25]

Onset after IV dosing is visible within 1 minute, with peak at approximately 5 minutes. It is important that clinicians monitor patients for 2 hours after administration of flumazenil as resedation can occur. However, significant resedation, requiring additional treatment, is very uncommon after clinical doses of midazolam. It specifically reverses effects of the benzodiazepines and therefore will not affect an opioid contribution to respiratory depression.

Ketamine

Ketamine is an arylcyclohexylamine that is structurally related to phencyclidine. The drug is highly water-soluble and is available in 1%, 5%, and 10% aqueous solutions. As with other water-soluble drugs, it cannot be mixed with diazepam or barbiturates. Ketamine does not cause pain on injection or tissue irritation. The molecule contains a chiral center producing two optical isomers. The S(+) isomer would appear to offer some clinical advantages over the racemic mixture [or the R(−) isomer] because it is a more potent anesthetic and analgesic isomer with a more rapid recovery and lower incidence of emergence delirium.[21] The S(+) isomer is available in Europe but not in the U.S.

Ketamine has a rapid onset of action, with clinical effects seen 30 to 60 seconds after a bolus injection. Clinical action is terminated by both redistribution and metabolism with hepatic metabolites about one third as active as the parent compound, and the metabolites are excreted via the renal route. Nystagmus, pupillary dilatation, detachment, increased muscle tone, extraneous movements, and increased lacrimation are commonly seen.

Ketamine acts an antagonist on the NMDA receptors. The incidence of psychosis when used alone is high, reported to be approximately 30% at 1–3 mg/kg. This incidence can be substantially reduced when combined with the benzodiazepines (e.g., midazolam). Ketamine is a stimulant on the cardiovascular and sympathetic nervous system. It causes hypertension and tachycardia. It is also a neurostimulant, resulting in increases in cerebral metabolic rate, cerebral blood flow, and intracranial and intraocular pressures, although subanesthetic doses appear to have minimal effects on these physiological changes. Ketamine has minimal respiratory depressant effect and is a bronchodilator.

Ketamine has been evaluated as an adjunct to other analgesics with inconsistent results. When low-dose ketamine (0.25 mg/kg) was given to surgical patients whose pain was poorly controlled with IV morphine, pain scores improved dramatically. Ketamine-treated patients also experienced less postoperative nausea and vomiting (PONV) and other side effects than those receiving placebo.[26]

Adding ketamine to a propofol infusion for sedation during breast surgery under local anesthesia reduced the requirement for supplementary opioids, but there was a dose-related increase in nausea, vomiting, and the need for airway support amongst patients receiving higher doses of ketamine.[27] Hwang and colleagues[28] recently compared the clinical efficacy of propofol/ketamine with propofol/alfentanil for patient-controlled sedation (PCS) during fiber optic bronchoscopy. The authors demonstrated that, although both techniques proved effective for sedation in patients undergoing fiber optic bronchoscopy, ketamine is superior to alfentanil when used in combination with propofol because of the high patient satisfaction and amnesia. The suggested dosing regimen for ketamine is presented in Table 7-3.

Methohexital

Methohexital is an oxybarbiturate and has pharmacokinetic properties more suitable for use in sedation than thiopental. It has more rapid clearance and shorter elimination half-life of 1.5 to 4 hours. This results in a more rapid recovery, especially with cumulative doses, and less drowsiness. However, methohexital is associated with such adverse effects as pain on injection, excitatory movements, hiccups, cough, antianalgesic properties, and an increase in the incidence of nausea and vomiting. One study reported methohexital to be more cost-effective than propofol.[29]

Methohexital compares favorably with propofol when used in a PCS setting. With a regimen of 2.5 mg (0.5 mL) bolus doses of methohexital and 5 mg (0.5 mL) doses of propofol, without a lockout, the procedure was completed satisfactorily in all patients. Patients in both groups achieved their desired levels of sedation, and no patient lost verbal contact. Immediately after the operation, patients in the methohexital group reported that they felt sleepier than those in propofol group but there were no differences at subsequent times. The results of the psychomotor tests were comparable for the two groups after operation.[30] The dosing regimen for methohexital is very similar to that of propofol (Table 7-3).

Dexmedetomidine

Dexmedetomidine is a highly selective alpha$_2$-adrenoceptor agonist with sedative and analgesic effects. Compared with clonidine, it is more selective for the alpha$_2$ adrenoceptor and acts as a full agonist in most pharmacologic test models. Potentially desirable effects include decreased requirements for other anesthetics and analgesics, a diminished sympathetic response to stress and the potential for cardioprotective effects against myocardial ischemia, and minimal effects on respiration. However, sympatholysis also may cause adverse clinical effects, such as hypotension and bradycardia. Although a primary indication for dexmedetomidine has been the sedation of the critically ill, it has also been used for intraoperative sedation[31,32] and sedation for fiber optic intubation.[33]

In patients undergoing hernia repair or hip or knee replacement under RA, Arain and Ebert[31] compared the cardio-respiratory effects of equi-sedative doses of dexmedetomidine or propofol for intraoperative sedation as well as postoperative analgesia and psychomotor performance. The average infusion rates were 0.7 μg/kg per hour for dexmedetomidine and 38 μg/kg per minute for propofol. There were no differences between groups in psychomotor performance and respiratory rate during recovery.

The dexmedetomidine group resulted in more sedation, lower blood pressure, and improved analgesia (less morphine use) in recovery. However, the time to eligibility for PACU discharge was similar.[31] When used as a sole agent for sedation for colonoscopy, dexmedetomidine was associated with distressing side effects, pronounced hemodynamic instability, prolonged recovery, and a complicated administration regimen when compared with meperidine/midazolam combination or fentanyl alone.[34] The sedative effects of dexmedetomidine are likely to limit its use in minor procedures such as colonoscopy and in office-based surgery.

Etomidate

Etomidate is a water-soluble imidazole compound and is often used for induction of anesthesia in medically complex ASA 3 or 4 outpatients due to its stability on hemodynamics. However, its use as a sedative is limited in the ambulatory setting due to its high incidence of adverse effects, including pain on injection, phlebitis, involuntary movements, emergence excitation, and high incidence of PONV. Table 7-4[35-39] illustrates commonly used IV sedation techniques.

Table 7-4. Commonly used intravenous sedation techniques

Procedure	Drug	Bolus	Infusion
Multiple procedures with local/regional anesthesia[35]	Midazolam	3–6 mg	3–14 mg/hour
	Propofol	45–95 mg	80–450 mg/hour
Ovum retrieval[36]	Mixture of 50 mL propofol (10 mg/mL) plus 4 mL alfentanil (500 μ/mL)		2 mL/kg per hour then 1 mL/kg per hour
Extracorporeal shock wave lithotripsy[37]	Midazolam	0.05 mg/kg	1 μg/kg per minute
	Alfentanil or	10 μg/kg	50 μg/kg per minute
	Fentanyl	1.5 μg/kg	
	Propofol	0.5 mg/kg	

(Continued)

Table 7-4. *Continued*

Procedure	Drug	Bolus	Infusion
Extracorporeal shock wave lithotripsy[38]	Midazolam Alfentanil *or* Midazolam Ketamine	4–9 mg 10 µg/kg 4–14 mg 0.4 mg/kg	0.5–2 µg/kg per minute 25–30 µg/kg per minute
Breast biopsy[27]	Propofol Ketamine	0.3 mg/kg	90 µg/kg per minute 9–18 µg/kg per minute
Breast biopsy[39]	Methohexital		30 µg/kg per minute
Hernia and orthopedic under regional anesthesia[30]	Dexmedetomidine	1 µg/kg	0.4–0.7 µg/kg per hour

Pharmacology of inhaled sedatives

Sevoflurane

Sevoflurane has a low blood/gas solubility that produces a rapid uptake and elimination of the agent.[40] In healthy volunteers, the alveolar F_A/F_I of sevoflurane (the rate at which fractional end-tidal alveolar concentration [F_A] approaches the fractional inspired concentration [F_I]) was 0.85 (i.e., "wash-in").[40] This increase was more rapid than that seen with isoflurane or halothane but somewhat slower than that seen with nitrous oxide and desflurane.[40] However, the clinical onset of effect of sevoflurane may be enhanced with the use of overpressure.

Sevoflurane has been investigated for providing sedation due to its rapid onset and offset as well as its nonpungent property, which makes inhalation of this agent tolerable. Sevoflurane produces dose-dependent depressant effects on the central nervous, respiratory, and cardiovascular systems.[40,41] In general, sedation with sevoflurane is associated with more rapid recovery and faster return of cognitive function compared with midazolam.[42] In a randomized, comparative study in patients receiving sedation for surgery, 76% of patients receiving sevoflurane had return of cognitive function 30 minutes postoperatively compared with 35% of midazolam-treated patients.[42]

The concentrations of sevoflurane required to produce sedation are variable. In patients who were slowly titrated to a moderate level of sedation with sevoflurane prior to surgery, there was a wide interindividual and intraindividual variability between end-tidal sevoflurane concentrations and depth of sedation as assessed by the bispectral index (BIS), unlike with propofol. Therefore, it is difficult to use the BIS to predict depth of sedation with sevoflurane, although objective clinical sedation scores (OAAS) remain valid.[43]

As with other inhalational anesthetics, sevoflurane can be associated with airway complications such as breath-holding, coughing, excitement, and laryngospasm,[40,41] although these events are less common than with other inhalational agents. Changes in hemodynamics are generally small, and the risk of fluoride-induced nephrotoxicity appears to be minimal. In a comparative trial in patients undergoing moderate sedation, sevoflurane compared to propofol or midazolam was associated with significantly faster return to baseline assessed by the Digit Symbol Substitution Test (76%, 48%, and 24%, respectively, at 10 minutes) but significantly more disinhibition-excitement (70%) compared with propofol (36%) or midazolam (5%).[43]

Nitrous oxide

Nitrous oxide is rarely used for sedation other than in dental anesthesia. It has a rapid onset and offset of action due to its low lipid/gas partition coefficient (0.47). Nitrous oxide in itself is not a full anesthetic but provides synergistic interactions when combined with another inhalational or IV sedative agent. It is discussed in greater detail in Chapter 9.

Pharmacology of opioids

Remifentanil

Remifentanil is a novel, ultrashort, mu-opioid receptor agonist with an analgesic potency similar to that of fentanyl. The preparation is in a form of crystalline white powder, readily soluble in water. The vial contains hydrochloric acid and glycine. Glycine is an inhibitory neurotransmitter that renders the preparation not suitable for extradural or subarachnoid injection. By virtue of predominant metabolism by nonspecific esterases, remifentanil is the first in the class of esterase-metabolized opioids within the 4-anilidopiperidine series of drugs. Because of the rapid systemic elimination of remifentanil (with a half-life of 8–10 minutes), it should have pharmacokinetic advantages in clinical situations requiring predictable termination of effect.[44]

The "context-sensitive" half-life time of remifentanil is estimated to be approximately 4 minutes and is independent of the infusion duration. In contrast, for alfentanil, sufentanil, and fentanyl, the context-sensitive half-time was much longer and was dependent on the infusion duration (Figure 7-1).

The hemodynamic response to remifentanil appears to be similar to that of other anilidopiperidines (i.e., mild bradycardia and a decrease of 15%–20% in arterial blood pressure may be observed). However, in elderly and dehydrated patients, significant hypotension may be observed. Hence, dose reductions of as much as 50%–70% may be required in these populations. Remifentanil is a potent respiratory depressant. In nonintubated patients, remifentanil produces respiratory depression in a dose-dependent fashion. However, because of remifentanil's lack of accumulation during continuous systemic administration, this effect is not expected to last for more than 10–15 minutes after discontinuation of the infusion.

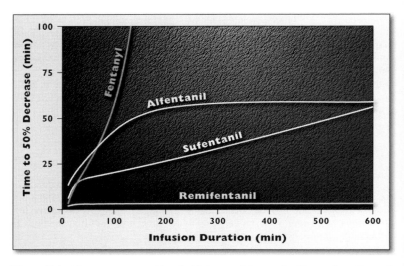

Figure 7-1. The context-sensitive half-times of fentanyl, alfentanil, sufentanil, and remifentanil. Defined as the time required to achieve a 50% decrease in concentration after termination of a continuous infusion targeted to maintain a steady-state concentration, the context-sensitive half-time has been used to compare the clinical behavior of individual drugs within a selected drug class. The context-sensitive half-time is a target controlled infusion (TCI) simulation. Reprinted from Egan TD.[59] Used with permission.

Systemically administered remifentanil does not release histamine. Remifentanil causes adverse effects typical of m-opioids (i.e., nausea, vomiting, pruritus, muscle rigidity, and cardiopulmonary suppression).[44] In a study of patients undergoing eye surgery, remifentanil had a lower frequency of postoperative nausea (8%) compared with fentanyl (54%).[45] However, other studies have shown no difference in the incidence of nausea or vomiting when remifentanil was compared with alfentanil[46] or fentanyl.[47] The incidence of muscle rigidity after IV delivery of remifentanil is similar to that with alfentanil, whereas onset may be more rapid. Although this side effect appears to be moderate, it might be prevented by slow injection of bolus doses of remifentanil over 60–90 seconds.

Fentanyl

Fentanyl, a piperidine derivative, is probably the most commonly used opioid for ambulatory anesthesia. It produces analgesia, sedation, drowsiness, and euphoria. The drug is injected in 25- to 50-µg increments at 1- to 5-minute intervals to a usual loading dose of 1–3 µg/kg. Its onset is approximately 5 minutes, with peak at approximately 10 minutes. Its clinical effects usually last approximately 45–60 minutes, although its effects are largely dependent on the total doses that have been administered, due to its exponential properties of its context-sensitive half-time (Figure 7-1). Hence, it is not recommended to be used as a continuous infusion for procedures under sedation. Doses administered should be reduced in elderly patients due to reduced clearance and more sensitive pharmacodynamic effects.[47]

Alfentanil

Alfentanil is shorter acting than fentanyl but longer lasting than remifentanil. Whereas sedation and euphoria may be more profound, respiratory depression is briefer than fentanyl. Similar to fentanyl, its clearance is reduced in the elderly, patients with liver disease, and in the obese. Following a bolus or an infusion leading dose of 5–10 µg/kg, onset is within 1 to 2 minutes, with a duration of approximately 20 minutes. The drug is conveniently administered via syringe pump titrated to clinical effects. A recent study compared bolus alfentanil 20 µg/kg and propofol 1 mg/kg versus bolus remifentanil 0.4 µg/kg and propofol 1 mg/kg in outpatients undergoing endometrial biopsy. The two groups were similar with regard to respiration and recovery profile.[48]

Emerging practice

Fospropofol

Fospropofol (Aquavan), a new sedative/hypnotic agent, is a water-soluble prodrug of propofol that is currently in clinical development in the U.S. After IV administration, propofol is released from this prodrug by the enzymatic action of alkaline phosphatases in the vascular endothelium.[49] This action provides predictable and controlled release of propofol with a smooth rise to therapeutic plasma propofol concentrations.

In healthy volunteers, fospropofol-delivered propofol is generally associated with a hemodynamic profile similar to that produced by propofol emulsion, but the onset of cardiovascular depression with fospropofol is delayed and smoother compared with propofol emulsion. However, recovery from fospropofol sedation is also longer than from propofol. Although it has the advantages of nonlipid formulation and minimal pain on injection, transient or mild to moderate pelvic/perianal tingling, itching, or burning sensations are common.[50]

Patient-controlled sedation

Bolus administration of IV propofol is usually used to provide sedation, but several problems exist. Patients vary widely in their requirement for sedation.

A refinement of the bolus dose technique is to administer sedation by a continuous infusion. However, the sedative effect of the drug varies until a steady-state concentration is reached and this may take considerable time. This can be overcome by the concept of target-controlled infusion (TCI).

The basic rationale for TCI of an IV anesthetic agent is to enable the anesthesia care providers to rapidly achieve a desired plasma concentration and alter the depth of sedation in as simple a manner as using standard volatile anesthetics delivered via calibrated vaporizers. The provider adjusts the target blood concentration of drug and titrates to clinical effect. A TCI system therefore improves both the convenience of administration and ease of control of anesthesia compared with conventional infusion techniques. A number of TCI devices are available and approved for clinical use in Europe and other parts of the world. However, these devices have not been approved in the U.S.

Recently, patient-controlled propofol for sedation using TCI has been compared with the same drug delivered by PCS using boluses. In a preliminary study, both techniques provided adequate sedation, good operating conditions, and stable physiological parameters. However, the TCI group achieved greater satisfaction, probably as a result of more rapid attainment of clinical effects.[51]

In one study, TCI propofol was started at a target concentration of $1\,\mu g/mL$. The patient was able to increase the C_T (target concentration) in $0.2\,\mu g/mL$ increments by double-pressing a demand button. There was a lock-out interval of 2 minutes and a maximum permissible C_T of $3\,\mu g/mL$. If no demands were made for 6 minutes, the system reduced the C_T by $0.2\,\mu g/mL$.

There was considerable interindividual variability in propofol consumption, with a mean of 39.3 mg/kg per minute (range, 3–131 mg/kg per minute). Optimum sedation was provided with a median C_T of 0.8–$0.9\,\mu g/mL$. A total of 89% of patients were happy to use the technique again. Reasons cited were comfort, self-titration, anxiolysis, and clear-headed recovery. One patient would not use the system again, because of pain at the site of infusion.[52]

Recently, several devices have demonstrated the potential to provide an objective measure of the level of sedation. These include the BIS, the Patient State Index (PSI) (SEDLine), and the auditory evoked potential index (AAI).[53–57] The BIS is a method of analyzing electroencephalogram (EEG) data based on the interfrequency phase relationships of the EEG.[53] A number of studies have evaluated the ability of the BIS to assess sedation levels.[53,54] For example, Bower and colleagues[54] evaluated the temporal relationship between the Modified Observer's Assessment of Alertness/Sedation (Modified OAA/S) scale and the BIS in 50 adults who received sedation with diazepam and meperidine for endoscopic procedures.

There was a significant temporal correlation between the BIS levels and the Modified OAA/S scores ($r = 0.59$; $P < 0.0001$), and BIS levels and Modified OAA/S scores corresponded with the need for additional sedation. It was estimated that a Modified OAA/S score of 3 corresponded to a BIS level of 81.5.[54] However, the correlation between the BIS and subjective sedation rating scales or sedative dose is variable, with some studies reporting a poor correlation.[53]

The PSI has been shown to correlate well with level of sedation in intensive care unit patients as measured by the Ramsay sedation score.[55] Trials comparing these objective measures of sedation (BIS with SEDLine, AAI) have demonstrated that there is a correlation between the methods; however, there is substantial variability in patient responses.[56,57] Thus, the role of sedation-monitoring techniques during endoscopic sedation remains to be determined by additional research.

Summary

Sedation techniques are increasingly useful in ambulatory anesthesia. The key to safe administration is an understanding of levels of sedation, from altered mood to loss of consciousness. Although sedation is often offered as "safer than general anesthesia," the literature easily demonstrates risks and adverse outcomes even when administered by skilled practitioners in all practice settings.

The success of sedation techniques depends on careful patient and procedure selection, patient preparation, appropriate monitoring, and attention to recovery and discharge. The safety of deep sedation given by nonanesthesiologists is controversial. Among sedatives, inhaled drugs, and analgesics, there are an array of drugs that can be used to achieve sedation, and achieving the desired outcomes requires a thorough knowledge of the onset and recovery of effects and side effects.

References

1. Philip BK. Monitored anesthesia. In: McGoldrick KE, ed. *Ambulatory Anesthesiology: A Problem Oriented Approach*. Baltimore, MD: Williams & Wilkins; 1995:387–398.

2. Bailey PL, Pace NL, Ashburn MA, et al. Frequent hypoxia and apnea after sedation with midazolam and fentanyl. *Anesthesiology*. 1990;73:826–830.

3. McNabb TG, Goldwyn RM. Blood Gas and hemodynamic effects of sedatives and analgesics when used as a supplement to local anesthesia in plastic surgery. *Plastic Reconstr Surg*. 1976;58:37–43.

4. Singer R, Thomas PR. Pulse oximeter in the ambulatory aesthetic surgical facility. *Plastic Reconst Surg*. 1988;82:111–114.

5. Greenberg CP, De Soto H. Sedation techniques. In: Twersky RS, ed: *The Ambulatory Anesthesia Handbook*. St Louis, MO: Mosby; 1995:301–359.

6. Kallar SK. Conscious sedation in ambulatory surgery. *Anesth Rev*. 1990;17(suppl 2):45–51.

7. Natof HE. FASA Special Study 1. Alexandria, VA: Federated Ambulatory Surgery Association; 1986.

8. Campbell RL. Prevention of complications associated with intravenous sedation and general anesthesia. *J Oral Maxillofac Surg*. 1986;44:289.

9. Daneshmend TK, Bell GD, Logan RFA. Sedation for upper gastrointestinal endoscopy: results of a nationwide survey. *Gut*. 1991;32:12–15.

10. Mackenzie N, Grant IS. Propofol for intravenous sedation. *Anaesthesia*. 1987;42: 3–6.

11. Bhananker SM, Posner KL, Cheney FW, Caplan RA, Lee LA, Domino KB. Injury and liability associated with monitored anesthesia care: a closed claims analysis. *Anesthesiology*. 2006;104:228–234.

12. Philip BK, Minzter BH. Intravenous sedation and monitored anesthesia care. In: White PF, ed. *Ambulatory Anesthesia and Surgery*. Philadelphia, PA: W.B. Saunders; 1997:349–367.

13. Walker JA, McIntyre RD, Schleinitz PF, et al. Nurse-administered propofol sedation without anesthesia specialists in 9152 endoscopic cases in an ambulatory surgery center. *Am J Gastroent*. 2003;98:1744–1750.

14. Rex DK, Overley C, Kinser K, et al. Safety of propofol administered by registered nurses with gastroenterologist supervision in 2000 endoscopic cases. *Am J Gastroent*. 2002;97:1159–1163.

15. Vargo JJ, Holub JL, Faigel DO, et al. Risk factors for cardiopulmonary events during propofol-mediated upper endoscopy and colonoscopy. *Aliment Pharmacol Ther*. 2006;24:955–963.

16. Green SM, Krauss B. Propofol in emergency medicine: pushing the sedation frontier. *Ann Emerg Med*. 2003;42:792–797.

17. Yagiela JA. Making patients safe and comfortable for a lifetime of dentistry: frontiers in office-based sedation. *J Dent Educ*. 2001;65:1348–1356.

18. Gan TJ, Glass PS, Howell ST, et al. Determination of plasma concentrations of propofol associated with 50% reduction in postoperative nausea. *Anesthesiology*. 1997;87:779–784.

19. Baker MT, Naguib M. Propofol: the challenges of formulation. *Anesthesiology*. 2005;103:860–876.

20. Rau J, Roizen MF, Doenicke AW, O'Connor MF, Strohschneider U. Propofol in an emulsion of long- and medium-chain triglycerides: the effect on pain. *Anesth Analg*. 2001;93:382–384.

21. Sneyd JR. Recent advances in intravenous anaesthesia. *Br J Anaesth*. 2004;93: 725–736.

22. Gan TJ, Glass PS. Pharmacokinetic and pharmacodynamic aspects of intravenous anesthesia. *Anesthetic Pharmacology Review*. 1995;3:28–36.

23. Glass PS, Gan TJ, Howell S, Ginsberg B. Drug interactions: volatile anesthetics and opioids. *J Clin Anesth*. 1997;9:18S–22S.

24. Horn E, Nesbit SA. Pharmacology and pharmacokinetics of sedatives and analgesics. *Gastrointest Endosc Clin N Am*. 2004;14:247–268.

25. Philip BK. Flumazenil: the benzodiazepine antagonist. *Anesthesiol Clin North Am*. 1993;11:799–814.

26. Weinbroum AA. A single small dose of postoperative ketamine provides rapid and sustained improvement in morphine analgesia in the presence of morphine-resistant pain. *Anesth Analg*. 2003;96:789–795.

27. Badrinath S, Avramov MN, Shadrick M, et al. The use of a ketamine-propofol combination during monitored anesthesia care. *Anesth Analg*. 2000;90:858–862.

28. Hwang J, Jeon Y, Park HP, et al. Comparison of alfetanil and ketamine in combination with propofol for patient-controlled sedation during fiberoptic bronchoscopy. *Acta Anaesthesiol Scand*. 2005;49:1334–1338.

29. Sun R, Watcha MF, White PF, et al. A cost comparison of methohexital and propofol for ambulatory anesthesia. *Anesth Analg*. 1999;89:311–316.

30. Hamid SK, McCann N, McArdle L, Asbury AJ. Comparison of patient-controlled sedation with either methohexitone or propofol. *Br J Anaesth*. 1996;77:727–730.

31. Arain SR, Ebert TJ. The efficacy, side effects, and recovery characteristics of dexmedetomidine versus propofol when used for intraoperative sedation. *Anesth Analg*. 2002;95:461–466.

32. Alhashemi JA, Kaki AM. Dexmedetomidine in combination with morphine PCA provides superior analgesia for shockwave lithotripsy. *Can J Anaesth*. 2004;51: 342–347.

33. Scher CS, Gitlin MC. Dexmedetomidine and low-dose ketamine provide adequate sedation for awake fibreoptic intubation. *Can J Anaesth*. 2003;50:607–610.

34. Jalowiecki P, Rudner R, Gonciarz M, et al. Sole use of dexmedetomidine has limited utility for conscious sedation during outpatient colonoscopy. *Anesthesiology*. 2005;103:269–273.

35. White PF, Negus JB. Sedative infusions during local and regional anesthesia: a comparison of midazolam and propofol. *J Clin Anesth*. 1991;3:32–39.

36. Sherry E. Admixture of propofol and alfentanil. *Anaesthesia*. 1992;47:477–479.

37. Monk TG, Boure B, White PF, et al. Comparison of intravenous sedative-analgesic techniques for outpatient immersion lithotripsy. *Anesth Analg*. 1991;72:616–621.

38. Monk TG, Rater JM, White PF. Comparison of alfentanil and ketamine infusions in combination with midazolam for outpatient lithotripsy. *Anesth Analg*. 1991;74: 1023–1028.

39. Sa Rego MM, Inagaki Y, White PF. The cost-effectiveness of methohexital versus propofol for sedation during monitored anesthesia care. *Anesth Analg*. 1999;88:723–728.

40. Patel SS, Goa KL. Sevoflurane. A review of its pharmacodynamic and pharmacokinetic properties and its clinical use in general anesthesia. *Drugs*. 1996;51:658–700.

41. Goa KL, Noble S, Spencer CM. Sevoflurane in paediatric anaesthesia: a review. *Paediatr Drugs*. 1999;1:127–153.

42. Ibrahim AE, Ghoneim MM, Kharasch ED, et al. Speed of recovery and side-effect profile of sevoflurane sedation compared with midazolam. *Anesthesiology*. 2001;94: 87–94.

43. Ibrahim AE, Taraday JK, Kharasch ED. Bispectral index monitoring during sedation with sevoflurane, midazolam, and propofol. *Anesthesiology*. 2001;95:1151–1159.

44. Glass PS, Gan TJ, Howell S. A review of the pharmacokinetics and pharmacodynamics of remifentanil. *Anesth Analg*. 1999;89:S7–S14.

45. Sator-Katzenschlager SM, Oehmke MJ, Deusch E, Dolezal S, Heinze G, Wedrich A. Effects of remifentanil and fentanyl on intraocular pressure during the maintenance and recovery of anaesthesia in patients undergoing non-ophthalmic surgery. *Eur J Anaesthesiol*. 2004;21:95–100.

46. Philip BK, Scuderi PE, Chung F, et al. Remifentanil compared with alfentanil for ambulatory surgery using total intravenous anesthesia. The Remifentanil/Alfentanil Outpatient TIVA Group. *Anesth Analg.* 1997;84:515–521.

47. Shafer SL, Varvel JR, Aziz N, et al. Pharmacokinetics of fentanyl administered by computer-controlled infusion pump. *Anesthesiology.* 1990;73:1091–1102.

48. Dogru K, Madenoglu H, Yildiz K, Boyaci A. Sedation for outpatient endometrial biopsy: comparison of remifentanil-propofol and alfentanil-propofol. *J Int Med Res.* 2003;31:31–35.

49. Fechner J, Ihmsen H, Hatterscheid D, et al. Pharmacokinetics and clinical pharmacodynamics of the new propofol prodrug GPI 15715 in volunteers. *Anesthesiology.* 2003;99:303–313.

50. Struys MM, Vanluchene AL, Gibiansky E, et al. FOSPROPOFOL injection, a watersoluble prodrug of propofol, as a bolus injection: a phase I dose-escalation comparison with DIPRIVAN (part 2): pharmacodynamics and safety. *Anesthesiology.* 2005;103: 730–743.

51. Rodrigo MR, Irwin mg, Tong CK, et al. A randomised crossover comparison of patient-controlled sedation and patient-maintained sedation using propofol. *Anaesthesia.* 2003;58:333–338.

52. Gillham MJ, Hutchinson RC, Carter R, Kenny GN. Patient-maintained sedation for ERCP with a target-controlled infusion of propofol: a pilot study. *Gastrointest Endosc.* 2001;54:14–17.

53. LeBlanc JM, Dasta JF, Kane-Gill SL. Role of the bispectral index in sedation monitoring in the ICU. *Ann Pharmacother.* 2006;40:490–500.

54. Bower AL, Ripepi A, Dilger J, Boparai N, Brody FJ, Ponsky JL. Bispectral index monitoring of sedation during endoscopy. *Gastrointest Endosc.* 2000;52:192–196.

55. Schneider G, Heglmeier S, Schneider J, Templ G, Kochs EF. Patient State Index (PSI) measures depth of sedation in ICU patients. *Intensive Care Med.* 2004:30;213–216.

56. Chen X, Tang J, White PF, et al. A comparison of patient state index and bispectral index values during the perioperative period. *Anesth Analg.* 2002;95:1669–1674.

57. Kreuer S, Bruhn J, Larsen R, Hoepstein M, Wilhelm W. Comparison of Alaris AEP index and bispectral index during propofol-remifentanil anaesthesia. *Br J Anaesth.* 2003;91:336–340.

58. Standards for Basic Anesthetic Monitoring. Park Ridge, IL: American Society of Anesthesiologists; October 25, 2005.

59. Egan TD. Target-controlled drug delivery: progress toward an intravenous "vaporizer" and automated anesthetic administration. *Anesthesiology.* 2003;99:1214–1219.

8. Regional anesthesia

Holly C. L. Evans, MD, FRCP(C)
Karen C. Nielsen, MD
Susan M. Steele, MD

Anesthesia for ambulatory surgery must facilitate home-readiness within hours of surgery. Regional anesthesia can fulfill this requirement by providing excellent intraoperative anesthesia while minimizing postoperative pain, sedation, nausea, and vomiting when compared to general anesthesia and opioid analgesia.[1-5] Single-injection peripheral nerve blocks with long-acting local anesthetic can prolong these benefits. Furthermore, continuous catheter techniques can facilitate same-day discharge of patients having more complex and painful surgical procedures.[6-8] When appropriate patient education and follow-up are provided, ambulatory discharge of a patient with an insensate extremity can be extremely safe and should be associated with very few complications.[9]

Preoperative preparation

Patient assessment

A comprehensive preoperative assessment should be performed for all patients who may receive regional anesthesia and should be focused on the specific considerations of these techniques. The physiologic effects of the specific regional technique must be considered in the context of the patient's underlying medical condition(s). In addition, patient comorbidities that increase the risk of regional anesthesia must be identified (Table 8-1). For example, published guidelines outline the risk of neuraxial anesthesia in anticoagulated patients.[10] When peripheral nerve blocks are considered for anticoagulated

Table 8-1. Conditions associated with increased risk following regional anesthesia

Significant coagulopathy
Perineural vascular malformation
Uncorrected hypovolemia
Significant aortic stenosis
Infection overlying needle puncture site
Systemic sepsis
Increased intracranial pressure
Unstable neurologic disease
Local anesthetic allergy
Patient refusal

patients, risk is determined on an individual basis according to the severity of the coagulation abnormality and the peripheral nerve block proposed (i.e., compressibility of the site, proximity to blood vessels, and consequences of hematoma). Anesthesia options, benefits, and risks should be discussed with all patients, and informed consent must be obtained.

Preoperative block area

The success of peripheral nerve blocks can be greatly enhanced when blocks are performed in a preoperative block room. This allows adequate time for placement of the block, onset of anesthesia, and supplementation if required. This approach can significantly improve operating room efficiency[11] and can be particularly beneficial in a rapid-paced ambulatory surgery center. A preoperative block area requires sufficient space, patient-monitoring facilities, appropriate resuscitation equipment, and trained health care providers. Using existing facilities and personnel (such as in the preadmission area or in the postanesthesia care unit) can minimize the cost of this approach.

Monitoring

All patients having regional anesthesia should have an intravenous line and appropriate monitoring during block performance as well as surgery. Essential monitors include a pulse oximeter, noninvasive blood pressure and electrocardiogram in addition to a trained anesthesia care provider. Supplemental oxygen should be applied, particularly when sedation is used.

Resuscitation equipment

Regional anesthesia can produce several physiologic changes. Consequently, resuscitative equipment must be available to manage conditions ranging from hypotension following spinal anesthesia to seizures or cardiorespiratory arrest as a result of local anesthetic toxicity. Resuscitative equipment should include oxygen, a positive-pressure bag and mask, suction, airway equipment, a cardiac arrest cart, and emergency medications (Table 8-2).

Local anesthetics and adjuvants

Local anesthetics achieve reversible neural conduction block by impeding movement of ions through sodium channels. A variety of local anesthetic agents are available with a range of potency, onset time, duration, and safety profiles.

Table 8-2. Resuscitative equipment required for regional anesthesia

Oxygen supply
Positive-pressure bag and masks (range of sizes)
Suction
Oral and nasal airways (range of sizes)
Endotracheal tube (range of sizes)
Laryngoscope handle and blades (range of shapes and sizes)
Defibrillator and pacemaker
Standard anesthesia medications
Resuscitation medications as recommended in ACLS protocols

ACLS, advanced cardiac life support.

The local anesthetic agent should be selected based on the intended clinical use and desired effects. Chloroprocaine, lidocaine, procaine, and mepivacaine have a rapid onset and a short duration of effect. Conversely, ropivacaine and bupivacaine have a more prolonged onset and duration of action. Table 8-3 summarizes the clinical profile of local anesthetics used for peripheral nerve blocks.

Many regional anesthesia techniques can involve injection of large volumes of local anesthetic solutions; consequently, local anesthetic toxicity should be considered a real risk. To minimize this risk, the recommended toxic dose of local anesthetic must not be exceeded (Table 8-3). In addition, the local anesthetic must be administered with slow, incremental injections and multiple aspirations to check for blood. Moreover, epinephrine should be used when appropriate to reduce systemic absorption and to act as a marker of intravascular injection. It is imperative that anesthesiologists recognize the presentation of local anesthetic toxicity (Table 8-4) and promptly initiate the required treatment. Management should include oxygenation, ventilation, termination of seizures, and treatment of cardiovascular collapse or arrhythmias according to advanced cardiac life support protocols.

Agents commonly added to local anesthetic solutions are summarized in Table 8-5. Epinephrine can be added to the local anesthetic solution to decrease systemic absorption and to limit the risk of systemic toxicity. This adjunct may prolong local anesthetic duration of action and improve the quality of anesthesia.

Table 8-3. Onset time, duration of effect, and maximum recommended dose of local anesthetic agents used for peripheral nerve blocks

	Onset (minutes)	**Duration (hours)**	**Maximum dose (mg/kg) of solution with epinephrine**
Chloroprocaine	10–20	1–2	14
Lidocaine	10–20	2–3	7
Mepivacaine	10–20	3–6	7
Bupivacaine	15–30	6–12	3
Ropivacaine	15–30	6–12	3.5

Table 8-4. Signs and symptoms of local anesthetic toxicity

Light-headedness
Perioral paresthesias
Tinnitus
Drowsiness
Confusion
Slurred speech
Muscle twitches
Grand mal seizure
Cardiac arrhythmias
Cardiorespiratory arrest

Phenylephrine has also been used for this purpose, although experience is much more limited. Bicarbonate may be added to hasten the onset of anesthesia and is particularly useful with the shorter-acting local anesthetics. Clonidine is an alpha-2 agonist with analgesic properties. This agent can be used to enhance the quality and duration of neuraxial and peripheral nerve blocks; however, associated hypotension, bradycardia, and sedation potentially limit its use in the ambulatory population.

Regional anesthesia equipment

Using a prepackaged sterile tray with disinfecting solution, drapes, syringes, needles, and gauze enhances efficiency of regional anesthesia and minimizes the risk of infectious complications.

A range of needle sizes and shapes are available for the various regional anesthesia techniques. A 10-cm, small-gauge, pencil-point spinal needle (i.e., 25- to 27-gauge Whitacre, Pencan, or Sprotte) is typically selected for spinal anesthesia in ambulatory patients in order to minimize the risk of postdural puncture headache. A 16- to 18-gauge Tuohy or Weiss needle and a 20-gauge catheter are used for epidural anesthesia.

Insulated, short-bevel needles are used for single-injection peripheral nerve blocks performed with the assistance of a nerve stimulator. Diameters range

Table 8-5. Dose of adjuvant in final solution according to site of administration

	Spinal	**Epidural**	**Peripheral nerve block**
Epinephrine	50–200 µg	2.5 µg/mL	2.5 µg/mL
Phenylephrine	1–5 mg		
Bicarbonate		0.1 mEq/mL	0.1 mEq/mL
Clonidine	150 µg	450 µg	50–100 µg

from 21 to 24 gauge, and a variety of lengths are available according to the type of block performed (i.e., 25–50 mm for interscalene, supraclavicular, and axillary; 75–100 mm for infraclavicular, lumbar plexus, and classic sciatic). Extension tubing (for injection and aspiration) and a stimulating cable are attached to the proximal end of needles used for single-injection and continuous nerve blocks. Continuous peripheral nerve blocks are accomplished using an insulated 16- to 18-gauge Tuohy needle of the appropriate length. Continuous catheters are 18–20 gauge in diameter and are available in two different varieties (nonstimulating and stimulating). A nonstimulating catheter is incapable of conducting current and often has centimeter markings and three distal orifices. A stimulating catheter has a single distal orifice and conducts current to the distal tip, allowing confirmation of perineural catheter placement.

Peripheral nerve stimulators for use in regional anesthesia are able to precisely generate a range of current from 0 to 5.0 mA and are capable of maintaining this current within the usual range of skin impedance. When starting a peripheral nerve block, the current should be set at 1.0–1.5 mA and gradually reduced once the appropriate motor endpoint is observed. It is generally accepted that the block needle is adequately close to the nerve(s) when the elicited motor response is present at a current of 0.5 mA. However, the nerve block needle may be dangerously close to the nerve(s) when the motor response is still present below a current of 0.2 mA. Most modern nerve stimulators provide the option of a 1- or 2-Hz pulse frequency. A frequency of 2 Hz (2 cycles or stimuli per second) provides greater real-time feedback of needle location compared to 1 Hz (1 cycle per second). In addition, many newer stimulators offer the ability to vary the pulse width from a length of 0.1 milliseconds, which is used to stimulate large, alpha motor fibers, up to a length of 1.0 milliseconds, which has a greater specificity for smaller, delta sensory fibers.

Recently, ultrasound has been used to guide localization of neural structures. This modality may prove advantageous for outpatients because a nerve block under direct ultrasound vision ensures perineural distribution of injectate and has the potential to limit adverse events such as intraneural injection, pneumothorax, and intravascular injection with resulting local anesthetic toxicity. Ultrasound machines used for regional anesthesia typically use a sound wave frequency of 10–14 MHz. This balances high-quality resolution (which is typically achieved with higher sound wave frequency) with adequate penetration depth from the skin (greater penetration depth is achieved with lower frequencies).

Sedation

Sedation for regional anesthesia should provide both anxiolysis as well as analgesia and should enable meaningful verbal communication with the patient. Symptoms such as paresthesias and early signs of systemic local anesthetic toxicity should be sought and when present should prompt alteration in technique in order to minimize complications. The combination of midazolam and fentanyl provides a comfortable and cooperative patient. Conversely, nonopioid analgesics such as ketamine or clonidine can provide analgesia in the absence

Table 8-6. Selected intravenous agents used for sedation

Class of agent	Mechanism of action	Systemic and side effects	Example
Benzodiazepines	GABA inhibitor	Anxiolysis Amnesia Anticonvulsant	Midazolam: 10–20 μg/kg IV prn
Opioids	Opioid receptor agonist	Analgesia Nausea, vomiting Respiratory depression	Fentanyl: 0.3–0.5 μg/kg IV prn Alfentanil: 2–5 μg/kg IV prn Remifentanil: 0.025–0.2 μg/kg per minute IV
Ketamine	NMDA antagonist	Dissociative state Analgesia Amnesia Bronchodilation Hallucinations	0.15–0.25 mg/kg IV prn
Alpha-2 Agonists	Alpha-2 agonist	Sedation Analgesia Hypotension Bradycardia	Clonidine: 1–2 μg/kg IV Dexmedetomidine: Bolus: 0.4–1 μg/kg IV over 10–20 minutes Infusion: 0.2–0.7 μg/kg per hour IV
Propofol	GABA inhibitor	Sedation Amnesia Anticonvulsant Antiemetic	25–50 μg/kg per minute IV

GABA, gamma-amino-butyric acid; IV, intravenous; NMDA, N-methyl-D-aspartate; prn, pro re nata (as necessary).

of opioid-related side effects. Table 8-6 describes a number of medications that can be used for nerve block placement and/or intraoperative sedation.

Neuraxial anesthesia

Spinal anesthesia

Spinal anesthesia involves injection of local anesthetic in the subarachnoid space caudal to the level of termination of the spinal cord. This technique can be used for lower extremity, urogenital, and lower abdominal surgery.

A number of local anesthetics and adjuvants can be used for spinal anesthesia, and selection is made based on the agent's onset, duration, baricity, and other characteristics (Table 8-7). Both lidocaine and mepivacaine provide rapid onset, short duration, and prompt return of ability to ambulate and void;[12,13] however, the use of these agents has been limited by the risk of transient neurological symptoms.[12,14] A 10% solution of procaine mixed with cerebrospinal fluid in a 1:1 ratio to generate a 5% solution can also provide spinal anesthesia of rapid onset and short duration. There exists a low risk of inadequate anesthesia and transient neurological symptoms with spinal procaine.[15] Longer-acting agents such as bupivacaine and ropivacaine rarely produce transient neurological symptoms; however, they can result in prolonged sensorimotor block with delayed ambulation and bladder function.[16,17] Consequently, if conventional doses of bupivacaine or ropivacaine are used, patients should be cautioned preoperatively about the possibility of a prolonged recovery. Lowering the dose of long-acting local anesthetic and adding a short-acting opioid such as fentanyl are modifications that can be used to minimize the density and duration of motor block;[18] however, the risk of inadequate anesthesia and block failure does exist. Recently, a preservative-free formulation of chloroprocaine was investigated for spinal anesthesia.[19] This agent was found to have a very short duration of action and few associated side effects, ideal qualities for many outpatient procedures.

The baricity of an agent represents its density relative to cerebrospinal fluid. This affects the spread of local anesthetic within the spinal column. Hyperbaric agents are denser than cerebrospinal fluid. With the patient in the supine position, these agents display greater cephalocaudad spread than isobaric agents. Anesthesia confined to the sacral dermatomes results when a patient maintains a sitting position after injection of a hyperbaric agent. Likewise, hyperbaric or hypobaric agents can be injected in the lateral decubitus position to obtain a unilateral block of the dependent or nondependent side, respectively.

Adjuvants to local anesthetics used for spinal anesthesia in ambulatory patients have been previously summarized (Table 8-5). Short-acting opioids such as fentanyl are commonly used; however, long-acting agents such as morphine should be avoided in outpatients due to the risk of delayed respiratory depression. Epinephrine prolongs the duration of spinal anesthesia and its use needs to be carefully considered for ambulatory patients. Because of the associated hypotension, bradycardia, and sedation, clonidine is not widely used.

Advantages of spinal anesthesia include ease of performance, rapid onset, and dense surgical anesthesia. Box 8-1 contains potential adverse effects of concern to ambulatory patients. Serious neurologic or infectious complications are rare.[20]

Epidural anesthesia

Epidural anesthesia involves the placement of a catheter and injection of local anesthetic into the epidural space. This block can be performed in the cervical, thoracic, lumbar, or sacral (i.e., caudal block) spine and provides bilateral block over several dermatomes. As a result, applications range from breast surgery to abdominal procedures to lower extremity cases.

Table 8-7. Characteristics of various local anesthetic agents used for spinal anesthesia

Local anesthetic agent and dose	Mean peak sensory block height	Mean time to 2-dermatome regression (minutes)	Mean time to complete sensory recovery (minutes)	Mean time to ambulation (minutes)	Mean time to voiding (minutes)
Chloroprocaine 30 to 60 mg[13,19]	T8 to T2	43–57	98 to 132	100 to 133	100 to 141
Lidocaine 40 to 60 mg[12,13]	T8	73	126 to 152	134	134 to 245
Mepivacaine 30 to 80 mg[12,41]	T9 to T4	73–96	158 to 203	180 to 242	180 to 252
Bupivacaine isobaric 7.5 to 10 mg[16,19]	T9 to T7	74–90	191	191	191 to 312
Bupivacaine hyperbaric 3.5 to 15 mg[18,42]	T9 to T4	47–151	74 to 343	110 to 395	110 to 428
Ropivacaine 8 to 22.5 mg[16,17]	T10 to T7	76–98	130 to 192	125 to 195	165 to 285

Box 8-1. Potential adverse effects of spinal anesthesia of concern to ambulatory patients
- Urinary retention
- Postdural puncture headache
- Transient neurologic symptoms
- Lack of prolonged postoperative analgesia

The local anesthetic solution should be selected based on the onset, duration, and other characteristics of the agent (Table 8-8). Unlike with spinal anesthesia, local anesthetic baricity and patient position have a minor effect on the spread of epidurally administered solutions. The mass and volume of local anesthetic injected as well as certain patient factors can affect onset, duration, quality, and cephalocaudad spread of epidural solutions.

Short-acting opioid adjuvants can be used to enhance the quality of anesthesia, and bicarbonate can be used to speed onset. Epinephrine increases duration, improves the quality of anesthesia, and limits systemic absorption of the local anesthetic. Whereas clonidine (100–200 μg) can also prolong duration of anesthesia, its use in outpatients is limited by its side effects.

Advantages of epidural anesthesia include ease of performance and the ability to prolong intraoperative anesthesia. Disadvantages of epidural compared to spinal anesthesia include a slower onset and a less reliable block. Despite the potential for prolonged postoperative analgesia, this technique has limited application for outpatients. Potential adverse effects include backache, urinary retention, and postdural puncture headache; however, local anesthetic toxicity, serious neurologic, or infectious complications are rare.[20]

Table 8-8. Characteristics of various local anesthetic agents used for epidural anesthesia

Agent and dose	Time to 2-segment regression (minutes)	Duration of sensory anesthesia (minutes)	Time to hospital discharge (minutes)
3% 2-chloroprocaine 20 to 22 mL[43,44]		73 to 133	130 to 269
1.5%–2% lidocaine 10 to 22 mL[43–45]	101.5	182	191 to 284
1.5%–2% mepivacaine 10 to 20 mL[43,45]	114.2	247	357
0.5%–0.75% bupivacaine		300–460	
0.5%–1% ropivacaine		240–420	

Caudal anesthesia

This technique involves injection of local anesthetic through the sacral hiatus into the sacral epidural space (Figure 8-1). Bilateral lower extremity and abdominal anesthesia is produced. Clinical applications include anorectal, perineal, genital, and lower extremity procedures. Caudal anesthesia is particularly well

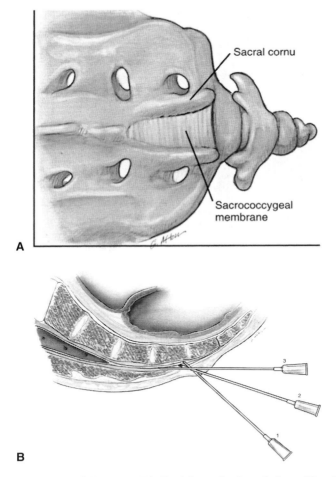

Figure 8-1. A) Sacral Anatomy; B) Caudal anesthesia technique. The skin is penetrated at a 60–90 degree angle (1), and the needle is redirected (2) and advanced 1–1.5 mm within the spinal canal (3). From Miller RD[46] with permission of publisher Elsevier Churchill Livingstone.

suited for pediatric patients. The patient should be placed in the lateral decubitus position with the hips and knees flexed. A 21- to 23-gauge needle should be inserted at 45 degrees to the skin and advanced through the sacral hiatus. A change in resistance can be appreciated as the sacrococcygeal membrane is penetrated and the caudal canal is entered. At this point, the needle should be flattened and advanced no more than 1–1.5 cm in order to avoid dural penetration. After negative aspiration, a volume of 0.75–1 mL/kg of local anesthetic should be injected incrementally to produce a mid- to upper-thoracic block. Risks include intrathecal injection and local anesthetic toxicity. Prolonged lower extremity motor block results; consequently, to prevent falls and injuries, ambulation should be avoided until block resolution occurs.

Combined spinal epidural anesthesia

This technique involves localization of the epidural space, insertion of a spinal needle through the Tuohy epidural needle to perform a spinal block, and subsequent threading of an epidural catheter into the epidural space. The use of this modality should be limited to the lumbar spine below the level of termination of the spinal cord. As such, clinical applications are confined to lower extremity, urogenital, and lower abdominal procedures. Rapid onset of surgical anesthesia is obtained from the spinal injection, and the epidural catheter provides the potential to prolong the duration of anesthesia. The goal is to minimize the extent and duration of motor block, thereby hastening recovery and discharge. For example, a small dose of local anesthetic can be given intrathecally (i.e., 5 mg of bupivacaine plus 15 μg of fentanyl); subsequently, epidural supplementation (i.e., with chloroprocaine) can be administered if the quality or duration of the spinal block proves inadequate.

Upper extremity peripheral nerve blocks

Interscalene brachial plexus block

The brachial plexus is composed of the C5 to T1 nerve roots (Figure 8-2). The interscalene block produces brachial plexus anesthesia following the injection of local anesthetic in close proximity to the C6 nerve root.

Figure 8-3 depicts the technique of interscalene block initially described by Winnie. The patient should be positioned supine with the head turned away from the side to be blocked and the arm in adduction. The skin should be disinfected and a local anesthetic skin wheal placed. The lateral border of the sternocleidomastoid muscle should be located and the palpating fingers rolled posteriorly into the groove between the anterior and middle scalene muscles. A 25- to 50-mm insulated needle should be inserted in the interscalene groove at the level of C6 (the cricoid cartilage) and directed slightly posterior and caudad. A nerve stimulator can be used to elicit contraction of the biceps muscle; subsequently,

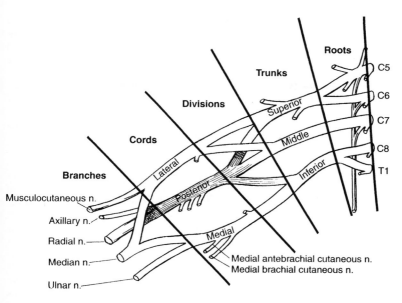

Figure 8-2. Roots, trunks, divisions, cords, and branches of the brachial plexus. n, nerve. From Miller RD[46] with permission of publisher Elsevier Churchill Livingstone.

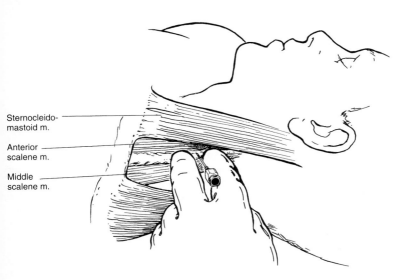

Figure 8-3. Interscalene brachial plexus block—Winnie's technique. m, muscle. From Miller RD[46] with permission of publisher Elsevier Churchill Livingstone.

a volume of 30–40 mL of local anesthetic solution should be injected incrementally after multiple negative aspirations for blood.

This technique produces excellent anesthesia and analgesia for shoulder and upper arm procedures. Interscalene block may not provide complete anesthesia of the inferior nerve roots of the brachial plexus (i.e., C8 and T1). Consequently, this block may not be well suited to distal upper extremity surgical procedures. In addition, the medial aspect of the upper arm innervated by the intercostobrachial nerve (from T2) is spared. Individual T1 and T2 paravertebral blocks can provide anesthesia of the medial upper arm and are useful additions to an interscalene block when extensive shoulder surgery is performed (i.e., shoulder arthroplasty).

When used for open rotator cuff repair, interscalene block can decrease pain scores, reduce opioid consumption, and lower the incidence of nausea and sore throat when compared to general anesthesia and opioid analgesia.[1] In addition, the peripheral nerve block can reduce both the time to home-readiness and the rate of unanticipated hospital admission. Continuous ambulatory interscalene block can further prolong these benefits.[6] Preliminary data also suggest that there can be a beneficial effect on postoperative cognitive function and quality of sleep.[21]

Phrenic nerve, cervical sympathetic ganglion, and recurrent laryngeal nerve blocks are commonly associated with interscalene block. This can produce dyspnea, Horner's syndrome (ptosis, miosis, and anhydrosis), and hoarseness, respectively. Symptoms are usually mild and rarely prevent same-day discharge of healthy ambulatory patients. Nevertheless, patients with more serious underlying pulmonary disease can be significantly affected by the transient reduction in lung volumes by up to 40% which typically occurs in association with a phrenic nerve block.[22] Serious complications such as vertebral artery injection, subarachnoid or epidural block, and nerve injury are rare when the proper technique is used.[23]

Supraclavicular brachial plexus block

The roots of the brachial plexus combine to form the superior, middle, and inferior trunks (Figure 8-2). A supraclavicular block involves injection of local anesthetic in close proximity to the trunks of the brachial plexus.

Figure 8-4 depicts the subclavian perivascular technique of supraclavicular block described by Winnie. The patient should be positioned supine with the head turned away from the side to be blocked. The skin should be disinfected and a subcutaneous wheal of local anesthetic administered. In the subclavian perivascular approach, a 50-mm needle should be inserted in the interscalene groove approximately 1 cm cephalad to the clavicle and superolateral to the subclavian artery. The needle should be advanced toward the ipsilateral axilla in a plane parallel to the bed. A nerve stimulator can be employed to elicit a distal upper extremity motor response (i.e., finger flexion or finger extension); subsequently, 30 mL of local anesthetic solution should be injected incrementally after multiple negative aspirations for blood.

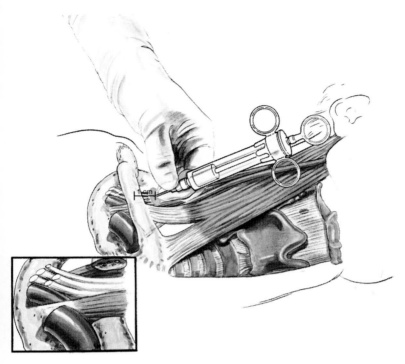

Figure 8-4. Supraclavicular brachial plexus block—subclavian perivascular approach of Winnie. From Brown DL[47] with permission of publisher W.B. Saunders Company.

The supraclavicular block can be used for plastic, orthopedic, and vascular procedures of the elbow, forearm, wrist, and hand. This block alone may not be sufficient for shoulder surgery since the axillary nerve is inconsistently anesthetized; however, more complete shoulder anesthesia can be obtained with the addition of a superficial cervical plexus block. A separate intercostobrachial nerve block can be performed for anesthesia of the medial upper arm sufficient for tourniquet application. This can be accomplished with a subcutaneous injection of 5–10 mL of local anesthetic deposited in a ring medial to the pulsation of the axillary artery at the level of the axilla. The supraclavicular block is performed where the brachial plexus is most compact; consequently, it produces reliable, rapid onset anesthesia and is particularly useful in a fast-paced ambulatory surgery center.

Although pneumothorax can occur, several large series[24,25] have shown a 0% incidence of pneumothorax following the subclavian perivascular technique. Other complications are also rare and include hematoma, intravascular injection of local anesthetic, and nerve injury.[24]

Infraclavicular brachial plexus block

As the brachial plexus passes over the lateral aspect of the first rib, the trunks branch to form the divisions that subsequently rejoin to form the medial, lateral, and posterior cords (Figure 8-2). The infraclavicular block involves the injection of local anesthetic in close proximity to the cords of the brachial plexus as they surround the subclavian artery.

The coracoid approach to the infraclavicular nerve block is illustrated in Figure 8-5. The patient should be positioned supine with the head in the neutral position. The skin should be disinfected and a subcutaneous wheal of local anesthetic administered. Using the coracoid approach, a 75- to 100-mm needle should be inserted 2 cm inferior and 2 cm medial to the coracoid process. The needle should be advanced perpendicular to the skin, and a nerve stimulator should be used to produce a distal upper extremity motor response (i.e., finger flexion with medial cord stimulation or finger extension with posterior cord stimulation). A volume of 30–40 mL of local anesthetic solution should be injected incrementally after multiple negative aspirations for blood.

This technique can be used for procedures of the elbow, forearm, wrist, and hand. The axillary nerve may be spared as this nerve exits the brachial plexus sheath proximal to the level of the infraclavicular block. In addition, supplemental block of the intercostobrachial nerve should be added for anesthesia of the medial arm sufficient for tourniquet application.

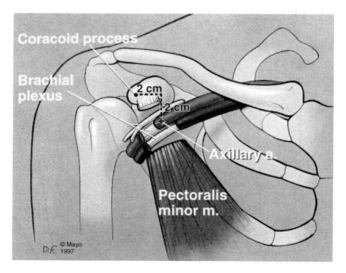

Figure 8-5. Infraclavicular brachial plexus block—coracoid approach. a, artery; m, muscle. From Wilson et al.[48] with permission from *Anesthesia & Analgesia*, published by Lippincott Williams & Wilkins.

When used for ambulatory hand and wrist surgery, the infraclavicular block can lower pain scores, reduce the incidence of postoperative nausea, vomiting, and sore throat, and hasten the achievement of discharge criteria when compared to general anesthesia with opioid analgesia.[2] Continuous ambulatory infraclavicular block may extend these advantages and can enhance day-time alertness while reducing night-time sleep disturbances on the day of surgery.[7] Additional advantages of the infraclavicular block include the ability to perform the block with the patient's head in neutral position as well as a relatively clean and immobile continuous catheter site. Complications may include vascular puncture due to the close proximity of the subclavian artery and the rare risk of pneumothorax and nerve injury.

Axillary brachial plexus block

The cords of the brachial plexus combine to form the axillary, musculocutaneous, median, radial, and ulnar nerves (Figure 8-2). The cutaneous distribution of these nerves is depicted in Figure 8-6. The axillary brachial plexus block involves injection of local anesthetic in close proximity to these terminal branches of the brachial plexus.

The patient should be positioned supine with the arm abducted and the elbow flexed. The skin should be disinfected and a wheal of local anesthetic placed subcutaneously. The axillary artery can be palpated high in the axilla (Figure 8-7). With the arm in this position, a 25- to 50-mm needle should be advanced superior, posterior, or inferior to the artery to elicit a median (finger flexion), radial (finger extension), or ulnar (supination) nerve motor response, respectively. The presence of fibrous septae within the axillary sheath can lead to nerve sparing if only a single injection of local anesthetic is carried out. As such, some practitioners advocate performing separate injections of multiple nerves (i.e., median and radial) to enhance block success and onset time. The musculocutaneous nerve exits the sheath proximal to the level of this block; consequently, a separate musculocutaneous nerve block should be performed. This can be achieved with a field block in which 5–10 mL of local anesthetic solution is injected into the substance of the coracobrachialis muscle. Alternatively, an insulated needle and nerve stimulator can be used to locate the musculocutaneous nerve (biceps contraction and elbow flexion) following which local anesthetic is injected. A separate intercostobrachial nerve block should also be performed to supplement an axillary brachial plexus block. A total volume of 40–50 mL of local anesthetic solution should be divided between the three to five injections required for a complete axillary brachial plexus block. Anesthesia of the elbow and the distal upper extremity is obtained; consequently, this block can be used for procedures of the elbow, forearm, wrist, and hand.

When used for ambulatory hand surgery, the axillary brachial plexus block can reduce pain scores, opioid consumption, and postoperative nausea and vomiting when compared to general anesthesia with opioid analgesia.[3] In addition, patients who receive this peripheral nerve block may achieve discharge criteria sooner. Continuous axillary blocks may be used to extend the duration of postoperative analgesia at home.[26]

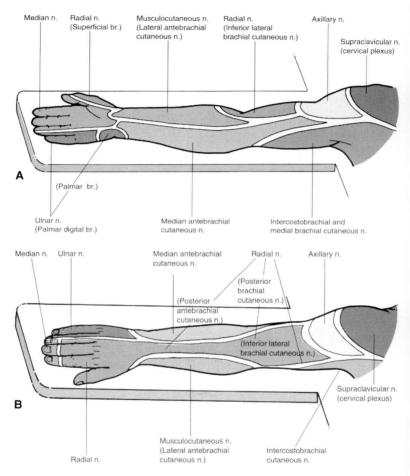

Figure 8-6. Anterior (A) and posterior (B) upper extremity peripheral nerve innervation. br, branch; n, nerve. From Brown DL[47] with permission of publisher W.B. Saunders Company.

The advantages of the axillary block include a readily identifiable pulsatile landmark, ease of performance, and low incidence of serious side effects. The needle insertion site in the axilla is accessible and externally compressible. Compression of the nerve block site can reduce the severity of hematoma when accidental or intended vascular puncture occurs or when this block is performed in patients with mild systemic coagulopathy.

Disadvantages of this block include the need for multiple injections, the risk of toxicity due to the large dose of local anesthetic used, and the prolonged onset

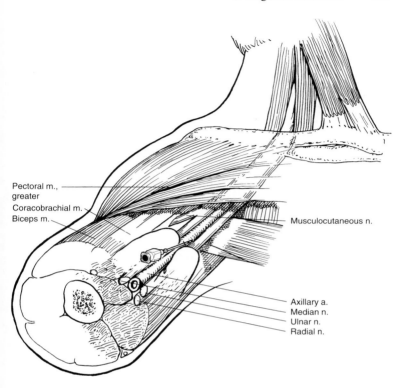

Pectoral m., greater
Coracobrachial m.
Biceps m.

Musculocutaneous n.

Axillary a.
Median n.
Ulnar n.
Radial n.

Figure 8-7. Axillary brachial plexus block technique. a, artery; m, muscle; n, nerve. From Miller RD[46] with permission of publisher Elsevier Churchill Livingstone.

time. Dislodgement and the maintenance of sterility are concerns when continuous axillary catheters are employed.

Distal upper extremity nerve blocks

The ulnar, median, and radial nerves can be blocked at the elbow and at the wrist. In combination, these blocks can provide excellent anesthesia for hand and finger surgery when a tourniquet is not required. In addition, individual nerve blocks may be valuable for supplementation of an incomplete brachial plexus block.

At the elbow, the median nerve is slightly medial to the brachial artery and the radial nerve courses more laterally between the brachialis and brachioradialis

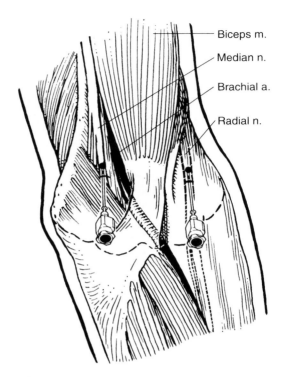

Figure 8-8. Technique of median and radial nerve blocks at the elbow. a, artery; m, muscle; n, nerve. From Miller RD[46] with permission of publisher Elsevier Churchill Livingstone.

muscles (Figure 8-8). To minimize the incidence of nerve injury after median and radial nerve block, a small volume of dilute local anesthetic should be used. The ulnar nerve is located in the ulnar groove at the elbow; however, due to the high risk of nerve injury, nerve block should rarely be performed here. At the wrist, the ulnar nerve is found lateral to the tendon of the flexor carpi ulnaris muscle and medial to the ulnar artery; the median nerve runs between the tendons of the palmaris longus and the flexor carpi radialis; and the radial nerve consists of subcutaneous branches that travel along the radial aspect of the wrist (Figure 8-9).

Intravenous regional anesthesia

This technique, also termed the Bier block, produces anesthesia following diffusion of local anesthetic from the venous system toward the nerves that run

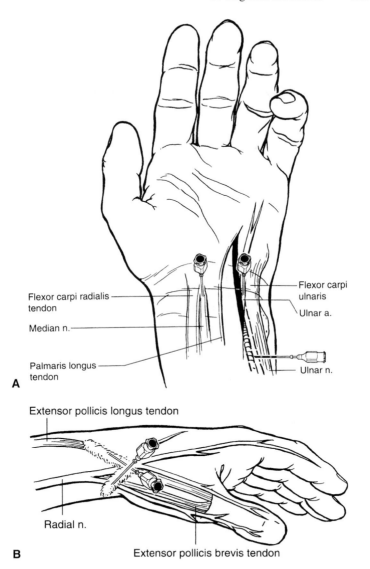

Figure 8-9. (A) Technique of median and ulnar nerve blocks at the wrist. (B) Technique of radial nerve block at the wrist. a, artery; n, nerve. From Miller RD[46] with permission of publisher Elsevier Churchill Livingstone.

close to the veins of the arm. A 22-gauge intravenous cannula should be placed in the operative hand and a double tourniquet on the upper arm. The arm should be exsanguinated using elevation, an Esmarch bandage, and the tourniquet. The proximal tourniquet should be inflated 100 mm Hg above the patient's systolic blood pressure and its integrity verified by the absence of a palpable radial artery pulse. Subsequently, an intravenous injection of 3–4 mg/kg of 0.5% lidocaine should be performed. With the onset of tourniquet pain at 30–45 minutes, the distal tourniquet can be inflated and the proximal tourniquet released. When the surgery is finished and when at least 30 minutes have elapsed since the injection of local anesthetic, the tourniquet can be sequentially deflated. This technique can be used for procedures of the forearm, wrist, and hand. The advantage of this technique includes the ease of performance. Its use is restricted by the time constraints imposed by the tourniquet as there should be no more than 120 minutes of limb ischemia. There is a risk of local anesthetic toxicity with improper tourniquet application or accidental tourniquet deflation. Proper tourniquet fit can be difficult to achieve in obese patients because the proximal arm of these patients is often conically shaped and not well suited to a cylindrically shaped tourniquet. Finally, no long-lasting postoperative analgesia is provided by this technique.

Lower extremity peripheral nerve blocks

Lumbar plexus block (posterior approach)

The L1 to L4 nerve roots combine to form the lumbar plexus and its terminal branches: the femoral, lateral femoral cutaneous, and obturator nerves (Figure 8-10). The cutaneous projection of these nerves and the sensory innervation of the lower extremity are depicted in Figure 8-11. The lumbar plexus block involves injection of local anesthetic close to the proximal part of the lumbar plexus in a paravertebral location.

The patient should be placed in the lateral decubitus position with the side to be blocked uppermost. The skin should be disinfected and a wheal of local anesthetic placed at the site of needle insertion. A line should be drawn through the posterior superior iliac spine, parallel to the long axis of the spine. A 100-mm needle should be inserted at the point where this line intersects the intercristal line. The needle should be directed slightly medial and advanced to contact the transverse process of the L4 vertebral body. This serves as a depth marker, and the needle should subsequently be redirected caudally and advanced between the transverse processes of L4 and L5. A nerve stimulator should be used to locate the lumbar plexus as it courses near the psoas muscle. Knee extension should be sought at a current of 0.5 mA, and 25–30 mL of local anesthetic solution should be injected incrementally after multiple negative aspirations for blood.

This nerve block will produce anesthesia of the three terminal branches of the lumbar plexus. This will result in sensory anesthesia of the anterolaterome-dial thigh and medial calf and motor block of the hip flexors, quadriceps, and

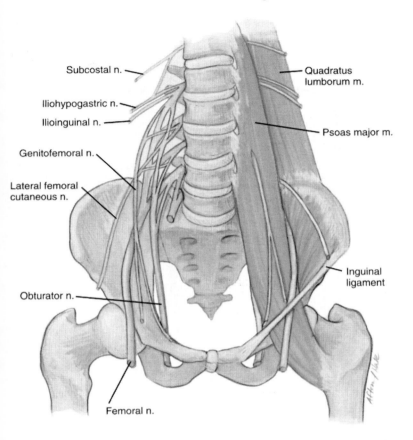

Figure 8-10. Location and components of the lumbar plexus. m, muscle; n, nerve. From Miller RD[46] with permission of publisher Elsevier Churchill Livingstone.

thigh adductor muscles. This block can be used for hip arthroscopy in conjunction with T11–12 paravertebral blocks. The lumbar plexus block can be combined with a sciatic nerve block to provide anesthesia for knee surgery such as arthroscopy or ligament reconstruction as well as for thigh tourniquet anesthesia. When used alone, the lumbar plexus block is effective for procedures of the anterior thigh such as muscle biopsy.

When performed with a sciatic nerve block for knee arthroscopy, a lumbar plexus block can reduce pain scores, lower the incidence of nausea and sore throat, and hasten the time until discharge criteria are achieved when compared to general anesthesia with opioid analgesia.[4]

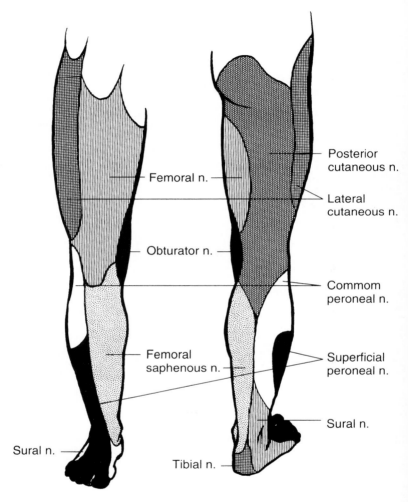

Figure 8-11. Lower extremity proximal and distal innervation. n, nerve. From Miller RD[46] with permission of publisher Elsevier Churchill Livingstone.

Hip flexor weakness can result from a lumbar plexus block, and early postoperative ambulation with a walker or crutches may be difficult for some outpatients. In addition, an epidural block can result from epidural spread of local anesthetic and this can significantly delay hospital discharge. Other serious complications occur in 1.3%[20] of patients and may include local anesthetic toxicity, retroperitoneal hematoma, nerve injury, and renal damage.

Femoral nerve block

This technique involves the injection of local anesthetic close to the femoral nerve below the inguinal ligament. At this level, the femoral nerve courses lateral to both the femoral vein and artery (Figure 8-12).

The patient should be positioned supine and the femoral artery should be palpated in the groin. The skin should be disinfected and a subcutaneous wheal of local anesthetic placed at the site of needle insertion. A 50- to 75-mm needle should be inserted lateral to the pulsation of the femoral artery at the level of the inguinal crease and advanced in a cranial direction. A nerve stimulator should be used to elicit quadriceps contraction at 0.5 mA, and 20 mL of local anesthetic solution should be injected incrementally after multiple negative aspirations for blood.

This nerve block can achieve sensory anesthesia of the anterior thigh, anterior knee, and medial calf as well as motor block of the quadriceps muscles. Associated block of the lateral femoral cutaneous nerve can occur and lead to sensory anesthesia of the lateral thigh. Accompanying obturator nerve block is infrequent, and consequently a "3-in-1" block is rarely achieved.[27] Despite the unilateral lower extremity weakness that results, most patients can ambulate and can achieve discharge criteria after a femoral nerve block. When compared to the more proximal lumbar plexus block, the femoral nerve block can retain hip flexor activity and this can facilitate the use of crutches or a walker. Other advantages of the femoral nerve block may include ease of performance and compressibility of the site.

Whereas femoral nerve block can provide effective analgesia following knee arthroscopy, no advantage was found compared to an intra-articular injection of local anesthetic.[28] When more painful anterior cruciate ligament reconstruction is considered, a femoral nerve block can provide superior analgesia compared to opioid analgesia[5] and intra-articular local anesthetic.[29]

A femoral nerve catheter and continuous infusion of local anesthetic can prolong postoperative analgesia. Catheter dislodgement and insertion site infection are potential drawbacks of continuous femoral nerve blocks; however, serious complications are rare (less than 0.03%).[20]

Fascia iliaca block

The fascia iliaca block involves injection of local anesthetic below the fascia iliaca in an attempt to produce a spread of solution to the lumbar plexus. Uses are the same as for the femoral nerve block. Advantages of the fascia iliaca block include the ease of performance. The patient should be positioned supine, the skin disinfected, and a wheal of local anesthetic placed at the site of needle insertion. A line representing the inguinal ligament should be drawn from the anterior superior iliac spine to the pubic tubercle and divided in three. A 22-gauge, 25- to 50-mm needle should be inserted 0.5–1 cm inferior to the junction of the lateral third and medial two thirds of the inguinal ligament. The needle should be advanced perpendicular to the skin, and loss of resistance can be felt

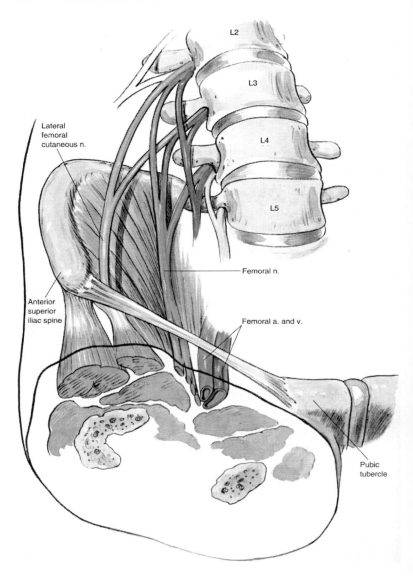

Figure 8-12. Femoral nerve anatomy at the inguinal ligament. a, artery; n, nerve; v, vein. From Brown DL[47] with permission of publisher W.B. Saunders Company.

twice as the needle passes through the fascia lata and the fascia iliaca. A volume of 30 mL of local anesthetic solution must be injected incrementally after multiple negative aspirations for blood.

Proximal sciatic nerve block

The sciatic nerve is formed from the L4 to S3 nerve roots. It is functionally and anatomically divided into the posterior cutaneous nerve of the thigh, the common peroneal nerve, and the tibial nerve. A proximal sciatic nerve block involves the injection of local anesthetic solution near the sciatic nerve in the gluteal region between the ischial tuberosity and the greater trochanter.

The patient should be placed in the lateral decubitus position with the operative leg uppermost. The dependent leg should be positioned straight and the nondependent leg should be flexed at the hip and knee. The skin should be disinfected and a wheal of local anesthetic administered at the site of needle entry. A line should be drawn from the posterior superior iliac spine to the midpoint of the greater trochanter (Figure 8-13). A perpendicular line should be extended caudally from the midpoint of this line. An additional line can be drawn from the posterior superior iliac spine to the sacral hiatus (as described by Labat) and a 100-mm needle inserted where this line intersects the perpendicular line. The

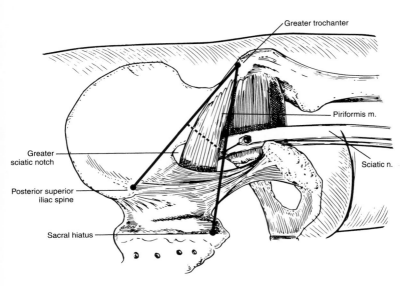

Figure 8-13. Anatomic landmarks for the posterior approach to the sciatic nerve block—Labat's technique. m, muscle; n, nerve. From Miller RD[46] with permission of publisher Elsevier Churchill Livingstone.

needle should be advanced perpendicular to all planes and a nerve stimulator used to elicit plantar flexion, dorsiflexion, toe flexion, toe extension, or foot inversion at 0.5 mA. A volume of 15–25 mL of local anesthetic solution should be injected incrementally after multiple negative aspirations for blood.

The sciatic nerve block produces sensory anesthesia of the posterior thigh, posterior knee, anteroposterolateral calf, ankle, and foot. It results in motor block of the hamstrings, the muscles involved in ankle movement, and the toe flexors and extensors.

The addition of a lumbar plexus or femoral nerve block to a sciatic nerve block can produce lower extremity anesthesia suitable for knee surgery or thigh tourniquet application. A combined femoral and sciatic nerve block can reduce pain following knee arthroscopy when compared to general anesthesia.[30] Furthermore, the addition of a sciatic nerve block to a femoral nerve block can enhance analgesia and reduce the incidence of unanticipated hospital admission following more invasive knee ligament repair when compared to femoral nerve block alone.[5]

The sciatic nerve block can be used with a femoral or saphenous nerve block for procedures of the ankle (i.e., ankle arthroscopy, fusion, or arthrodesis), foot (i.e., fracture reduction and hallux valgus repair), or toes. The saphenous nerve is the terminal branch of the femoral nerve. It provides sensation to the medial calf and can be blocked by subcutaneous infiltration medial to the tibial tuberosity or by injection of local anesthetic deep to the sartorius muscle at the level of the proximal patella.

The proximal sciatic nerve block produces more extensive lower extremity weakness than block of the sciatic nerve in the popliteal fossa. Consequently, ambulation is more significantly affected following a proximal sciatic nerve block. Serious complications are rare (less than 0.05%).[20]

Distal sciatic nerve block (popliteal fossa approach)

The sciatic nerve divides into the common peroneal and tibial nerves in the popliteal fossa. The popliteal sciatic nerve block is achieved by injection of local anesthetic near the sciatic nerve as it courses behind the knee at a point proximal to division into its terminal branches.

The patient should be positioned prone with the operative knee slightly flexed. The skin should be disinfected and a wheal of local anesthetic placed at the site of needle entry. The margins of the superior half of the popliteal fossa must be identified—the biceps femoris muscle laterally and semitendinosus/semimembranosus muscles medially (Figure 8-14). A 50- to 75-mm needle should be inserted superolaterally in the popliteal fossa, 7–10 cm proximal to the popliteal crease and 1 cm lateral to the midpoint of the fossa. The needle should be advanced in a cephalad direction and a nerve stimulator used to elicit toe flexion or extension or foot inversion at 0.5 mA. A volume of 40 mL of local anesthetic solution should be injected incrementally after multiple negative aspirations for blood.

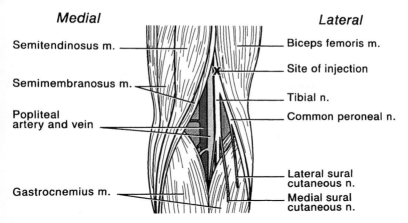

Figure 8-14. Popliteal sciatic nerve block technique. m, muscle; n, nerve. From Benzon et al.[49] with permission from *Anesthesiology* published by Lippincott Williams & Wilkins.

Sensory anesthesia is produced in the distribution of the common peroneal and tibial nerves. This correlates to the posterior knee, anteroposterolateral calf, ankle, and foot. A supplementary femoral or saphenous nerve block can be used to produce comprehensive anesthesia distal to the knee. The popliteal sciatic nerve block provides motor block to the muscles involved in ankle movement as well as the toe flexors and extensors. The hamstring muscles are spared and so ambulation should be less affected than with the proximal sciatic nerve block.

The popliteal sciatic nerve block can provide excellent anesthesia for foot surgery (i.e., fracture reduction and forefoot reconstruction). A continuous popliteal sciatic nerve block can prolong postoperative analgesia and reduce the incidence of unanticipated hospital admissions when compared to opioid analgesia for ambulatory foot and ankle surgery.[8] Serious complications from the popliteal sciatic nerve block are rare.[8,20,31]

Distal lower extremity nerve blocks

The ankle block is the most common application of distal lower extremity nerve blocks. This block involves injection of local anesthetic close to the terminal nerves of the lower extremity at the ankle. At this level, the saphenous nerve is the terminal branch of the femoral nerve. The superficial and deep peroneal nerves are from the common peroneal nerve in the sciatic system. The tibial nerve is also from the sciatic system. The sural nerve is formed from branches of the common peroneal and tibial nerves in the sciatic system.

The patient should be positioned supine and the skin disinfected. Due to the risk of distal ischemia, epinephrine-containing local anesthetic should be avoided. The saphenous nerve block can be performed with subcutaneous injection of 5 mL of local anesthetic solution anterior to the medial malleolus, close to the saphenous vein. The superficial peroneal nerve block can be carried out with a subcutaneous injection of 10 mL of local anesthetic solution in a ring around the anterior aspect of the ankle from the medial to the lateral malleolus. The deep peroneal nerve block can be executed with an injection of 5 mL of local anesthetic solution lateral to the pulsation of the dorsalis pedis artery. The tibial nerve block can be done with infiltration of 5–10 mL of local anesthetic solution posterior to the pulsation of the tibial artery behind the medial malleolus. A nerve stimulator can be used to localize this nerve by eliciting toe flexion. A sural nerve block can be accomplished with infiltration of 5 mL of local anesthetic posterior to the lateral malleolus. All or selected nerves can be blocked according to the location of the surgical procedure.

Advantages of the ankle block include ease of performance and preservation of lower extremity motor function. Drawbacks include a lack of tourniquet anesthesia and the inability to prolong analgesia by catheter techniques. Serious complications are rare.

Continuous ambulatory peripheral nerve blocks

Continuous peripheral nerve blocks using catheters can extend the duration of postoperative analgesia beyond that obtained with single-injection blocks. As a result, opioid use and opioid-related side effects can be deferred for a longer period of time and often avoided.[6-8] In addition, continuous peripheral nerve blocks may enable the ambulatory management of surgical procedures that previously required prolonged hospital admission for adequate postoperative pain control.

Dilute local anesthetic can be used in order to reduce the risk of systemic toxicity as well as to minimize motor block. The safety profile of 0.2% ropivacaine makes it a suitable drug for this purpose. A continuous infusion of local anesthetic (i.e., 5–8 mL/hour) can be coupled with intermittent patient-controlled boluses (i.e., 2 mL every 15–20 minutes) in order to provide continuous analgesia with the ability to supplement if required. Disposable pumps are frequently used and mitigate concerns about transmission of infection between patients. Elastomeric or more sophisticated electronic disposable infusion pumps are available for ambulatory use. Elastomeric pumps are simple to use and inexpensive. The potential advantages of the electronic pumps include greater accuracy and reprogrammability.[32]

Appropriate patient selection and education is crucial for the success of ambulatory continuous peripheral nerve blocks. Patients must have a reliable caregiver present for the duration of the local anesthetic infusion. In addition, patients and their caregivers must demonstrate a thorough understanding of the issues important for the safe use of home perineural infusions. They must be aware of the sensorimotor effects of regional anesthesia and their consequences. For example, they must recognize the importance of padding and protecting the insensate extremity in order to avoid nerve injury. In addition, they must understand that weight-bearing on a numb lower extremity is strictly prohibited due to the risk of falling. Patients with lower extremity nerve blocks must demonstrate competency ambulating and negotiating stairs with a walker or crutches prior to discharge home. Furthermore, it is imperative that patients and their caregivers appreciate the risk, signs, and symptoms of local anesthetic toxicity and the actions to take should this complication occur. As such, patients and their caregivers must comprehend basic ambulatory infusion pump functions, including how to stop the infusion. It must be emphasized that maintaining catheter site cleanliness and sterility is important in order to reduce the likelihood of infection. Patients and caregivers must receive instructions for removal and disposal of the catheter and pump. A plan must be established for the use of supplemental oral opioid analgesia should breakthrough pain occur. Finally, adequate medical support must be available to patients with ambulatory perineural infusions. All patients must be provided with telephone and/or pager number(s) to contact an anesthesiologist in case of emergency. In addition, a health care worker must perform daily telephone follow-up to ensure patient well-being.

Truncal peripheral nerve blocks

Paravertebral nerve block

A paravertebral nerve block involves injection of local anesthetic in close proximity to a segmental spinal nerve as it courses through the paravertebral space. The paravertebral space is a wedge-shaped region on either side of the vertebral column bounded at each segmental level by the parietal pleura, vertebral body, and the superior costotransverse ligament that extends from the transverse process above to the rib below.

The patient can be positioned sitting, prone, or lateral decubitus with the side to be blocked uppermost. The levels to be blocked should be chosen according to the surgical procedure performed, bearing in mind that the thoracic spinal nerves exit below their respective transverse processes, which, in turn, are located at the same horizontal level as the spinous process of the vertebra above. An 8-cm, 22-gauge Tuohy needle should be attached to extension tubing and a syringe containing local anesthetic. This skin should be disinfected and a local anesthetic skin wheal placed at the sites of needle entry. The needle should be inserted 2.5 cm lateral to the cephalad border of the appropriate spinous process (i.e., needle inserted beside T5 spinous process to effect block of T6 spinal nerve). The needle should be advanced perpendicular to all planes until the transverse process is contacted. Subsequently, the needle should be withdrawn and redirected caudad to the transverse process (Figure 8-15). The needle should be advanced approximately 1 cm deep to the depth of the transverse process until a change in resistance is appreciated as the superior costotransverse ligament is pierced. Aspiration must be performed to rule out intrathecal or intravascular placement; subsequently, a volume of 3–5 mL of local anesthetic solution can be injected at each thoracic level or 5–7 mL injected at each lumbar level.

Paravertebral blocks can produce unilateral or bilateral thoracic or lumbar anesthesia according to the levels blocked. Block with long-acting local

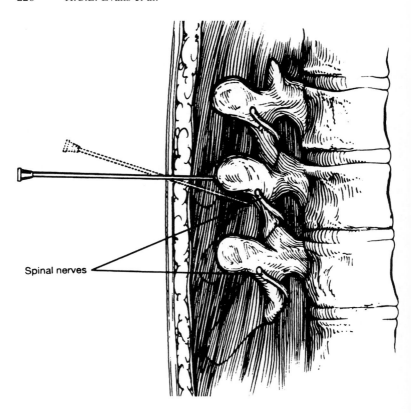

Figure 8-15. Paravertebral nerve block technique. From Greengrass et al.[50] Reprinted with permission from Elsevier.

anesthetic can provide up to 23 hours of analgesia.[33] When used for breast biopsy or lumpectomy, blocks should be performed at the level of the lesion, one level above and one level below. Mastectomy requires T2 to T6 blocks on the affected side and the addition of T1 when an axillary dissection is performed. Bilateral blocks from T9-T11 are required for umbilical hernia repair, whereas unilateral T11-L2 blocks are effective for inguinal hernia repair. Paravertebral blocks of T1-T3 can be used with an interscalene block to provide complete shoulder anesthesia, T11-T12 blocks can be used to supplement a lumbar plexus block for hip surgery, and T11-L1 can achieve an effective block for iliac crest bone harvesting.

Paravertebral blocks have been compared to general anesthesia with opioid analgesia for breast surgery. The nerve blocks were associated with lower pain scores, reduced opioid consumption, decreased incidence of nausea and vomiting, shorter hospital stay, and improved arm motion.[34,35] Similar benefits were observed in studies involving patients having inguinal[36,37] and umbilical[38] hernia repair. Nevertheless, the administration of opioids either for nerve block or intraoperative sedation can mitigate some of these advantages.

In two large series, pneumothorax occurred in 0.3%–2.1% of patients.[39,40] This complication can occur postdischarge, which has obvious implications for outpatients. The risk of local anesthetic toxicity can be minimized by using a precalculated dose of local anesthetic based on the patient's weight and by adding epinephrine to the local anesthetic solution. Other potential adverse effects are extremely rare and include epidural or intrathecal injection with associated hypotension, total spinal anesthesia, or postdural puncture headache.[39,40]

Iliohypogastric and ilioinguinal nerve blocks

These nerves are branches of the lumbar plexus and can be blocked in the anterior abdominal wall as they course between the external and internal oblique muscles. The iliohypogastric nerve supplies sensation to the suprapubic area; the ilioinguinal nerve innervates the superomedial thigh and part of the genitals. Ilioinguinal and iliohypogastric nerve block can be used for analgesia following inguinal hernia, orchidopexy, and hydrocele repairs and is advantageous in its simplicity. The patient should be positioned prone, the skin disinfected, and local skin infiltration performed. A needle should be inserted 1–2 cm medial and 1–2 cm superior to the anterior superior iliac spine along a line drawn from it to the umbilicus (Figure 8-16). A loss-of-resistance can be appreciated as the needle

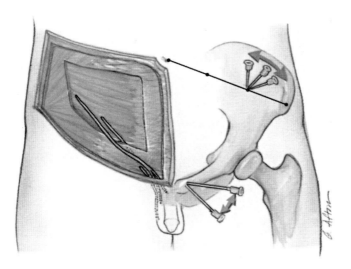

Figure 8-16. Ilioinguinal and iliohypogastric nerve block technique. From Miller RD[46] with permission of publisher Elsevier Churchill Livingstone.

pierces the external oblique muscle. After negative aspiration for blood, local anesthetic should be injected in a fan-wise manner. Side effects include inadvertent femoral nerve block, which may impair the mobility of an outpatient.

Head and neck nerve blocks

Ophthalmologic blocks

Retrobulbar block involves placement of local anesthetic inside the cone of the extraocular muscles. The peribulbar block involves deposition of local anesthetic exterior to this cone. According to the technique used, block of the nerves within the cone (optic, oculomotor, abducens, and nasociliary) or those outside the cone of extraocular muscles (lacrimal, frontal, infraorbital and trochlear) is achieved. The patient should be positioned supine and directed to look straight forward. A 23- to 25-gauge, 25-mm needle should be inserted at the inferolateral border of the orbital bone (Figure 8-17). When performing the retrobulbar block,

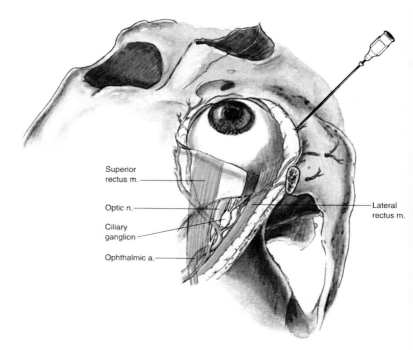

Figure 8-17. Retrobulbar (peribulbar) block technique. a, artery; m, muscle; n, nerve. From Brown DL[47] with permission of publisher W.B. Saunders Company.

the needle should initially be advanced posteriorly until it has passed the equator of the globe. The needle should then be redirected slightly posteromedially and advanced through the cone of the extraocular muscles. When performing the peribulbar block, the needle should be directed posteriorly and advanced parallel to the cone of the extraocular muscles without penetrating it. After a negative aspiration for blood and cerebrospinal fluid, a volume of 2–4 or 4–8 mL of local anesthetic can be used for the retrobulbar and peribulbar blocks, respectively. These blocks are typically supplemented with block of the facial nerve branch that supplies the orbicularis oculi muscle in order to provide complete orbital anesthesia. Risks include hematoma from ophthalmic artery penetration, brady-cardia caused by the oculocardiac reflex, globe puncture, intrathecal injection with associated total spinal anesthesia, and optic nerve damage. More recently, ophthalmologists administer topical anesthesia to the cornea, in lieu of the tra-ditional retrobulbar or peribulbar blocks, providing only sensory but not motor block to the globe.

Superficial cervical plexus block

This nerve block involves injection of local anesthetic near the superficial cervical plexus as it emerges posterior to the lateral border of the sternocleido-mastoid muscle (Figure 8-18). The patient should be positioned supine with the

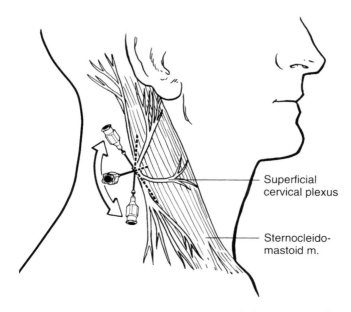

Superficial
cervical plexus

Sternocleido-
mastoid m.

Figure 8-18. Superficial cervical plexus block technique. m, muscle; From Miller RD[46] with permission of publisher Elsevier Churchill Livingstone.

head turned away from the side to be blocked. A 25-gauge needle should be used to deposit 5 mL of local anesthetic solution at the midpoint of the posterior border of the sternocleidomastoid, and an additional 5 mL should be injected subcutaneously cephalad and caudad along the posterior border of the muscle. This will achieve a sensory block of the anterolateral neck and can be useful for cervical lymph node biopsies and as a supplement to paravertebral blocks for breast surgery. Significant complications are rare, but caution should be taken to avoid penetration of the external jugular vein.

Summary

Regional anesthesia has numerous benefits for ambulatory patients. In many cases, general anesthesia can be avoided and associated side effects such as sore throat and drowsiness are reduced.[1,2,4] Peripheral nerve blocks provide excellent postoperative analgesia and can reduce opioid consumption as well as associated nausea and vomiting.[1-4,34,35] Furthermore, excellent postoperative pain control with minimal associated side effects can result in fewer nursing interventions, reduced hospital length of stay, and cost savings.[1-4,34,35] Finally, regional anesthesia and its associated benefits can lead to high patient satisfaction.

References

1. Hadzic A, Williams BA, Karaca PE, et al. For outpatient rotator cuff surgery, nerve block anesthesia provides superior same-day recovery over general anesthesia. *Anesthesiology.* 2005;102:1001–1007.

2. Hadzic A, Arliss J, Kerimoglu B, et al. A comparison of infraclavicular nerve block versus general anesthesia for hand and wrist day-case surgeries. *Anesthesiology.* 2004;101:127–132.

3. McCartney CJ, Brull R, Chan VW, et al. Early but no long-term benefit of regional compared with general anesthesia for ambulatory hand surgery. *Anesthesiology.* 2004;101:461–467.

4. Hadzic A, Karaca PE, Hobeika P, et al. Peripheral nerve blocks result in superior recovery profile compared with general anesthesia in outpatient knee arthroscopy. *Anesth Analg.* 2005;100:976–981.

5. Williams BA, Kentor ML, Vogt MT, et al. Femoral-sciatic nerve blocks for complex outpatient knee surgery are associated with less postoperative pain before same-day discharge: a review of 1,200 consecutive cases from the period 1996–1999. *Anesthesiology.* 2003;98:1206–1213.

6. Klein SM, Grant SA, Greengrass RA, et al. Interscalene brachial plexus block with a continuous catheter insertion system and a disposable infusion pump. *Anesth Analg.* 2000;91:1473–1478.

7. Ilfeld BM, Morey TE, Enneking FK. Continuous infraclavicular brachial plexus block for postoperative pain control at home: a randomized, double-blinded, placebo-controlled study. *Anesthesiology.* 2002;96:1297–1304.

8. White PF, Issioui T, Skrivanek GD, Early JS, Wakefield C. The use of a continuous popliteal sciatic nerve block after surgery involving the foot and ankle: does it improve the quality of recovery? *Anesth Analg.* 2003;97:1303–1309.

9. Klein SM, Nielsen KC, Greengrass RA, Warner DS, Martin A, Steele SM. Ambulatory discharge after long-acting peripheral nerve blockade: 2382 blocks with ropivacaine. *Anesth Analg.* 2002;94:65–70.

10. Horlocker TT, Wedel DJ, Benzon HP, et al. Regional anesthesia in the anticoagulated patient: defining the risks (the second ASRA consensus conference on neuraxial anesthesia and anticoagulation). *Reg Anesth Pain Med.* 2003;28:172–197.

11. Armstrong KP, Cherry RA. Brachial plexus anesthesia compared to general anesthesia when a block room is available. *Can J Anaesth.* 2004;51:41–44.

12. Liguori GA, Zayas VM, Chisholm MF. Transient neurologic symptoms after spinal anesthesia with mepivacaine and lidocaine. *Anesthesiology.* 1998;88:619–623.

13. Kouri ME, Kopacz DJ. Spinal 2-chloroprocaine: a comparison with lidocaine in volunteers. *Anesth Analg.* 2004;98:75–80.

14. Salazar F, Bogdanovich A, Adalia R, Chabas E, Gomar C. Transient neurologic symptoms after spinal anaesthesia using isobaric 2% mepivacaine and isobaric 2% lidocaine. *Acta Anaesthesiol Scand.* 2001;45:240–245.

15. Hodgson PS, Liu SS, Batra MS, Gras TW, Pollock JE, Neal JM. Procaine compared with lidocaine for incidence of transient neurologic symptoms. *Reg Anesth Pain Med.* 2000;25:218–222.

16. Kallio H, Snall EV, Kero MP, Rosenberg PH. A comparison of intrathecal plain solutions containing ropivacaine 20 or 15 mg versus bupivacaine 10 mg. *Anesth Analg.* 2004;99:713–717.

17. Gautier PE, De Kock M, Van Steenberge A, et al. Intrathecal ropivacaine for ambulatory surgery. A comparison between intrathecal bupivacaine and intrathecal ropivacaine for knee arthroscopy. *Anesthesiology.* 1999;91:1239–1245.

18. Liu SS, Ware PD, Allen HW, Neal JM, Pollock JE. Dose-response characteristics of spinal bupivacaine in volunteers. Clinical implications for ambulatory anesthesia. *Anesthesiology.* 1996;85:729–736.

19. Yoos JR, Kopacz DJ. Spinal 2-chloroprocaine: a comparison with small-dose bupivacaine in volunteers. *Anesth Analg.* 2005;100:566–572.

20. Auroy Y, Benhamou D, Bargues L, et al. Major complications of regional anesthesia in France: The SOS Regional Anesthesia Hotline Service. *Anesthesiology.* 2002;97: 1274–1280.

21. Nielsen KC, Greengrass RA, Pietrobon R, Klein SM, Steele SM. Continuous interscalene brachial plexus blockade provides good analgesia at home after major shoulder surgery-report of four cases. *Can J Anaesth.* 2003;50:57–61.

22. Urmey WF, Gloeggler PJ. Pulmonary function changes during interscalene brachial plexus block: effects of decreasing local anesthetic injection volume. *Reg Anesth.* 1993;18:244–249.

23. Borgeat A, Ekatodramis G, Kalberer F, Benz C. Acute and nonacute complications associated with interscalene block and shoulder surgery: a prospective study. *Anesthesiology.* 2001;95:875–880.

24. Franco CD, Vieira ZE. 1,001 subclavian perivascular brachial plexus blocks: success with a nerve stimulator. *Reg Anesth Pain Med.* 2000;25:41–46.

25. Vaghadia H, Chan V, Ganapathy S, Lui A, McKenna J, Zimmer K. A multicentre trial of ropivacaine 7.5 mg × ml(−1) vs bupivacaine 5 mg × ml(−1) for supra clavicular brachial plexus anesthesia. *Can J Anaesth.* 1999;46:946–951.

26. Rawal N, Axelsson K, Hylander J, et al. Postoperative patient-controlled local anesthetic administration at home. *Anesth Analg.* 1998;86:86–89.

27. Parkinson SK, Mueller JB, Little WL, Bailey SL. Extent of blockade with various approaches to the lumbar plexus. *Anesth Analg.* 1989;68:243–248.

28. Goranson BD, Lang S, Cassidy JD, Dust WN, McKerrell J. A comparison of three regional anaesthesia techniques for outpatient knee arthroscopy. *Can J Anaesth.* 1997;44:371–376.

29. Mulroy MF, Larkin KL, Batra MS, Hodgson PS, Owens BD. Femoral nerve block with 0.25% or 0.5% bupivacaine improves postoperative analgesia following outpatient arthroscopic anterior cruciate ligament repair. *Reg Anesth Pain Med.* 2001; 26:24–29.

30. Casati A, Cappelleri G, Berti M, Fanelli G, Di Benedetto P, Torri G. Randomized comparison of remifentanil-propofol with a sciatic-femoral nerve block for out-patient knee arthroscopy. *Eur J Anaesthesiol.* 2002;19:109–114.

31. Zaric D, Boysen K, Christiansen J, Haastrup U, Kofoed H, Rawal N. Continuous popliteal sciatic nerve block for outpatient foot surgery–a randomized, controlled trial. *Acta Anaesthesiol Scand.* 2004;48:337–341.

32. Ilfeld BM, Enneking FK. Continuous peripheral nerve blocks at home: a review. *Anesth Analg.* 2005;100:1822–1833.

33. Weltz CR, Greengrass RA, Lyerly HK. Ambulatory surgical management of breast carcinoma using paravertebral block. *Ann Surg.* 1995;222:19–26.

34. Naja MZ, Ziade MF, Lönnqvist PA. Nerve-stimulator guided paravertebral blockade vs. general anaesthesia for breast surgery: a prospective randomized trial. *Eur J Anaesthesiol.* 2003;20:897–903.

35. Klein SM, Bergh A, Steele SM, Georgiade GS, Greengrass RA. Thoracic paravertebral block for breast surgery. *Anesth Analg.* 2000;90:1402–1405.

36. Klein SM, Pietrobon R, Nielsen KC, et al. Paravertebral somatic nerve block compared with peripheral nerve blocks for outpatient inguinal herniorrhaphy. *Reg Anesth Pain Med.* 2002;27:476–480.

37. Naja MZ, el Hassan MJ, Oweidat M, Zbibo R, Ziade MF, Lönnqvist PA. Paravertebral blockade vs general anesthesia or spinal anesthesia for inguinal hernia repair. *Middle East J Anesthesiol.* 2001;16:201–210.

38. Naja Z, Ziade MF, Lönnqvist PA. Bilateral paravertebral somatic nerve block for ventral hernia repair. *Eur J Anaesthesiol.* 2002;19:197–202.

39. Naja Z, Lönnqvist PA. Somatic paravertebral nerve blockade. Incidence of failed block and complications. *Anaesthesia.* 2001;56:1184–1188.

40. Lönnqvist PA, MacKenzie J, Soni AK, Conacher ID. Paravertebral blockade. Failure rate and complications. *Anaesthesia.* 1995;50:813–815.

41. Pawlowski J, Sukhani R, Pappas AL, et al. The anesthetic and recovery profile of two doses (60 and 80 mg) of plain mepivacaine for ambulatory spinal anesthesia. *Anesth Analg.* 2000;91:580–584.

42. Ben-David B, Levin H, Solomon E, Admoni H, Vaida S. Spinal bupivacaine in ambulatory surgery: the effect of saline dilution. *Anesth Analg.* 1996;83:716–720.

43. Kopacz DJ, Mulroy MF. Chloroprocaine and lidocaine decrease hospital stay and admission rate after outpatient epidural anesthesia. *Reg Anesth.* 1990;15:19–25.

44. Neal JM, Deck JJ, Kopacz DJ, Lewis MA. Hospital discharge after ambulatory knee arthroscopy: A comparison of epidural 2-chloroprocaine versus lidocaine. *Reg Anesth Pain Med.* 2001;26:35–40.

45. Terai T, Yukioka H, Fujimori M. A double-blind comparison of lidocaine and mepivacaine during epidural anaesthesia. *Acta Anaesthesiol Scand.* 1993;37:607–610.

46. Miller RD. *Miller's Anesthesia.* 6th ed. Philadelphia, PA: Churchill Livingstone; 2005.

47. Brown DL. *Atlas of Regional Anesthesia.* 2nd ed. Philadelphia, PA: W.B. Saunders Company; 1999.

48. Wilson JL, Brown DL, Wong GY, Ehman RL, Cahill DR. Infraclavicular brachial plexus block: parasagittal anatomy important to the coracoid technique. *Anesth Analg.* 1998;87:870–873.

49. Benzon HT, Kim C, Benzon HP, et al. Correlation between evoked motor response of the sciatic nerve and sensory blockade. *Anesthesiology.* 1997;87:547–552.

50. Greengrass R, Steele S. Paravertebral blocks for breast surgery. *Techniques in Regional Anesthesia and Pain Management.* 1998;2:8–12.

9. General anesthesia

Ralph Gertler, MD
Girish P. Joshi, MB, BS, MD, FFARCSI

Patients eligible for ambulatory anesthesia must achieve discharge criteria rapidly after completion of the surgery. Therefore, the anesthetic technique used should allow early recovery and reduce common postoperative complications, in particular pain, nausea, and vomiting. The choice of anesthetic technique (i.e., general versus regional anesthesia) can be an important determinant of the recovery after ambulatory surgery.[1] A recent meta-analysis suggests that regional anesthesia techniques reduce postanesthesia care unit (PACU) use and post-operative nausea and pain; however, they do not reduce the time to home-readiness.[2] Overall, general anesthesia continues to be the mainstay of ambulatory anesthesia practice.

An ideal general anesthetic technique should provide smooth and rapid induction, optimal operating conditions, and rapid recovery with minimal (if any) side effects. In addition, it would be beneficial if the anesthetic technique allowed for "fast-tracking" (i.e., patients can be moved through the recovery process rapidly to facilitate early discharge home). Furthermore, an ideal anesthetic technique should allow the patients to return to their daily living (i.e., preoperative level of functioning) as soon as possible.

The introduction of shorter-acting intravenous anesthetics (e.g., propofol), inhaled anesthetics (e.g., desflurane and sevoflurane), and opioid analgesics (e.g., remifentanil) has allowed practitioners to more consistently achieve a recovery profile that facilitates fast-tracking. In addition, the use of brain function monitoring (or depth of hypnosis monitoring) may improve ease of titration of anesthetics and thereby facilitate the early recovery process. Furthermore, less invasive airway management (i.e., supralaryngeal) devices may also contribute to early recovery. This chapter will highlight current general anesthesia techniques that facilitate these goals.

Premedication

Benzodiazepines are often used to provide anxiolysis and sedation prior to transferring the patient to the operating room. Anxiolysis prior to surgery may reduce the perioperative stress response as well as reduce postoperative pain. Midazolam (1–2 mg, intravenous) administered just prior to induction of total intravenous general anesthesia has been used to reduce the incidence of intra-operative awareness.[3] Although there is a concern that midazolam may delay recovery, a meta-analysis using data largely from hospital facilities did not find a significant delay in discharge after premedication with midazolam.[4]

Induction of anesthesia

Intravenous

Induction of general anesthesia can be achieved by either intravenous or inhaled anesthetics. In adult patients, intravenous induction of anesthesia is most commonly used. Since the introduction of propofol, older intravenous anesthetics such as thiopental, methohexital, and etomidate are rarely used and therefore will be discussed only briefly. Commonly used doses for induction and their side effect profile are summarized in Tables 9-1 and 9-2. Numerous studies have

Table 9-1. Dosing of intravenous sedative-hypnotic agents

Drug	Dose	Indication
Midazolam	0.2–0.5 mg/kg	Induction
Propofol	1.0–2.5 mg/kg	Induction
	50–200 μg/kg per minute	TIVA maintenance
Etomidate	0.2–0.3 mg/kg	Induction
Sodium thiopental	2–5 mg/kg	Induction
Ketamine (give with	1–2 mg/kg	Induction (IV)
benzodiazepine)	3–4 mg/kg	Induction (IM)

Doses should be titrated starting with the lower recommented dose.
IM, intramuscular; IV, intravenous; TIVA, total intravenous anesthesia.

Table 9-2. Nonanesthetic side effects of intravenous hypnotic-sedative agents

Side effects (percentage)	Thiopental	Propofol	Etomidate	Ketamine
Change in blood pressure	−8	−17	−2	+28
Change in heart rate	+14	+7	+8	+33
Induction pain	0	5–10	30	0
Induction movement	0	5	20	Very little
Induction hiccups	0	5	20	Very little
Induction apnea	6	40	20	Rare
Recovery restlessness	10	5	35	Common
Recovery nausea	7–10	5	20	Common
Recovery vomiting	7–10	5	20	Common

Adapted from Evers and Maze.[47] Used with permission from Churchill Livingstone © 2004.

reported the superior recovery with propofol as compared with thiopental. Raeder and Misvaer[5] evaluated recovery profile with the use of thiopental 4 mg/kg, methohexital 2 mg/kg, and propofol 2.2 mg/kg for short (10-minute) surgical procedures and found that the recovery after thiopental was slower than methohexital and propofol at 45 minutes and remained significantly slower throughout the 4-hour postanesthesia observation. Induction of anesthesia with methohexital is associated with a higher incidence of excitatory movements and hiccupping as well as increased incidence of bronchospasm in asthmatic patients, making it a less attractive alternative compared with propofol.[6] Because of its unique recovery profile, propofol is considered the sedative-hypnotic drug of choice for induction of anesthesia in ambulatory patients, despite higher acquisition cost. The rapid redistribution and metabolic clearance of propofol facilitates a faster emergence from anesthesia and return to a baseline state. Propofol also offers an advantage over other intravenous anesthetics because of its antiemetic properties and associated euphoria on emergence.

Because it maintains hemodynamic stability, etomidate may be preferable for the induction of anesthesia in patients with significant cardiac disease. De Grood et al.[7] compared induction of anesthesia with propofol and etomidate followed by isoflurane maintenance. They found that propofol was superior with respect to early and intermediate recovery. Overall, etomidate remains an acceptable choice in selected outpatients with significant cardiac disease.

Inhalational

Inhalational induction may be used as an alternative to intravenous propofol induction if intravenous access is difficult, if the patient is "needle-phobic," or if maintenance of spontaneous ventilation is preferred (e.g., in patients with an anticipated difficult airway).[8] In addition, the use of sevoflurane for induction as well as maintenance may be less expensive than a propofol-based anesthetic. Because of its nonpungent, nonirritant properties, sevoflurane has become the inhaled anesthetic of choice for inhalational induction of anesthesia. In contrast, desflurane, because it is pungent and an irritant, is not suitable for inhalational induction. The techniques for inhalation induction with sevoflurane include progressive increases in inspired concentration (incremental induction) or use of high-inspired concentrations (vital capacity induction).[9]

Several studies have compared sevoflurane induction to propofol, with differing results. These differences might be related to the specific inhalation induction technique used. In a study in adult volunteers, induction with sevoflurane 8% (rather than 3%) significantly reduced the "second stage" of anesthesia without adversely affecting hemodynamic stability.[10] In this study, single-breath vital-capacity sevoflurane induction resulted in shorter induction times, with more than 50% of the patients losing consciousness after the first breath. Spontaneous movements and hemodynamic changes occurred more often with propofol, whereas coughing occurred more often with sevoflurane. One study comparing induction with propofol and sevoflurane using a tidal volume breath technique reported that induction with propofol was more rapid (57 versus 84 seconds), but the incidence of apnea was higher (65% versus 16%) and the time to settled respiration was longer (126 versus 94 seconds) in the propofol group.[11] The mean arterial pressure was better maintained and the incidence of adverse respiratory events was lower with sevoflurane induction. Although both groups received sevoflurane for maintenance of anesthesia, the time to emergence (eye opening to command) was shorter in patients with sevoflurane induction.[11] Another study comparing induction with propofol and sevoflurane using a vital-capacity primed-circuit technique reported that induction with sevoflurane was more rapid overall (51 versus 81 seconds), with the time to loss of consciousness after a single breath of 39 seconds. Induction side effects were different in the two groups (cough and hiccough for sevoflurane versus movement and blood pressure changes for propofol), but overall incidences were similar. There were no significant differences in any index of early or intermediate recovery or in patients' assessments of quality of induction or wakeup.[9] Inhalation induction of anesthesia may be facilitated with supplementation of anesthetic drug with potent opioids. Use of remifentanil (1 μg/kg intravenous bolus, followed by 0.25 μg/kg per minute infusion) reduced the end-tidal sevoflurane concentration required for tracheal intubation from 4.5% to 2.5%.[12]

Maintenance of anesthesia

Maintenance of anesthesia with inhaled anesthetics remains the mainstay of modern anesthesia practice, probably because of the ease of titratability. Doses should be age-adjusted as shown in Table 9-3. Song et al.[13] assessed the recovery times and ability to fast-track with desflurane, sevoflurane, or propofol total intravenous anesthesia (TIVA). Compared with propofol TIVA, maintenance of anesthesia with desflurane or sevoflurane resulted in shorter times to awakening, tracheal extubation, and orientation. Fast-track eligibility was significantly lower

Table 9-3. Age-dependent minimal alveolar concentration (MAC) values

Age	Desflurane O$_2$ 100%/N$_2$O 60%	Sevoflurane O$_2$ 100%/N$_2$O 65%	Isoflurane O$_2$ 100%/N$_2$O 67%
25 years	7.3/4.0	2.6/1.4	1.3/0.55
45 years	6.0/2.8	2.1/1.1	1.15/0.4
70 years	5.2/1.7	1.5/0.7	1/0.2

in the propofol group compared to desflurane or sevoflurane (26% versus 90% and 75%, respectively). However, there were no differences between the groups with respect to the times to oral intake and home-readiness. Earlier emergence with desflurane and sevoflurane was reported when electroencephalogram (EEG)-based bispectral index (BIS) monitoring was used to titrate the anesthetic agents.[14] BIS titration reduced the times to verbal responsiveness by 30%–55%. Similar to previous studies, there were no differences in later recovery times. A study comparing desflurane- and sevoflurane-based anesthesia reported that recovery indices and psychomotor functions were marginally superior with sevoflurane than with desflurane, but this did not reach statistical significance.[15] A comparison of the advantages of the volatile inhaled anesthetics to propofol for anesthesia can be found in Box 9-1.

Juvin et al.[16] evaluated the recovery characteristics among morbidly obese patients receiving desflurane, isoflurane, and propofol. Immediate recovery occurred faster and was more consistent, and oxygen saturations were higher, after desflurane than after propofol or isoflurane; however, these differences persisted only in the early recovery phase (up to 2 hours after surgery). Another study in morbidly obese patients found no differences in emergence (i.e., time to follow command and extubation) and recovery (i.e., cognitive function and psychomotor performance) profile between desflurane and sevoflurane.[17] When concentrations of inhaled anesthetics are titrated down toward the end of surgery, the differences between inhaled anesthetics are reduced.[18]

Box 9-1. Inhaled anesthetics compared to propofol for maintenance of ambulatory anesthesia

Advantages of volatile inhaled anesthetics (desflurane, sevoflurane)
- Better titratabilty of anesthetic depth both up and down, facilitating faster early recovery
- Less risk of intraoperative awareness
- Simplicity of administration
- Lower drug cost

Advantages of propofol
- Reduced postoperative nausea and vomiting
- Residual euphoria and patient satisfaction
- Lack of need for scavenging

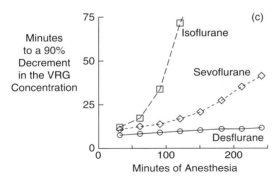

Figure 9-1. Time to a 90% decrement in the concentration in the vessel rich group (VRG) of tissues differs among desflurane, sevoflurane, and isoflurane as a function of their different solubilities. The graph for isoflurane deviates from the other two anesthetics when anesthesia exceeds 60 minutes, and the graph for sevoflurane deviates after 120 minutes. Adapted from Eger and Shafer.[18] Used with permission from Lippincott Williams & Wilkins.

Juvin et al.[19] investigated recovery characteristics in elderly patients and found a more rapid recovery with desflurane, when compared with isoflurane and propofol. In addition, a significantly larger percentage of patients receiving desflurane were judged to be fast-track-eligible compared with those receiving either isoflurane or propofol (73% versus 43% and 44%, respectively). A recent study evaluated the ability to swallow water without coughing or drooling after desflurane and sevoflurane anesthesia and found that patients receiving desflurane were able to swallow water without coughing or drooling significantly earlier.[20] Based on these findings, the authors concluded that desflurane allowed an earlier return of protective airway reflexes. Interestingly, a systematic review of randomized trials found that early recovery, characterized by opening eyes and obeying commands, was statistically significantly different, but of doubtful clinical relevance, in patients given desflurane or sevoflurane compared with those who received isoflurane.[21]

The concept of context-sensitive half-time can be applied to the recovery phase of inhalational anesthetics as it is for opioids; the context-sensitive half-times for isoflurane, sevoflurane, and desflurane are all shorter than remifentanil. The difference between desflurane and sevoflurane becomes apparent after 120 minutes if a 90% decrement in depth is needed for recovery (Figure 9-1).

Total intravenous anesthesia

With the introduction of propofol and newer delivery systems (e.g., target-controlled infusion, which is not yet available in the U.S.), there is increased interest in TIVA. Compared to inhaled anesthetic techniques, the propofol-based TIVA maintenance technique is associated with a lower incidence of postoperative nausea and vomiting (PONV).[22,23] However, PONV after inhaled anesthetics may be reduced by the use of prophylactic antiemetics.[23] Other benefits of TIVA include the ability to provide general anesthesia without the need for an anesthesia machine (e.g., vaporizers and scavenging systems), which can be useful in office-based and out-of-OR locations. Although inhaled anesthetic techniques allow for earlier emergence, which may facilitate fast-tracking (i.e., bypassing the PACU), this does not translate into an earlier time to home-readiness.[8] It is well recognized that propofol TIVA may be more expensive than an inhaled anesthesia technique. However, certain high-risk patients may benefit from TIVA techniques despite higher costs.

Nitrous oxide

Nitrous oxide has a rapid onset and offset of action due to its blood/gas partition coefficient (0.47). Although not a full anesthetic by itself, it provides synergistic interactions when combined with other inhalational or intravenous agents. Because of its amnestic and analgesic properties, as well as its ability to reduce the requirements of expensive inhaled and intravenous anesthetic drugs, N_2O is commonly used as part of a balanced anesthesia technique. Although several studies have suggested that N_2O increases the incidence of PONV, a meta-analysis of randomized controlled trials found that the emetic effect of N_2O is not significant and that omitting N_2O may increase the risk of awareness.[24] A recent review acknowledged that the use of N_2O remains controversial but that the literature does not support a reason to avoid N_2O.[25]

Brain function (hypnosis) monitoring

Among the conventional indicators used to assess depth of consciousness (or depth of hypnosis) are response to verbal commands, eyelash reflex, pupil size, muscle tone, hemodynamic changes (increase in heart rate and arterial blood pressure), purposeful movement, end-tidal anesthetic analyzer, and capnography. Although these indicators are not specific or sensitive, they are valuable and are recommended for assessing intraoperative consciousness.[26] Currently, a wide spectrum of brain activity monitors are available on the market. These devices record and process EEG, auditory evoked potential, and electromyographic activity.[27] All monitors display the information in a simple way with descriptive values assigned to the results of the processed signals.[27] Although there are a variety of monitors currently available, the properties of an ideal monitor are yet to be achieved (Box 9-2). These brain function monitors may improve the ability to titrate anesthetic drugs and thus facilitate recovery from general anesthesia. A meta-analysis of randomized controlled trials and a cost analysis included 1,380 subjects from 11 trials.[28] The use of BIS monitoring

Box 9-2. Ideal depth of anesthesia monitor

Provide valid and reliable measure of anesthetic depth
Help individualize anesthesia by integrating technology and pharmacology
  principles
Link accurate drug administration with measured state of arousal
Help detect and prevent awareness
Help avoid excessive anesthetic depth
Use processed analysis of electroencephalogram or midlatency auditory-
  evoked potentials
Cost-effective

modestly reduced anesthetic consumption (by 19%), risk of PONV (32% versus 38%; odds ratio, 0.77), and PACU time (by 4 minutes). However, these benefits did not lead to a significant reduction in time to discharge home. Furthermore, cost analysis showed that the cost of BIS electrodes exceeded any cost savings.[28]

Although brain function monitoring may shorten emergence and phase I recovery, they do not have uniform sensitivity across all anesthetic drugs and patients and therefore do not reflect the state of hypnosis nor prevent intraoperative recall or awareness.[26,27,29] Of note, a recent American Society of Anesthesiologists' Practice Advisory for Intraoperative Awareness and Brain Function Monitoring concluded that brain function monitoring is not routinely indicated for patients undergoing general anesthesia, either to reduce the frequency of intraoperative awareness or to monitor depth of anesthesia.[26]

Opioids

Opioids continue to play an important role in anesthesia practice in general; however, opioid-related side effects, including nausea, vomiting, sedation, bladder dysfunction, and respiratory depression, may contribute to a delayed recovery and interfere with the ability to fast-track. Therefore, opioids should be used sparingly in patients undergoing ambulatory surgery. The usual doses and intervals of use are displayed in Table 9-4.

Fentanyl is the most commonly used intraoperative opioid in ambulatory anesthesia. Remifentanil, a fentanyl derivative, is an ultrashort-acting opioid with a context-sensitive half-time of approximately 3 minutes (regardless of the duration of its administration) and elimination half-time of approximately 10 minutes (Figure 9-2). The methyl-propionic acid ester side chain of remifentanil is hydrolyzed by plasma and tissue esterase to a less potent (1/4,600 potency of the parent compound) carboxylic acid derivative. Remifentanil has a rapid onset. Its blood-brain equilibration time is 1 minute. It has a small central volume of distribution, fast clearance, and rapid offset of effect.

Remifentanil infusion provides profound intraoperative analgesia and hemodynamic stability and reduces the requirements of inhaled anesthetics or

Table 9-4. Perioperative analgesics in the ambulatory setting-adults

Analgesic	Dose	Duration of effect
Fentanyl	0.5–2 µg/kg	30 minutes
Remifentanil	0.015–0.2 µg/kg/min	5 minutes after end infusion
Acetaminophen	10–15 mg/kg PO	4 hours
	40 mg/kg PR	
Propacetamol	20–30 mg/kg IV	4 hours
Ketorolac	15–30 mg/IV	6–8 hours
	30–60 mg/IM	
Celecoxib	400 mg PO, then 200 mg PO	12 hours

Dose should be titrated starting with the lower recommended dose. IM, intramuscular; IV, intravenous; PO, per os; PR, per rectum.

propofol. Both dose-finding and comparative studies of remifentanil in ambulatory anesthesia show rapid and smooth recovery. In the ambulatory setting, remifentanil in combination with propofol allows synergism, cost savings, and ease of use.[30] Remifentanil was studied as the opioid component of TIVA for ambulatory laparoscopic surgery, compared to the older opioid alfentanil. Remifentanil doses were chosen to provide maximal suppression of response to intubation and intraoperative stimuli: 1 µg/kg bolus with 0.5 µg/kg per minute until trocar insertion, then 0.25 µg/kg per minute titrated to response. Remifentanil

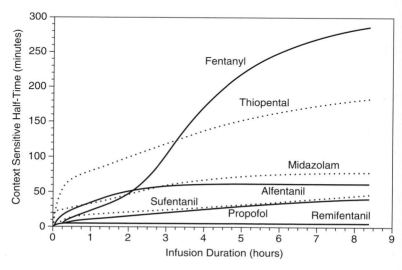

Figure 9-2. Context-sensitive half-times. Adapted from Hughes et al.[48] Used with permission from Lippincott Williams & Wilkins.

infusion, given at non-equipotent higher doses, provided better suppression of intraoperative responses with fewer adjustments to correct light anesthesia yet maintained comparable recovery profiles. The overall incidence of PONV was similar but earlier with remifentanil.[31] Overall, remifentanil has replaced alfentanil in the current ambulatory anesthesia practice. There is a learning curve with the use of remifentanil. Because the incidence of adverse events (rigidity, respiratory depression, and bradycardia) is dose-related, avoidance of bolus dosing and use of low infusion rate of remifentanil 0.125–0.25 µg/kg per minute may be more appropriate.[32] Because of its rapid offset of analgesic effect, it is necessary that a longer acting opioid (such as fentanyl) or nonopioid (nonsteroidal anti-inflammatory drugs or local anesthetics) be used to provide postoperative analgesia. The use of longer-acting opioids in the postoperative period may reduce the potential advantages of remifentanil in ambulatory anesthesia.

Anesthetic adjuvants

Sympatholytic drugs (e.g., esmolol), as an alternative to opioids, have been reported to maintain hemodynamic stability during surgery. Use of esmolol as an alternative to remifentanil during outpatient laparoscopic gynecological surgery reduced anesthetic requirements and postoperative pain as well as decreased the incidence of PONV from 35% to 4%.[33] However, there was no difference in the PACU bypass rates and times to home-readiness. Use of α_2-adrenergic agonists (e.g., dexmedetomidine) with hypnotic, sedative, sympatholytic, and analgesic properties reduces anesthetic and opioid requirements.[34] Therefore, dexmedetomidine has potential benefits in morbidly obese patients as well as patients with sleep apnea in whom opioid-related respiratory depression is of significant concern. The commonly used dosage consists of a loading dose of 0.5–1 µg/kg over 10 minutes followed by 0.2–0.7 µg/kg per hour. However, there is a need for further research evaluating the benefits of dexmedetomidine in the ambulatory setting. The duration of action may be long for ambulatory anesthesia use.

Neuromuscular blocking drugs

Muscle relaxants are commonly used as a part of a balanced anesthetic technique to facilitate tracheal intubation and improve surgical conditions. With increased emphasis on using minimal concentrations of hypnotic-sedatives (i.e., propofol or inhaled anesthetics), it is tempting to use muscle relaxants to ensure patient immobility. However, even minimal postoperative residual paralysis could cause distressing residual symptoms such as visual disturbances, inability to sit without assistance, facial weakness, and generalized weakness.[35] Importantly, these symptoms can prolong the recovery time and decrease the ability to fast-track. Residual paralysis may be present despite the use of reversal drugs and signs of clinical recovery from neuromuscular blockade. Therefore, the use

Table 9-5. Neuromuscular blocking agents and reversal agents in clinical practice

Agent	Intubation dose (2× ED95) mg/kg	Onset time (minutes)	Duration of action until train of four (TOF) > 0.9 after intubation dose (minutes)	Common side effects
Rocuronium	0.6	1.5–2.5	55–80	Mild vagolytic
Vecuronium	0.1	2–3	50–80	None
Mivacurium*	0.15–0.2	2.5–4.5	25–40	Histamine
Atracurium	0.5	2–3	55–80	Histamine
Cisatracurium	0.1–0.2	3–6	60–90	None
Neostigmine	0.05–0.07 µg/kg	2–5	60–90	Cholinergic
Edrophonium	0.5–1 mg/kg	1–2	60–90	Cholinergic
Glycopyrrolate	10 µg/kg	1–2	30	Tachycardia
Sugammadex	2–4 mg/kg	1.5–6.5	Unknown	No known side effects

*No longer available in the U.S.

of muscle relaxants should be avoided whenever possible. Doses commonly used in clinical practice are summarized in Table 9-5. Some investigators have proposed intubation without muscle relaxation as an alternative. Bulow et al.[36] found consistent and satisfactory intubating conditions using propofol, alfentanil, and topical lidocaine. Similarly, tracheal intubation may be accomplished with a combination of remifentanil and propofol.[37] However, higher doses (2–4 µg/kg) of remifentanil are necessary to achieve satisfactory intubating conditions in all patients.

If muscle relaxant use is deemed necessary, a shorter-acting muscle relaxant should be preferred. Succinylcholine is an ultrashort-acting relaxant but has been associated with postoperative muscle pain in patients ambulating shortly after their procedure. However, eliminating succinylcholine may not eliminate postoperative muscle pain in outpatients. Pretreatment with different nondepolarizing relaxants did not reduce the incidence of succinylcholine-induced myalgia but may have potential adverse effects.[38] Succinylcholine may still be a valuable muscle relaxant after carefully considering contraindications and side effect profile.

Because propofol may depress laryngeal and pharyngeal reflex, lower doses of muscle relaxants may be adequate to accomplish tracheal intubation. The optimal dose of rocuronium to achieve acceptable intubating conditions, after induction of anesthesia with propofol 2–2.5 mg/kg and remifentanil 0.5 µg/kg per minute, was 0.3 mg/kg, whereas increasing the dose to 0.45 and 0.6 mg/kg did not improve the conditions.[37] Reducing the intubating dose of rocuronium (0.3 mg/kg) shortened the duration of spontaneous recovery to a train-of-four ratio of 0.8, which was reduced further by reversal of the neuromuscular blockade with neostigmine. It is suggested that muscle relaxants for intubation should be administered based on clinical needs rather than on the train-of-four response.

Many practitioners avoid the use of reversal drugs because of their potential to increase the incidence of PONV. However, other studies report that the incidence of PONV and the need for antiemetics did not increase with the use of neostigmine-glycopyrrolate for reversal of residual muscle paralysis.[39,40] Because of the potential for detrimental effects of residual neuromuscular paralysis, the use of neuromuscular blocking drugs should be minimized in an ambulatory setting, but reversal drugs should be used (in appropriate doses) when necessary without hesitation. Newer reversal agents like sugammadex are undergoing clinical evaluation.[41] Sugammadex is a modified g-cyclodextrin, a cyclic oligosaccharide carbohydrate that acts by rapidly encapsulating a steroidal neuromuscular blocking agent such as rocuronium or vecuronium and forming a stable complex that prevents the pharmacological action of the neuromuscular blocking agent at the neuromuscular junction. This provides a completely novel mechanism for reversal of neuromuscular block which is independent of acetylcholinesterase inhibition and does not require the coadministration of anticholinergic agent. In the near future, this drug at 2–4 mg/kg may provide specific antagonism of the steroidal muscle relaxants rocuronium and vecuronium. So far, its use appears to be safe with minor side effects and provides effective use of muscle relaxants and their antagonism in ambulatory anesthesia.

Airway management

The laryngeal mask airway (LMA) has gained widespread popularity as a general-purpose airway device and is currently used for routine elective surgical procedures at least as frequently as the tracheal tube. General indications and contraindications for use can be found in Box 9-3. Compared with the tracheal

---

Box 9-3. General indications and contraindications for use of laryngeal mask airways

Indications
- As an alternative to face mask ventilation, for achieving and maintaining control of the airway
- Routine and emergency anesthetic procedures
- Known or unexpected difficult airways
- Establishing an airway during resuscitation in profoundly unresponsive patients

Contraindications
- Patients who are not fasted or where fasting cannot be confirmed
- Patients who may have retained gastric contents
- Patients who have fixed decreased pulmonary compliance

tube, the LMA is easy to place, does not require muscle relaxation and laryngoscopy, and thus may prevent complications associated with tracheal intubation. The LMA is tolerated at lower anesthetic concentrations than the tracheal tube and therefore allows titration of anesthetic concentrations to the surgical stimulus rather than for airway device tolerance. With the patient breathing spontaneously, dosing requirements of hypnotic anesthetics (intravenous or inhaled) can be titrated using a brain function monitor or recommended end-tidal concentrations of inhaled anesthetics known to prevent awareness. This may allow earlier emergence from anesthesia and improve perioperative efficiency. There are different LMAs to meet different clinical situations (Table 9-6); other supraglottic airways and laryngeal tubes (Combitube™) are also available. Having a choice of devices for managing difficult airways in ambulatory patients is essential in all practice locations. See Chapter 6 for a discussion of the difficult airway algorithm.

Junger et al.[42] were able to show that the discharge times from the operating room were shortest in the patients who had received regional anesthesia and a propofol TIVA using an LMA compared to balanced anesthesia with tracheal intubation. In contrast, Hartmann et al.[43] reported that although the induction of anesthesia was shorter when LMA was used, emergence from anesthesia was similar. The LMA should be avoided in patients with laryngeal

Table 9-6. Different LMA™ devices for adult ambulatory patients

Device	Indication	Sizes available
LMA Classic™	Routine use; reusable; typical maximum airway seal pressure 20 cm H_2O	3, 4, 5, 6
LMA Unique™	Routine use; disposable	3, 4, 5
LMA Proseal™	Positive-pressure ventilation, with or without muscle relaxants; typical maximum airway seal pressure 30 cm H_2O	3, 4, 5
LMA Flexible™	Wire-reinforced tube, for head and neck procedures	3, 4, 5, 6
LMA Fastrach™	For anticipated or unanticipated difficult airway situations and for cardiopulmonary resuscitation, to facilitate continuous ventilation during intubation	3, 4, 5; ETT 6.0, 6.5, 7.0, 7.5, 8.0
LMA CTrach™	To increase intubation success rates during difficult airways, by providing a direct view of the larynx while enabling ventilation during intubation	3, 4, 5; ETT 6.0, 6.5, 7.0, 7.5, 8.0

Single-use models of Flexible™ and Fastrach™ as well as pediatric sizes for the Classic™, Unique™, Proseal™, and Fastrach™ are also available. ETT, endotracheal tube.

pathology or decreased lung compliance as well as in those at high risk of regurgitation.

Optimal LMA insertion requires an adequate "depth of anesthesia" to obtund pharyngeal reflexes, which can be achieved either with intravenous induction with propofol or inhalation induction with sevoflurane.[44] Of the available intravenous induction drugs, propofol 2.5–3 mg/kg provides the best conditions, due to the pharyngeal and laryngeal relaxation associated with its use. Intravenous lidocaine may further improve conditions for LMA insertion because it provides additional pharyngeal relaxation. Other intravenous induction drugs (e.g., thiopental) do not produce conditions that are as satisfactory, and it may be necessary either to give a larger induction dose or to "deepen" anesthesia with an inhaled anesthetic prior to LMA insertion. Because co-administration of remifentanil 0.5–1 μg/kg with propofol facilitates tracheal intubation without the use of muscle relaxants,[45] it should also facilitate placement of the LMA but may carry the risk of apnea or rigidity.

Sevoflurane is generally considered to be the inhaled anesthetic of choice for patients breathing spontaneously through an LMA. However, one study suggests that desflurane can be safely used in patients breathing spontaneously through an LMA.[45] This study reported a higher incidence of transient movements to surgical stimulus (40% versus 5%) with propofol-N_2O as compared with a desflurane-N_2O anesthetic technique in patients breathing spontaneously through the LMA. In addition, the emergence from anesthesia and time to home-readiness were earlier with desflurane.

The LMA can be used for controlled ventilation during general anesthesia and may be easier to manage than the tracheal tube in the absence of neuromuscular blockers. The use of pressure support ventilation (PSV) allows more effective ventilation and carbon dioxide elimination. Other potential advantages of PSV include shorter time to awakening, possibly due to improved elimination of inhaled anesthetics after they are discontinued. When compared with patients receiving continuous positive airway pressure, those receiving PSV have improved gas exchange, lower end-tidal carbon dioxide concentrations, slower respiratory rates, lower work of breathing, and higher expired tidal volume.[46]

Summary

The most important aspect of a general anesthetic technique is its ability to consistently achieve rapid recovery to patients' normal functioning after termination of surgery. Intravenous induction of anesthesia with propofol remains the technique of choice, but inhalational induction with sevoflurane may be useful. Maintenance of anesthesia with shorter-acting inhaled anesthetics (i.e., desflurane and sevoflurane) allows easy titrability of hypnotic depth and provides a more rapid immediate recovery as compared to TIVA with propofol. However, there are no differences between inhaled anesthesia and TIVA with respect to late recovery (e.g., PACU stay and home-readiness). Titration of hypnotic-sedatives with brain function monitoring may reduce the time to emergence. Opioid-related adverse effects may be associated with delayed recovery and thus opioids should be used judiciously and nonopioid analgesics should be used whenever possible. Avoidance or use of judicious amounts of muscle relaxants as well as use of reversal drugs are critical in achieving a rapid recovery. Prophylactic multimodal analgesia and antiemetic therapy should reduce postoperative complications such as pain, nausea, and vomiting and allow rapid recovery and discharge home.

References

1. Chung F, Mezei G. Factors contributing to a prolonged stay after ambulatory surgery. *Anesth Analg*. 1999;89:1352–1359.
2. Liu SS, Strodtbeck WM, Richman JM, Wu CL. A comparison of regional versus general anesthesia for ambulatory anesthesia: a meta-analysis of randomized controlled trials. *Anesth Analg*. 2005;101:1634–1642.
3. Miller DR, Blew PG, Martineau RJ, Hull KA. Midazolam and awareness with recall during total intravenous anaesthesia. *Can J Anaesth*. 1996;43:946–953.
4. Smith AF, Pittaway AJ. Premedication for anxiety in adult day surgery. *Cochrane Database Syst Rev*. 2003:CD002192.
5. Raeder JC, Misvaer G. Comparison of propofol induction with thiopentone or methohexitone in short outpatient general anaesthesia. *Acta Anaesthesiol Scand*. 1988;32: 607–613.
6. Pizov R, Brown RH, Weiss YS, et al. Wheezing during induction of general anesthesia in patients with and without asthma. A randomized, blinded trial. *Anesthesiology*. 1995;82:1111–1116.
7. de Grood PM, Harbers JB, van Egmond J, Crul JF. Anaesthesia for laparoscopy. A comparison of five techniques including propofol, etomidate, thiopentone and isoflurane. *Anaesthesia*. 1987;42:815–823.
8. Joshi G, Gertler R. Is one general anesthetic technique associated with faster recovery? In: Fleisher L, ed. *Evidence-Based Practice of Anesthesiology*. Philadelphia, PA: Elsevier Science; 2004:236–240.
9. Philip BK, Lombard LL, Roaf ER, et al. Comparison of vital capacity induction with sevoflurane to intravenous induction with propofol for adult ambulatory anesthesia. *Anesth Analg*. 1999;89:623–627.
10. Hall JE, Ebert TJ, Harmer M. Induction characteristics with 3% and 8% sevoflurane in adults: an evaluation of the second stage of anaesthesia and its haemodynamic consequences. *Anaesthesia*. 2000;55:545–550.
11. Thwaites A, Edmends S, Smith I. Inhalation induction with sevoflurane: a double-blind comparison with propofol. *Br J Anaesth*. 1997;78:356–361.
12. Cros AM, Lopez C, Kandel T, Sztark F. Determination of sevoflurane alveolar concentration for tracheal intubation with remifentanil, and no muscle relaxant. *Anaesthesia*. 2000;55:965–969.
13. Song D, Joshi GP, White PF. Fast-track eligibility after ambulatory anesthesia: a comparison of desflurane, sevoflurane, and propofol. *Anesth Analg*. 1998;86:267–273.

14. Song D, Joshi GP, White PF. Titration of volatile anesthetics using bispectral index facilitates recovery after ambulatory anesthesia. *Anesthesiology*. 1997;87:842–848.

15. Tarazi EM, Philip BK. A comparison of recovery after sevoflurane or desflurane in ambulatory anesthesia. *J Clin Anesth*. 1998;10:272–277.

16. Juvin P, Vadam C, Malek L, et al. Postoperative recovery after desflurane, propofol, or isoflurane anesthesia among morbidly obese patients: a prospective, randomized study. *Anesth Analg*. 2000;91:714–719.

17. Arain SR, Barth CD, Shankar H, Ebert TJ. Choice of volatile anesthetic for the morbidly obese patient: sevoflurane or desflurane. *J Clin Anesth*. 2005;17:413–419.

18. Eger EI 2nd, Shafer SL. Tutorial: context-sensitive decrement times for inhaled anesthetics. *Anesth Analg*. 2005;101:688–696.

19. Juvin P, Servin F, Giraud O, Desmonts JM. Emergence of elderly patients from prolonged desflurane, isoflurane, or propofol anesthesia. *Anesth Analg*. 1997;85:647–651.

20. McKay RE, Large MJ, Balea MC, McKay WR. Airway reflexes return more rapidly after desflurane anesthesia than after sevoflurane anesthesia. *Anesth Analg*. 2005;100:697–700.

21. Gupta A, Stierer T, Zuckerman R, et al. Comparison of recovery profile after ambulatory anesthesia with propofol, isoflurane, sevoflurane and desflurane: a systematic review. *Anesth Analg*. 2004;98:632–641.

22. Visser K, Hassink EA, Bonsel GJ, et al. Randomized controlled trial of total intravenous anesthesia with propofol versus inhalation anesthesia with isoflurane-nitrous oxide: postoperative nausea with vomiting and economic analysis. *Anesthesiology*. 2001;95:616–626.

23. Apfel CC, Korttila K, Abdalla M, et al. A factorial trial of six interventions for the prevention of postoperative nausea and vomiting. *N Engl J Med*. 2004;350:2441–2451.

24. Tramer M, Moore A, McQuay H. Omitting nitrous oxide in general anaesthesia: meta-analysis of intraoperative awareness and postoperative emesis in randomized controlled trials. *Br J Anaesth*. 1996;76:186–193.

25. Smith I. Nitrous oxide in ambulatory anaesthesia: does it have a place in day surgical anaesthesia or is it just a threat for personnel and the global environment? *Curr Opin Anaesthesiol*. 2006;19:592–596.

26. Practice Advisory for Intraoperative Awareness and Brain Function Monitoring. American Society of Anesthesiologists, 2005. Available at: http://www.asahq.org/publicationsAndServices/practiceparam.htm#brain. Accessed July 5, 2007.

27. Bruhn J, Myles PS, Sneyd R, Struys MM. Depth of anaesthesia monitoring: what's available, what's validated, and what's next? *Br J Anaesth*. 2006;97:85–94.

28. Liu SS. Effects of Bispectral Index monitoring on ambulatory anesthesia: a meta-analysis of randomized controlled trials and a cost analysis. *Anesthesiology*. 2004;101:311–315.

29. White PF. Use of cerebral monitoring during anaesthesia: effect on recovery profile. *Best Prac Res Clin Anaesthesiol*. 2006;20:181–189.

30. Rognas LK, Elkjaer P. Anaesthesia in day case laparoscopic female sterilization: a comparison of two anaesthetic methods. *Acta Anaesthesiol Scand.* 2004;48:899–902.

31. Philip BK, Scuderi PE, Chung F, et al. Remifentanil compared with alfentanil for ambulatory surgery using total intravenous anesthesia. *Anesth Analg.* 1997;84:515–521.

32. Joshi GP, Warner DS, Twersky RS, Fleisher LA. A comparison of the remifentanil and fentanyl adverse effect profile in a multicenter phase IV study. *J Clin Anesth.* 2002;14:494–499.

33. Coloma M, Chiu JW, White PF, Armbruster SC. The use of esmolol as an alternative to remifentanil during desflurane anesthesia for fast-track outpatient gynecologic laparoscopic surgery. *Anesth Analg.* 2001;92:352–357.

34. Gertler R, Brown HC, Mitchell DH, Silvius EN. Dexmedetomidine: a novel sedative-analgesic agent. *Proc (Bayl Univ Med Cent).* 2001;14:13–21.

35. Kopman AF, Yee PS, Neuman GG. Relationship of the train-of-four fade ratio to clinical signs and symptoms of residual paralysis in awake volunteers. *Anesthesiology.* 1997;86:765–771.

36. Bulow K, Nielsen TG, Lund J. The effect of topical lignocaine on intubating conditions after propofol-alfentanil induction. *Acta Anaesthesiol Scand.* 1996;40: 752–756.

37. Schlaich N, Mertzlufft F, Soltesz S, Fuchs-Buder T. Remifentanil and propofol without muscle relaxants or with different doses of rocuronium for tracheal intubation in outpatient anaesthesia. *Acta Anaesthesiol Scand.* 2000;44:720–726.

38. Joshi GP, Hailey A, Cross S, et al. Effects of pretreatment with cisatracurium, rocuronium, and d-tubocurarine on succinylcholine-induced fasciculations and myalgia: a comparison with placebo. *J Clin Anesth.* 1999;11:641–645.

39. Joshi GP, Garg SA, Hailey A, Yu SY. The effects of antagonizing residual neuro-muscular blockade by neostigmine and glycopyrrolate on nausea and vomiting after ambulatory surgery. *Anesth Analg.* 1999;89:628–631.

40. Nelskyla K, Yli-Hankala A, Soikkeli A, Korttila K. Neostigmine with glycopyrrolate does not increase the incidence or severity of postoperative nausea and vomiting in outpatients undergoing gynaecological laparoscopy. *Br J Anaesth.* 1998;81:757–760.

41. Shields M, Giovannelli M, Mirakhur RK, et al. Org 25969 (sugammadex), a selective relaxant binding agent for antagonism of prolonged rocuronium-induced neuromus-cular block. *Br J Anaesth.* 2006;96:36–43.

42. Junger A, Klasen J, Hartmann B, et al. Shorter discharge time after regional or intra-venous anaesthesia in combination with laryngeal mask airway compared with balanced anaesthesia with endotracheal intubation. *Eur J Anaesthesiol.* 2002;19:119–124.

43. Hartmann B, Banzhaf A, Junger A, et al. Laryngeal mask airway versus endotracheal tube for outpatient surgery: analysis of anesthesia-controlled time. *J Clin Anesth.* 2004;16:195–199.

44. Molloy ME, Buggy DJ, Scanlon P. Propofol or sevoflurane for laryngeal mask airway insertion. *Can J Anaesth.* 1999;46:322–326.

45. Tang J, White PF, Wender RH, et al. Fast-track office-based anesthesia: a comparison of propofol versus desflurane with antiemetic prophylaxis in spontaneously breathing patients. *Anesth Analg.* 2001;92:95–99.
46. Brimacombe J, Keller C, Hormann C. Pressure support ventilation versus continuous positive airway pressure with the laryngeal mask airway: a randomized crossover study of anesthetized adult patients. *Anesthesiology.* 2000;92:1621–1623.
47. Evers AS, Maze M. *Anesthetic Pharmacology. Physiologic Principles and Clinical Practice. Companion to Miller's Anesthesia.* Philadelphia, PA: Churchill Livingstone; 2003.
48. Hughes MA, Glass PS, Jacobs JR. Context-sensitive half-time in multicompartment pharmacokinetic models for intravenous anesthetic drugs. *Anesthesiology.* 1992;76:334–341.

10. Anesthesia outside the operating room

Steven C. Hall, MD

The provision of anesthetic services outside the traditional operating room environment is a challenge to both the adaptability and sensibility of the anesthesiologist. In an effort to increase the comfort and safety of patients and to assist other physicians, we are increasingly asked to provide services for a variety of diagnostic and therapeutic procedures. These services are variably called "anesthesia" or "sedation" or "monitored anesthesia care" (MAC). No matter what the service is called, the basic principle is that the anesthesiologist is entrusted to provide the best in patient care, no matter what drugs or techniques we use.

Because of our unique capabilities and experience, these cases performed throughout the facility offer an opportunity to improve patient care and satisfaction with their overall experience, increase the awareness of the services that anesthesiologists can provide, and serve as an additional source of revenue. This chapter discusses these considerations within an ambulatory or hospital-based facility. Chapter 11 will focus exclusively on office-based surgery and anesthesia.

General principles

Site evaluation

The most important lesson about site evaluation is this: you must perform a thorough site evaluation and, if necessary, alteration before agreeing to provide anesthesia services in the site. This is your single best opportunity to ensure both that the site is appropriately prepared and that adequate policies, procedures, and agreement regarding coverage are in place. Once you start providing care, it is much harder to change any of these issues. In terms of the physical environment, space requirements, electrical service, communications system, lighting, traffic control, personnel, and potential hazards should be evaluated (Box 10-1).

If it is not possible to deliver safe and effective care at the site, the clinician should reevaluate the decision to make a commitment to provide service. The survey of the site should be undertaken in the presence of the personnel who will be providing the diagnostic or therapeutic activity, so that they can be asked questions about space, time constraints, personnel, and traffic. The anesthesia department should also enlist the help of the facility's biomedical engineers or other technical personnel to determine whether the electrical outlet supply, ventilation, and scavenging capability are adequate for the additional demands of anesthetic equipment.

Box 10-1. Principles of site evaluation

- Space
- Electrical services
- Communications
- Lighting
- Traffic control
- Personnel
- Hazards

Box 10-2. Traffic control
- Patient reception area
- Family waiting and consultation area
- Patient introduction area
- Patient transport
- Recovery

All local or state government building codes or safety codes must be considered in evaluating a potential site. Storage of oxygen and nitrous oxide cylinders, use of enriched oxygen, area ventilation, hazardous waste storage, lighting, and several other matters might be subject to local codes. The safety director or similar administrative officer of the facility should assist in these determinations. Of interest, two issues that are often overlooked, but are of great concern to local building inspectors, are corridor width and fire exits.

Most municipalities have specific ordinances on these two issues in areas where general anesthesia is administered. Although the service in charge of the area where you are looking think that "sedation" is all that will be given, it is best to assume that general anesthesia will be administered at least occasionally, mandating that the area be prepared for the higher standard. Consequently, it is useful to think of these as "procedure" areas or suites instead of "sedation" suites, focusing on the potential to provide a spectrum of anesthetic care.

Patient traffic flow should be considered (Box 10-2). The manner in which the patient (and accompanying responsible adult) is admitted and registered for the procedure, the area where the patient can change clothes and be examined by the anesthesiologist, the place where the accompanying adult can wait and converse with a treating physician, and the recovery and discharge area should be evaluated. A routine for efficient admission and preparation of the patient should be developed before the first anesthetic is given. There will often be adjustments to this routine as experience is gained, but a reasonable approach should be in place before embarking on the coverage of care.

Although most of the efforts in assessing and preparing a space focus on clinical care, it is worthwhile to give some consideration to the attractiveness of the patient and family spaces as well as the convenience of the traffic flow. The patient satisfaction with the experience and likelihood of returning to the institution for other care can be influenced by how attractive and comfortable the clinical spaces are as well as how convenient and efficient they find the clinical care. Good signage, short distances to walk, comfortable seating, well-equipped waiting areas, and other conveniences can have a meaningful impact on the satisfaction of the patient with the entire experience.

Space and equipment considerations

Each area will have its own unique requirements and restrictions (Box 10-3). However, there are certain basics that should be present for every anesthetizing

Box 10-3. Principles of site evaluation

Space
- Room for anesthesia equipment
- Room for anesthesia personnel
- Access to patient and anesthesia equipment
- Storage
- Interference from imaging or other equipment

Electrical service
- Adequacy of number of outlets
- Line fault protection
- Emergency, uninterrupted outlets
- Isolated power supplies or ground fault circuit interrupters for "wet" locations

Communications
- Dedicated, two-way system versus dedicated telephone

Lighting
- Room light
- Procedure light
- Emergency light

location. This is necessary not only for provision of basic anesthesia care, but also for response to a reasonable range of potential emergencies. Remember, not all emergencies that may be encountered are medical in nature. There can also be problems such as loss of electricity, loss of lighting, absence of assisting personnel, or fire. The traditional operating room is designed and engineered with multiple safety systems in place,[1] and personnel in the operating room have been educated in safety procedures.

In distant locations, however, this may not be the case. Therefore, one of the first items to identify is a reliable method of communication used to summon help. This can be a telephone, intercom, or other system, but it must be present before delivering anesthetic care. Additionally, all personnel who may be participating in the procedure and the sedation/anesthetic care must be identified. In particular, the qualifications and responsibility of the nonanesthesia personnel should be delineated, and appropriate training should be provided.

The area should be sufficiently spacious to allow the anesthesiologist immediate access to anesthetic machinery and other equipment that may be needed. There should be adequate room to prepare and administer the anesthetic, and there should be unimpeded patient access. A well-lit area is crucial, but the room should also have the capability of bright illumination of the patient for tasks such as obtaining vascular access. The anesthesia equipment and monitors must be easily seen at all times during the procedure. If equipment (such as C-arm fluoroscopy unit) must be moved during the procedure, the access to the patient should be maintained. In some situations (e.g., radiation oncology), all personnel must leave the area during part of the procedure. If this is the case, the anesthesiologist must clearly understand when these periods will occur and what options exist for quick access to the patient.

There should be enough electrical outlets to accommodate all of the anesthetic and monitoring equipment without unduly overtaxing the circuits. Clearly labeled outlets to an uninterrupted emergency power supply should be designated for the sole use by the anesthesiologist. All outlets should be properly grounded and within easy reach. It is desirable to position equipment such that the electrical cords are not a potential source of tripping.

Equipment needs vary with location; however, certain requirements must be met (Box 10-4). A reliable supply of oxygen adequate not only for the length of the intended procedure, but also for emergencies, is essential in all sites. Although a piped source of oxygen (and other gases like nitrous oxide) is ideal, it may be impractical. If piped gases are used, the anesthesiologist must be familiar with the source of the gas, its capabilities, and the procedure for enlisting backup sources. Likewise, if tanks of oxygen are the local source, there must be at least one full backup tank immediately available. It is prudent to have a freestanding tank-based backup system available, even if a piped source of oxygen is used.

Whenever anesthesia or MAC is administered, suction must be available. This suction must be adequate to deal with any reasonable expected needs during anesthesia. Piped suction systems have the advantage of reliable power that is usually superior to small, independently powered machines that may be used in remote locations. The anesthesiologist must confirm that the available suction apparatus will be suitable for patient needs.

Box 10-4. Equipment evaluation

Anesthesia equipment
- Anesthesia machine and ventilator
- Monitors
- Backup nitrous oxide tanks
- Airway equipment, drugs, intravenous fluid storage
- Anesthesia work surface
- Lighting
- Self-inflating resuscitation bag

Oxygen source
- Presence of piped oxygen (strongly encouraged)
- Backup oxygen systems and alarms
- Additional tank backup

Suction

Scavenging
- Validation of scavenging effectiveness

Emergency cart and defibrillator

Based on American Society of Anesthesiologists' Guidelines for Nonoperating Room Anesthetizing Locations.[51]

If administration of anesthetic gases or vapors is a possibility at the site, provisions must be made for adequate scavenging of waste gases. If a suction apparatus is used, the gases must not only be removed from the area, but also be directed out of contact with all personnel in the facility. If a passive system is used, the anesthesiologist must ensure that all waste gases are contained within the passive system. It is useful to test the area's atmosphere for appropriate trace anesthetic gases during an actual case to confirm that the system works and that the trace gas concentrations are within accepted standards. In addition, there are likely to be local building ordinances about room ventilation if volatile anesthetic agents are used in an area, especially a number of minimum total room air exchanges per hour.

Emergency equipment should be present whenever sedation or anesthesia is given. The minimum equipment should include a self-inflating, positive pressure ventilating resuscitation bag that is capable of delivering at least 90% oxygen;[2] airway supplies, such as a full range of sizes of airways, endotracheal tubes, and stylets; standard resuscitation drugs; a battery-powered source of lighting; a defibrillator; and any other usual equipment for resuscitation. There should be a clear policy about whose responsibility it is to check and maintain this emergency equipment.

Lastly, the functioning and safety of the anesthesia machine, monitors, and other equipment used in a remote location should be equivalent to those of equipment used in the traditional operating room. The American Society of Anesthesiologists (ASA) Standards for Basic Anesthetic Monitoring and Guidelines for Nonoperating Room Anesthetizing Locations apply no matter where in the facility the sedation/anesthetic is given.[3]

Distant sites should not be a "dumping ground" for outdated equipment. This equipment should be checked and maintained in the same manner as the operating room equipment. If this equipment is to be brought from the operating room area each time it will be used, excess equipment should be minimized and less bulky machines should be used. If some or all of the anesthesia equipment is stored on-site, both maintenance and security of the equipment and supplies should be guaranteed.

Scheduling

If anesthesia services are to be supplied to remote locations, each area will have multiple unique problems that should be addressed. These relate, in general, to three specific questions.

- Which patients and procedures are suitable candidates?
- When will anesthetic services be provided?
- Who is responsible for admission, preparation, and discharge of the patient?

It is common practice to establish policies for suitability of patients which mirror policies already in place for operative procedures. However, the physicians and others requesting anesthesia services may not commonly be involved in patient preparation for operative procedures and may not easily understand the anesthesiologist's concerns about extensive preprocedure evaluation, fasting guidelines, and written informed consent, among others. Consequently, it is important that clear policies and guidelines be provided and explained to radiologists, endoscopists, and others involved in requesting anesthesia services for their patients. The clerical and nursing staff involved in scheduling services can be especially useful in ensuring that needed preprocedure requirements are met. It is important that those involved in scheduling understand the policies involving patient suitability.

Patient suitability

There must be a clear understanding of which patients are suitable for this care (Box 10-5). In general, if the patient would normally be an appropriate candidate for an outpatient surgical procedure, he or she would also be a suitable candidate for a therapeutic or diagnostic procedure of similar length and intensity outside the operating room. This will vary by institution, and the anesthesiologist must feel comfortable with both the patient status and the procedure before agreeing to provide service.

If only a few patients are to be covered, it is often possible to provide service on short notice at the convenience of those outside the operating room. However, if requests are frequent, a more formal arrangement is necessary. Because of the potential for having to provide multiple coverages with only limited anesthesia personnel, there should be specific guidelines concerning the times at which service will be provided. When giving anesthesia far from the operating room, it is usually necessary to devote experienced personnel who are usually covering only that case.

If attending staff are usually assigned to more than one case simultaneously, this will alter the normal pattern of personnel allocation. For this reason, it is more efficient to assign specific times when coverage will be provided and then ensure that adequate anesthesia personnel are available. Emergency coverage outside the operating room should be handled in the same fashion as emergency coverage in the operating room environment. There may be need for third-party payor insurance approval.

Box 10-5. Patient suitability policies

Age limitations
American Society of Anesthesiologists physical limitations
Duration and intensity of procedure
Necessity of preanesthetic visit
  • Specific medical conditions
  • Specific procedures

Box 10-6. Patient preparation policies

Preanesthetic instructions
- Fasting requirements
- Responsible accompanying adult
- Chronic medications

Method of obtaining medical consultation and clearance
Informed consent
History and physical examination
Laboratory studies

The routines and policies for patient admission, evaluation, and preparation must be established and clearly understood before accepting coverage of the procedure. If there are facility, departmental, or state requirements for fasting, history, physical examination, laboratory, or consultation, these must be organized and obtained from assigned personnel (Box 10-6). For instance, if informed consent is necessary, it should be clear who is to obtain the consent. Likewise, after the patient recovers from the anesthetic, it should be clear who has the responsibility to check the patient and approve discharge from the facility (Box 10-7).

Quality management activities (such as postanesthetic phone check) that are used for patients who have undergone surgery in the operating room should be used for patients having surgery outside the operating room. It is useful for the Department of Anesthesiology to routinely compare the quality assurance experiences outside the operating room with those in the operating room suites to determine whether there are unique issues, problems, or improvements in these areas that need different solutions than applied in the main operating room areas.

Some settings may have a preponderance of pediatric patients. The need for cooperation or compliance is usually harder to obtain in pediatric patients, leading to the need for anesthesia services in pediatric patients whereas an adult would require only reassurance or some sedation. Because of this, special care must be used in designing scheduling, evaluation, and equipment for procedures and areas that will address the needs of pediatric patients. General guidelines, such as those of the Committee on Pediatric Anesthesia of the ASA (http://www.

Box 10-7. Recovery and discharge policies

- Dedicated recovery staff or operating room facility
- Responsibility for discharge from recovery area
- Responsibility for discharge from institution
- Postanesthetic follow-up
- Continuing quality management activities

asahq.org/clinical/PediatricAnesthesia.pdf), are helpful in developing an adequate system that addresses the unique needs of children.

Radiology suite

Radiation safety

Whenever anesthesia personnel work in the radiology suite, computerized tomography (CT) scanner, nuclear medicine laboratory, or radiation therapy facility, they must be cognizant of the basics of radiation safety. Ionizing radiation can cause direct tissue damage, chromosomal damage, and an increased risk of malignancy.[4,5] Although it is the responsibility of the radiology personnel to help anesthesia staff understand what measures are needed to minimize exposure, it is the responsibility of the anesthesia staff to strictly adhere to safety guidelines.

The most basic concept in understanding radiation safety is that the closer the anesthesiologist is to the source of radiation, the higher the level of exposure. Because it is unusual for the anesthesiologist to be placed directly in the radiation beam, scatter radiation is the biggest danger. Because scatter radiation increases significantly when the power output of the beam increases or when the size of the imaged field increases, exposure is much higher when larger areas are imaged or techniques such as fluoroscopy are used.

Techniques with a high-intensity, focused beam (e.g., CT scanning) have lower scatter. Scatter radiation falls off with the inverse square of the distance from the field. For instance, the exposure 1 meter away is usually less than 1/1,000 the exposure at the field. Radiation exposure limits, as established by the National Council on Radiation Protection and Measurements, have been based primarily on studies of civilians exposed to atomic bomb blasts during World War II.[6] This risk of genetic damage appears to be less than previously thought, although the risk of cancer is higher. Indeed, the risk of cancer is of greatest concern to those who have been repeatedly exposed to radiation. The primary cancer risks after excessive exposure include leukemia and thyroid cancer. However, this kind of excessive exposure rarely occurs.[7]

For anesthesiology personnel who are more likely to have multiple, smaller exposures, there are two important factors: the total amount of radiation exposure and the rate of exposure. A large total dose received over a long period of time is less likely to produce significant change than is the same dose received in a single exposure. There is special concern about not only total body exposure, but also localized skin or extremity exposure as well as optic lens exposure because of the susceptibility of the lens to form cataracts.

Safety precautions observed by radiology staff should also be observed by anesthesiologists. They should wear a lead apron that covers the front, back, and sides. A thyroid collar should also be worn if prolonged exposure is expected. Leaded glass screens or treated glasses and goggles should be used for eye protection if there is repeated exposure to high scatter levels.

If personnel have repeated exposures, it may be useful to use the same radiation monitoring devices that the radiology department uses. However, the most important safety precaution is to avoid exposure. This includes not only planning and using protective gear, but also having the radiologist inform anesthesia personnel when exposure is possible. Distance is important, because being 6 feet away from the beam decreases scatter exposure to the same level as having 2.5 millimeters of lead (the equivalent of five lead aprons) or 9 inches of concrete between the beam and the anesthesiologist.

Angiography and embolization procedures

The angiography suite is often a difficult place to administer an anesthetic because of limited space and access to the patient. Patients often have prolonged procedures on a hard table; proper attention to positioning, padding, access to the airway, lack of stretch on the brachial plexus or pressure on peripheral nerves, and adequate lighting of the patient and equipment are important. The patient may be repositioned or tilted during the procedure, and after repositioning, the patient must be reevaluated for all of these factors.

Angiography is usually performed to identify the extent of peripheral or central vascular disease or malignancy. Central nervous system (CNS) angiography is indicated for a variety of tumors, aneurysms, and arteriovenous malformations, whereas peripheral vascular angiography is used to identify both arterial and venous lesions, usually those associated with atherosclerosis. Whereas patients with CNS lesions may otherwise be healthy, those with peripheral atherosclerotic lesions often have other vascular problems.

Anesthesiologists may be asked to provide either MAC or general anesthesia during these procedures because of the discomfort of the procedure, problems with patient cooperation, or significant medical conditions that require monitoring and treatment. This last category is exceptionally challenging because the patient may acutely decompensate and require aggressive resuscitation at the same time that the procedure is done. Because of this, the anesthesiologist must both understand the procedure and know the status of the patient before committing to providing coverage so that proper preparations of equipment and personnel can be made.

Monitoring for the patient undergoing angiography is based on the patient's medical condition and the anticipated procedure. For short procedures, sedation and monitoring may be the best choice. For longer procedures, it may be prudent to provide the ventilatory and hemodynamic control that general anesthesia gives. If there are special problems (e.g., increased intracranial pressure), both monitoring and anesthetic approaches will need to be tailored to address them specifically. Some of the medical problems that are common in the angiography suite include the following:[8]

- Increased intracranial pressure (vascular and malignant lesions)
- Seizure disorder
- Coronary artery insufficiency
- Renal and peripheral vascular insufficiency

- Cardiac failure (low output, coronary artery disease; high output, arteriovenous malformation)

Proper preanesthetic evaluation, determination of whether the patient is an outpatient candidate, and preprocedure preparation should be the same for these patients as for a similar patient coming to the operating room. Contrast media used in angiography can cause significant cardiovascular, CNS, and renal complications. The older high-osmolality agents (1,400 to 1,500 mOsm/L) have a higher incidence of reactions compared to newer low-osmolality agents (660 to 700 mOsm/L). There are direct myocardial depressant, arrhythmic, and vasodilating actions that can cause transient hypertension followed by hypotension, as well as diuresis followed by hypovolemia. The agents can also cause seizures, cerebral edema, and renal damage.

The total amount of dye used should be recorded and monitored, and the amount is usually limited to 4 to 6 mL/kg. There can also be systemic responses, such as histamine release and complement activation. Reactions range from mild histamine release to life-threatening bronchospasm, angioneurotic edema, and anaphylaxis. These reactions must be treated promptly with diphenhydramine, steroids, oxygen, fluids, and, if necessary, epinephrine.[9] Pretreatment with prophylactic steroids and antihistamines has been used in patients having previous reactions to dye.

Embolization is occasionally used for lesions such as arteriovenous malformation. Although these patients are usually admitted after the procedure, some adults with a stable medical status and no evidence of postprocedure instability may be sent home the same day after an extended observation period. This is especially appropriate if the embolization was in a superficial location; if the site was an extremity, distal perfusion should be checked and clearly be unimpaired before the patient is discharged. If materials such as pledgets or coils are used for the embolization, there is always the chance of bleeding or of migration of the object to a distal location that could require surgical intervention to remove. If toxic chemicals are used for sclerosing the area, there may be either local or systemic reactions.

Radiation therapy

Radiation therapy treatment with high-energy beams is useful for treatment of specific tumors (e.g., retinoblastoma) and for total body irradiation before bone marrow transplantation. Although the exposure time is only a few minutes, usually multiple exposures are administered over the course of a few weeks. Anesthesiologists usually become involved only when the patient is a child because, even though the exposures are short, the patient must stay very still.

The radiation levels are so high that the anesthesiologist cannot be in the room during exposure. The heavily shielded door is sealed during the exposure, and usually it takes a couple of minutes to reopen the door and gain access to the room and the patient. The patient is appropriately sedated or anesthetized and then monitored with the usual monitors and two cameras, one focused on the patient and the other on the monitors. The patient is immobilized with padding and sandbags or a specially designed frame. The sedation or anesthetic is individually tailored to each patient, but the goal is immobility, maintenance of the airway and ventilation, and rapid emergence so that the patient can return home.

Several regimens have been used, including intravenous benzodiazepines or propofol, rectal methohexital, and volatile agents by mask.[10,11] It is desirable to develop a consistent routine of sedation or anesthesia which involves significant interaction with the patient and family. If the anesthesiologist develops a positive rapport with them, the provision of daily care is easier, and the negative effects of multiple hospital visits can be minimized. If an intravenous technique is chosen, it may be prudent to have a permanently implanted central line available to eliminate the discomfort of punctures with each procedure.

Computerized tomography and magnetic resonance imaging scanner

Both CT and magnetic resonance imaging (MRI) scanners are important diagnostic tools. They differ in the images they provide and the challenges they raise for the anesthesiologist. In general, it is much easier to provide care in the CT scanner suite. Although it may be a challenge to keep the patient still while the examination bed is moved in and out of the imager, the equipment and mechanical problems are straightforward.

All the usual monitoring and anesthetic equipment used in the operating room are suitable for use in the CT suite; the only problem is the relatively small size of the room. As CT scanning times continue to become shorter, the following are among the most common reasons the anesthesiologist is asked to assist:

- The patient (often a child) is insufficiently cooperative
- The patient is medically compromised and requires constant attention
- A diagnostic or therapeutic procedure is going to be performed under CT guidance

Magnetic resonance imaging equipment considerations

Unlike CT scanners, MRI scanners have several important equipment considerations that influence anesthetic management. For an MRI, the patient is inserted into a tube that is surrounded by a powerful electromagnet. The generated field, which is 10,000 to 30,000 times as powerful as the earth's magnetic field, orients hydrogen molecules in the body so that they face one direction. The addition of radiofrequency signals alters the orientation of these molecules for a short time before they return to the baseline, during which they release a signal that is used to build the MRI picture.[12] Both components of this process have significance for anesthetic equipment.[13]

The magnetic field is so strong that it can draw ferromagnetic objects into the core of the magnet's bore, injuring the patient or anyone else that is between the object and the center of the magnetic field. The magnetic force, measured in gauss units (G), markedly decreases in strength the farther from the magnet the object is, with the 5 G and 50 G limits most commonly used.[12] Five gauss and below are considered "safe" levels of static magnetic field exposure for the general public and is the minimum perimeter around the MRI system beyond which all non-MRI safe equipment and unscreened individuals should remain. Items with high ferromagnetic content are drawn into a 50 G easily; pacemakers may not function properly in fields as low as 1 to 2 G.[13]

The functional ferromagnetic capability of an object can be assessed by placing a pacemaker magnet on the object and watching for noticeable attraction. Known ferromagnetic items should be kept at least 15 feet away from the magnet and, if at all possible, outside the scanning room.[12,14] Objects that can be drawn into the magnet include hemostats, keys, pens, ferromagnetic gas tanks, clipboards, and scissors; the magnetic field also can demagnetize watches and destroy the magnetic data strips on credit cards and magnetic tapes.

The magnetic field can displace ferromagnetic vascular clips inside a patient (especially in the CNS, where scar tissue does not form).[15] Cardiac pacemakers can be converted to the asynchronous mode or inactivated by the magnetic field.[16] Bioimplants made of stainless steel (high grades only), tantalum, aluminum, nickel, and most alloys are not attracted by the magnet and are safe.[17,18] If there is concern about possible internal metal, such as surgical implants or metal fragments, an initial x-ray or CT scan will identify the presence of a radio-opaque object. The decision to proceed should be made with the radiologist and managing service.

The magnetic field can also draw anesthetic equipment into the magnet and can interfere with its function. Therefore, all anesthetic equipment in the scanning room should have a low ferromagnetic content. Also, any anesthetic equipment that can induce a radiofrequency signal can disrupt the patient's signal, producing an inadequate MRI picture. Monitors, in particular, can emit a radio frequency signal that degrades the image. Because of this, many monitors have been evaluated for suitability to use in the MRI suite (Table 10-1).[14,18]

Table 10-1. Anesthesia equipment for magnetic resonance imaging

Problematic	Can be compatible
Electrocardiogram	Blood pressure measuring equipment
Anesthesia machines	Pulse oximetry
Automated intravenous infusion devices	Capnography
Laryngoscopes and alkaline batteries	Laryngeal mask airway
	Plastic stethoscopes
	Other miscellaneous plastic devices

Box 10-8. Electrocardiogram monitoring in the MRI suite

Safety precautions
- Use four-lead, two-ground system
- Place all four electrodes close to center of trunk
- Check lead wires for fraying
- Place towel or sheet under lead wires
- Braid lead wires together to prevent loop formation
- Recheck wires periodically

Some models of commonly available monitors have been found to work well in the MRI, but some models are not suitable. Now, specially built monitors are available that contain low ferromagnetic content, extensive shielding, and in-line filters to prevent both degradation of the MRI picture and interference with the monitor's function. There are also a wide variety of pulse oximeter, capnograph, and noninvasive blood pressure monitors available that have been shown to work well in the MRI suite.[19] Plastic stethoscopes and mercury plastic film thermometers are also safe in the MRI suite.

Of all the standard monitors, the electrocardiograph (ECG) has been the source of most difficulty.[20] This monitor has been a source of patient burns, MRI signal degradation, and inadequate monitoring signal. Most of the attention has focused on the electrodes and lead wires. Because the lead wires are ferromagnetic, the strong magnetic field can distort the ECG signal. Also, there is a risk of burns at the site of the lead or over the course of the lead wires (Box 10-8). If the wire loops on itself, the loop acts as an antenna, and current is induced in this loop that leads to heat build-up and subsequent burn.[20] In our institution, we have used the following advice from engineers to decrease the risk of current generation:

- Use a four-lead, two-ground system instead of a three-lead system. Four-leads are standard, as supplied by most MRI-compatible ECG monitors, because the extra ground wire facilitates draining away extraneous current quickly, minimizing both the risk of patient burn and MRI signal degradation.
- All electrodes should be placed close to the center of the patient's trunk. Lead wires are checked before each use for evidence of fraying of the insulation. A towel or sheet should be placed under the lead wires. The lead wires should not come in contact with the skin, which prevents burning even if the lead wires become heated.
- Lead wires should be braided together as soon as possible. This prevents loop formation and subsequent induction of current.
- The position of the lead wires should be rechecked each time the patient is moved, ensuring that a loop has not formed.

The positioning of anesthetic equipment, as well as monitors, is an important issue. It is possible either to have the monitors inside the MRI scanning room or, if so designed, to have the sensors in the scanning room and the monitor display in the control room.[13,21] Likewise, if an anesthesia machine or other piece of anesthetic equipment is used, it can be placed in the scanning room or in the control room. If equipment is used inside the scanning room, the anesthesiologist must ensure that it has low ferromagnetic content and works efficiently in the environment.

There currently is a commercially available anesthesia machine that has had the ferromagnetic content markedly reduced to allow it to function in the scanning room. There also are a variety of ventilators that have been shown to work effectively in the scanning room. Remember that there is other anesthetic equipment besides an anesthesia machine, ventilator, and monitors that may be ferromagnetic. Fittings on the anesthetic circuit, the laryngoscope and its batteries, stylets, and other small equipment may be ferromagnetic and may need to be replaced.[14,18]

There are two alternatives to having anesthesia equipment in the scanning room.[22] The first alternative is to use standard anesthesia equipment and leave it in the control room. The anesthesia circuit must enter the room through a shielded conduit through the wall or door and be at least 20 to 25 feet long to reach the patient in the scanner. Two advantages of this approach are the ability to use an unmodified anesthesia machine and the lack of need for equipment or personnel to be in the scanner at all times. The disadvantage of this approach is the need to place the conduit at the time of initial construction or to have it retrofitted.

An alternative is to administer sedation or anesthesia without the use of an anesthesia machine. A vaporizer can be mounted on the piped oxygen source in the room and be used as an anesthetic source. Another possible technique involves intravenous or rectal medications. If an infusion pump is used, both its ferromagnetic content and ability to work in proximity to the magnet must be checked. Specific intravenous sedation techniques are discussed in Chapter 9.

Anesthetic techniques

An MRI scan often takes considerably longer to obtain than a CT scan, up to an hour (Box 10-9). If the patient is cooperative, it may be possible to use sedation alone to provide adequate conditions. However, prolonged scanning is disturbing to many patients because of the loud noise produced by the scanning process and a sense of claustrophobia that may develop, especially in adults. As a practical matter, the anesthesiologist is usually summoned only when standard sedation regimens do not result in the desired immobility or if a child is medically unstable.[13]

A general anesthetic technique using any of a wide variety of agents is suitable in this setting. It is important to decide on the method used to provide a clear airway during the scan. Many institutions prefer to place an endotracheal tube or laryngeal mask airway (LMA) to maintain a secure airway, especially when the patient is out of sight in the scanner.[22] The anesthetic regimen is planned to provide an adequate level of anesthesia but rapid awakening when the scan is finished. The scan does not produce pain, and deep levels of anesthesia are not needed.

Box 10-9. Anesthetic care in the MRI suite

General anesthesia versus monitored anesthesia care issues

Nonpainful procedure
Varying degrees of patient cooperation (children are particularly difficult)
Prolonged scan time
Availability of anesthesia or other trained personnel
Inhalation, intravenous, or rectal-based techniques possible

Control of the airway

Spontaneous ventilation
  • Unsecured airway
  • Laryngeal mask airway
  • Endotracheal intubation
Controlled ventilation

Anesthesia equipment—specifically designed or tested for compatibility

In-room nonferromagnetic equipment
  • Modified anesthesia machine
  • Monitors
  • Intravenous pumps
  • Ventilators
Out-of-room equipment
  • Shielded conduit through wall or door
Scavenging

Alternative methods include total intravenous anesthesia, such as a propofol infusion, or bolus intravenous or rectal drugs to maintain sedation or anesthesia.[22,23] Box 10-10 provides recommendations for the use of propofol. It is important to note that drip devices will creep over time, providing varying levels of drug administration. If the airway is unprotected, the patient must be closely observed; this is difficult when a small patient disappears from ready sight inside the bore of the magnet. It is possible to use an unsecured airway as long as the anesthesiologist is meticulous in monitoring and stops the scan if there is concern that the patient is not breathing adequately or has inadequate airway.

The need for the constant presence of an observer in the scanning room is controversial. The anesthesiologist must be certain that observation by monitors is adequate to assess the patient if there is no observer present in the scanning room. Concern has been raised about the potential danger of exposure to intense electromagnetic fields, but there is no definitive scientific evidence of an adverse effect from exposure to MRI fields.[24]

Recovery from anesthesia should be done in the same manner as for other anesthetized patients. The MRI scanner may be located far from the postanesthesia care unit. The anesthesiologist must decide whether it is better to transport

268   S.C. Hall

> **Box 10-10. Suggested propofol infusion rates for MRI[23]**
>
> Induction: 2 mg/kg of propofol or inhalation induction
> Maintenance: Pediatrics 100 µg/kg per minute; adults 50 µg/kg per minute
>
> *Suggested dilution and infusion rates for nonautomated infusions*
> 1. 200 mg propofol (20 mL) is diluted to total volume of 66 mL (final concentration 3 mg/mL). Use only those solutions deemed compatible (i.e., dextrose lactated Ringer)
> 2. Using calibrated drip chamber so that 60 drops = 1 mL; 1 drop per kg per minute = 50 µg/kg per minute
>
> Titrate accordingly
> Example: For a 20-kg patient, count 20 drops per minute = 50 µg/kg per minute.
>
> For smaller children and infants:
> 1. 100 mg propofol (10 mL) is diluted to total volume of 66 mL (final concentration 2 mg/mL).
> 2. Using calibrated drip chamber so that 60 drops = 1 mL; 2 drops per kg per minute = 50 µg/kg per minute.

the patient to this area for recovery or to develop the capability to recover these patients in the vicinity of the scanner. If recovery is done locally, the same personnel training, equipment, and discharge criteria should be used as are used after other anesthetics. Responsibility for discharge from the institution must be delineated.

Invasive cardiology

There is an increasing presence of anesthesiologists during various invasive cardiology procedures, such as cardiac catheterizations. This allows the cardiologist to perform longer and more aggressive procedures on sick patients and to concentrate solely on the procedure, knowing that the anesthesiologist is providing sophisticated monitoring and evaluation of the patient. In addition, cardiologists commonly insert and evaluate pacemakers and automated internal cardiac defibrillators (AICDs) in the cardiac catheterization lab. The anesthesia service may be asked to provide care for these patients, also.

As with most areas outside the operating room, the catheterization and electrophysiology laboratory provides challenges to the anesthesiologist to ensure that there is adequate space, access to the patient, lighting, temperature control, electrical outlets, and radiation protection. However, the two biggest challenges are caring for patients with significant medical disease and interacting and anticipating the special needs of the cardiologist.

Patient considerations

Providing anesthesia in the cardiac catheterization and other invasive cardiology laboratories is a good example of the challenges we meet outside the operating room which are primarily related to the medical condition of the patient. Most pediatric patients scheduled for catheterization procedures have heart disease that requires further evaluation, meaning that the anesthesiologist has some uncertainty about the exact anatomic and physiologic status of the patient.[25]

Most of these patients have congenital heart disease that may be uncorrected, partially corrected, or repaired at the time of catheterization. These three anatomic conditions can be associated with a wide variety of functional states. Even a patient who has undergone surgical repair can have significant myocardial dysfunction, arrhythmias, pulmonary hypertension, or failure to thrive. The anesthesiologist should be familiar with anesthetic management of patients with these lesions and be comfortable caring for the patient in an environment that is not as well designed for anesthetic care as the operating room.

There is sometimes a tendency to send the junior-most staff to give anesthesia in remote locations. When dealing with patients with significant medical disease, it is crucial that the staff be confident and experienced in the care of patients with these conditions. Additionally, only patients with stable cardiac disease should be catheterized as outpatients. Anesthetic management can significantly alter the hemodynamics of a patient with congenital heart disease.[25] The anesthesiologist must have a clear understanding of the patient's current clinical status and probable anatomic lesion and the likely consequences of anesthetic agents. Although a provisional evaluation based on clinical examination and echocardiography is made before the catheterization, the practitioner must be aware that the working diagnosis may not fully define the patient's pathophysiologic state. The preanesthetic evaluation is performed primarily to determine the functional status of the patient.[25] This includes the following:

- Identifying the probable anatomic lesion
- The presence and magnitude of shunting, arrhythmias, dynamic or fixed obstruction, or valvular insufficiency
- Adequacy of current cardiac output
- Recent changes in the patient's exercise tolerance

Obtaining information about medications, allergies, previous anesthetic experiences, and other medical problems is also an important part of the evaluation. The anesthetic evaluation and preparation are the same as those done when preparing a patient for surgery in the operating room. Consultation with the cardiologist is useful in determining the patient's current status.

After assessing and preparing the patient, the anesthesiologist administers an anesthetic tailored to the patient's probable anatomic lesion and functional status. Experience has clearly demonstrated that it is possible to provide general anesthesia for virtually all patients safely. A wide variety of anesthetics, such as ketamine, propofol, narcotics, and volatile agents, have been used successfully.[25,26]

The patient monitoring, evaluation, and management that are done by experienced practitioners are more important than the specific agents chosen.

However, some anesthetic agents may be better suited to an individual patient, depending on his or her anatomic lesion, degree of shunting, and reserve. Careful titration of agents, coupled with meticulous monitoring and evaluation, is the basis of successful management. Although the anesthetic technique used for the eventual cardiac repair may be used for the catheterization, it is desirable to have the patient awake and extubated at the end of the procedure.

Cardiac catheterization considerations

During the cardiac catheterization, there are certain matters that the anesthesiologist should understand (Box 10-11). The cardiologist, who often works without other physicians present, may not be familiar with direct communication with other physicians. There should be a continual exchange between the anesthesiologist and the cardiologist so that both understand the other's concerns. For instance, the cardiologist may cause considerable blood loss from cannulation of femoral vessels and withdrawal of samples.

The anesthesiologist needs to keep close track of this loss and anticipate the need for transfusion. The cardiologist may not understand the hemodynamic consequences of dysrhythmias during anesthesia, since these do not have the same significance in the nonanesthetized patient. Finally, the measurement of pressures and saturations in the heart can be altered by the anesthetic. Enriched oxygen can invalidate shunting and pulmonary artery pressure studies, whereas volatile agents, hyperventilation, and muscle relaxants can change baseline values for heart rate, rhythm, and myocardial contractility. These matters should be discussed with the cardiologist as the case proceeds.

Many new procedures have dramatically expanded the scope of cardiac interventionalists. These procedures are more likely to be done on an inpatient or 23-hour observation basis. Radiofrequency and cryotherapy ablation of accessory pathways are techniques that often entail a prolonged catheterization and rhythm evaluation. An important anesthetic consideration in these cases is that conduction through the pathways can be altered by anesthetic agents, making induction of dysrhythmias difficult. The anesthesiologist may have to change the technique to provide optimal conditions for the study and ablation. In addition, the cardiologist may need to induce prolonged periods of tachycardia during the procedure, necessitating fluid loading and inotropic support to maintain adequate blood pressure and cardiac output.

Box 10-11. Cardiac catheterization considerations

- Communication with cardiologist and other nonanesthesia personnel
- Blood loss
- Dysrhythmias
- Effect of anesthesia on measured hemodynamic parameters

Balloon dilations of stenotic pulmonary and aortic valves, as well as aortic coarctations, are increasingly performed in the catheterization suite.[27] These procedures produce a short, sudden cessation of blood flow during the expansion of the balloon and may result in significant disruptions in forward flow and subsequent hypotension. This brief period of absent cardiac output is usually well tolerated, but malignant arrhythmias or cardiac decompensation may occur in some patients, such as the infant with aortic stenosis and a small left ventricle. Although rupture is a rare complication, it can occur. Because of the potential for difficulty, the anesthesiologist must be prepared to deal with the range of complications quickly and efficiently; cardiostimulatory medications must be immediately available at the time of dilation.

In pediatrics, other useful procedures are transcatheter closures of septal defects, patent ductus arteriosus, and the fenestrated Fontan using a percutaneously inserted device.[28] Two joined plastic umbrellas are introduced through the femoral sheath and positioned on either side of the septal defect. After ensuring proper placement by transesophageal echocardiography or fluoroscopy, the umbrellas are locked together, obliterating the defect. Complications have included dysrhythmias, significant cardiac decompensation, and embolism of the umbrellas. Nonetheless, this procedure may become an important method of closing defects without the use of cardiopulmonary bypass.

As with anesthesia in other areas, it is useful to design the anesthetic technique to allow rapid awakening. Although most children stay in the facility after catheterization, some may be discharged. As with other remote surgical locations, it must be decided whether to transport the patient to the postanesthesia care unit or to establish a recovery facility closer to the catheterization lab.

Automated implantable cardiac defibrillators and pacemakers

In the past, both pacemakers and AICDs were inserted by cardiac surgeons in the operating room. Today, these devices are routinely inserted and checked by cardiologists in the cardiac catheterization or electrophysiology lab instead. With both devices, permanent transvenous leads are inserted into the right atrium, right ventricle, or both, followed by tunneling of the leads to a subcutaneous pocket, where the generator is installed. Although this can sometimes be performed using just local anesthesia, it is common to use sedation or general anesthesia to make the experience more pleasant for the patient.

General anesthesia is needed when the AICD is being tested, either during initial insertion or on follow-up. Testing of the AICD consists of inducing ventricular tachycardia or fibrillation and determining whether the device senses the arrhythmia and then delivers an appropriate energy level for cardioversion or defibrillation. Vulnerable periods include both the time of arrhythmia and treatment as well as the immediate recovery period because of potential prolonged cardiac dysfunction after the arrhythmia in some patients.

There is no evidence that one general anesthetic drug or technique is innately superior to another for these cases. The most important determinant is the underlying myocardial function of the patient. In the early experience with AICDs, most of the patients had the devices inserted during surgery because of recognized continuing arrhythmias and often had poor myocardial function.

In these patients, any anesthetic technique can cause significant hypotension and decreased cardiac output. Consequently, it is reasonable to closely monitor with direct arterial pressures patients who have shown hemodynamic instability in the past and patients who currently have low left ventricular ejection fraction, especially those with fractions less than 20%, although it might be better for these patients to stay overnight or to be inpatients.

Electroconvulsive therapy

Electroconvulsive therapy (ECT) is used in the treatment of patients with affective disorders (e.g., depression) and schizophrenia. A grand mal seizure is induced by electrical current, and this seizure is accompanied by a wide range of cardiac and respiratory side effects. The duration of the seizure has been thought to be a determinant of effectiveness, with 30 seconds considered a minimum. However, the threshold may change with treatments. There are several anesthetic considerations for patients having this procedure.[29]

The grand mal seizure starts with a short tonic phase followed by a clonic phase. Initially, there is vagally mediated bradycardia and hypotension, followed by several minutes of sympathetically mediated tachycardia and hypertension. This may be accompanied by significant dysrhythmias, myocardial ischemia, and, rarely, myocardial failure. There may also be apnea, hypoventilation, and increased cerebral blood flow and pressure in this period. Because clinical depression is more common in the elderly, these patients have reduced functional reserve to withstand the dramatic changes in hemodynamics during ECT. Their medical status, with an emphasis on the cardiac system, should be clear before administering anesthesia.

Before undergoing ECT, the patient should be questioned about the use of psychotropic medications. Tricyclic antidepressants and monoamine oxidase inhibitors have significant anesthetic significance. They affect not only adrenergic tone, but also the response to sympathomimetic drugs. Because of the cardiac effects of lithium therapy, it has been suggested that patients should be off lithium therapy before receiving ECT. Because of the increase in cerebral blood flow, ECT usually has not been done on patients with intracranial masses or elevated pressure but may be useful under some circumstances.[30]

The goal of anesthetic management is to prevent injury (such as fractures) during the seizure, to provide amnesia but rapid emergence, to control the airway and ventilation, and to treat significant cardiovascular disturbances. After pre-oxygenation, a short-acting anesthetic and succinylcholine are administered to provide anesthesia and prevent injury from muscle spasms. Methohexital (0.5 to 1.0 mg/kg) was often the traditional agent because of its short length of action.

The associated hypertension commonly required treatment, especially in patients with cardiovascular disease. A short-acting beta blocker or direct vasodilator is usually sufficient for this purpose.[31] The use of propofol has been met with favor, despite some concerns about shorter seizure duration.[32-35] It may be particularly useful for ambulatory ECT. However, recovery may be more influenced by the postictal state than by the anesthetic agent. Postanesthetic care should be given in the same manner as it is to other patients receiving general anesthesia.

Lithotripsy

The use of lithotripsy as a noninvasive surgical approach for the disintegration of urinary tract stones is common. The management of urinary tract stones has changed from open removal from the kidney and the ureter, to the application of ultrasound for their disintegration, as well as laser removal of the stones from the ureter.[36,37] Placement of stents to maintain ureteral patency following removal of calculi or dilation of strictures has proven to be another great advancement in ureterolithotomy. The majority of renal calculi can now be managed by extracorporeal shock-wave lithotripsy (ESWL), which may be considered the treatment of choice for renal stones smaller than 2 cm and for the majority of ureteral calculi, with success rates approaching 80% to 90%. The majority of these procedures are done on an ambulatory basis.

The principal underlying ESWL is the application of generated high-pressure shock waves to the flank focused on the target stone. The shock wave is repeated several thousand times, causing the stone to disintegrate. All lithotriptors share four main features (Box 10-12): an energy source, a focusing device, a coupling medium, and a stone localization system. The earlier form of ESWL provided by the original Dornier HM3 used a spark plug energy generator and required patients to be submerged in water in a hydraulically operated chair-like support.

The water bath acted as the coupling medium to transmit the shock waves to the patient, with stone localization provided by biplanar fluoroscopy. Although the basic principles of shock-wave lithotripsy remain unchanged, modifications of the four basic components of the first-generation lithotripter have provided newer-generation lithotriptors that are more effective with less physiologic trespass. Although ESWL is considered a noninvasive procedure, the impact of the shock waves at the entry site may cause a sharp stinging pain or visceral pain. Whereas single low-impulse shock waves are easily

Box 10-12. Components of lithotriptors
- Energy source
- Focusing device
- Coupling medium
- Stone localization system

tolerated, administration of multiple shocks usually requires pharmacologic intervention.

Because of the modification to shock-wave generation, focusing devices, coupling medium, and stone localization system, some form of analgesia, sedation, or local anesthesia is usually required with the majority of the latest generation of lithotriptors.[38] As the shock-wave pressure (power) and focal region of the recent generation machines have been reduced, so has the requirement for anesthesia or analgesia. However, the price paid for anesthesia-free lithotripsy is a reduction in stone fragmentation efficiency. Some patients treated with the current generation lithotriptors occasionally require a second treatment.

Complications

Effectiveness of treatment is determined by eradication of calculus with a minimal number and severity of complications. Complications of ESWL have been reported to occur in less than 3% of all cases and include the following:[39]

- Medical problems (e.g., myocardial infarction, pulmonary embolism, and congestive failure)
- Nausea, pain, or fever
- Ureteral obstruction with colic and infection
- Perirenal hematoma
- Urosepsis

In addition, hemorrhage blisters of the skin and the area where the shock waves enter and leave the body can occur, as well as edema of the kidney and bleeding into the renal pelvis or calices.

There is an 8% incidence of new-onset hypertension reported; the etiology is unknown. Cardiac complications include arrhythmias (e.g., benign supraventricular and ventricular premature beats). The possibility of ventricular tachycardia or fibrillation by shock waves placed in the vulnerable period of the ECG led to the development of technology by which the shock wave is linked to the R wave of the ECG: The shock waves are delayed to avoid the vulnerable period of the cardiac cycle. The newer second-generation lithotriptors have further reduced these complications.[39]

Sedation and anesthetic techniques

Newer lithotriptors require little or no anesthesia as shock-wave pain is reduced by lower voltage and a broader shock entry site pattern.[40] However, some patients still experience deep visceral pain and require intravenous sedation or analgesia. In addition, patients presenting for repeat ESWL may already have experienced the procedure under a certain anesthetic technique and be highly anxious. Patients requiring multiple anesthetics for repeated treatments and stent procedures related to ESWL may benefit from the use of continuous infusion techniques involving a combination of short-acting analgesics (remifentanil or fentanyl), a sedative-hypnotic (propofol), and anxiolytics/amnestics (midazolam).[41]

There are variations between institutions in the use of sedation versus general anesthesia for these procedures, although general anesthesia is most commonly used if there is an endosurgical procedure (ureteroscopic laser lithotripsy) used. General anesthesia with an LMA is a common technique, with a propofol infusion or sevoflurane being used as the primary anesthetic. Some adults and older children will tolerate ESWL without general anesthesia but do receive sedation/analgesia intravenously.[42]

Spinal and epidural anesthesia[43] and intercostal blocks[44] have been used in this setting. Eutectic mixture of local anesthesia (EMLA) has also been evaluated. Variability in the success of EMLA cream compared to a placebo or intravenous sedation[45,46] has been reported; however, this may be due to differences in the models of lithotriptors used. EMLA must be applied at least 45 to 60 minutes before the procedure for adequate onset of dermal analgesia.

The lithotripter and fluoroscopy do not interfere with the anesthesia machine or equipment; however, they force the patient to become positioned a distance from the anesthesiologist. Therefore, infusion pumps, supplemental nasal oxygen, precordial stethoscopes, blood pressure cuffs, ECG leads, capnography, and other equipment will require that sufficient extension tubing be used to reach the patient. Immersion-type lithotriptors, which are used less frequently, are associated with potential access problems because only the patient's head and arms are above the water level. Immersion itself is associated with compression of peripheral blood vessels and the subsequent increase in cardiac preload may be poorly tolerated in patients with cardiovascular disease.[38]

During the procedure, the patient is repositioned constantly as fluoroscopy or ultrasonography is used to check the success of the stone disintegration. If fluoroscopy is used, exposure of the patient and staff to ionizing radiation becomes a hazard. Easy access to the patient, intravenous fluids and the applied monitors, and adequate ventilation and circulation should be ensured.

Miscellaneous procedures

Other medical and surgical procedures, such as bronchoscopy, gastrointestinal endoscopy, and emergency room procedures, may require anesthesia services. General principles of monitored care or general anesthesia are discussed below and may be applied to any setting provided that policies are in place and that the roles of the various providers are understood. In addition, open communication between the physicians, nurses, and ancillary personnel is vital for the provision of safe, high-quality services.

Sedation, monitored anesthetic care, and anesthesia for procedures outside the operating room

Applicable techniques

There is increasing recognition of the benefits of analgesia and sedation for diagnostic and therapeutic procedures. In the past, both the analgesic and sedative needs of patients, especially children, have been underappreciated. In an effort to provide humane but safe patient care, a wide variety of drugs and techniques has been used. For instance, local anesthetic field blocks, local infiltration, and regional blocks are easy to administer, have a short duration, and are relatively safe. However, many patients require additional sedation to comfortably withstand the procedure.

Although there is increased appreciation of the benefits of sedation of patients for procedures and diagnostic studies, there is also recognition of the potential dangers of sedation. Practitioners have asked their anesthesia colleagues both for help with choice of drugs and for recommendations on how to provide analgesia and sedation safely. Anesthesiologists can have a positive impact on the care of both adults and children in their facility by helping to institute reasonable practices.

Universal guidelines

Anesthesiologists approach MAC with the same rational approach that they use with patients scheduled for general or regional anesthesia. It is second nature for anesthesiologists to evaluate and prepare patients, institute proper monitoring, titrate medication to effect, and ensure proper recovery before discharge. However, these basics of the anesthesiologist's approach are not necessarily appreciated by other clinicians who may provide sedation.[47]

The anesthesia staff can have an important role in making sedation safer by participating in the development of institutional guidelines for sedation administration.[48] Guidelines that promote proper patient evaluation, monitoring, and documentation are powerful tools for improving care of these patients. The anesthesia staff may participate in setting medication dosage regimens, but the focus should be on patient evaluation and monitoring, which can have a significant impact on recovery. Guidelines and techniques for sedation are discussed in more detail in Chapter 7.

There are several organizations that have developed standards and guidelines for sedating patients. The anesthesia staff can use these as a basis when assisting its institution to develop its own. An example of a published program that can be used as a resource is the 2002 version of sedation guidelines published by the American Academy of Pediatrics (AAP) (Box 10-13).[2] These guidelines are specifically tailored to the pediatric patient but have many elements that will be part of any guidelines, whether pediatric or adult.

Box 10-13. Guidelines for monitoring and management

Resuscitation cart
Oxygen source
Positive-pressure oxygen-delivery system that can deliver at least 90%
  oxygen for at least 60 minutes
Suction
Monitors:
  • Continuous measurement of O_2 saturation, heart rate
  • Intermittent respiratory rate
  • Blood pressure
Person other than the one performing the procedure to monitor the patient
Documentation of vital signs and medication
Preanesthesia evaluation
Informed consent
Recovery parameters
Discharge instructions

Based on American Academy Pediatrics Guidelines Committee on Drugs.[2]

In these guidelines, a distinction is made between conscious sedation and
deep sedation, with conscious sedation considered a state of depressed consciousness in which the patient retains a patent airway and protective reflexes
and is arousable by verbal command or physical stimulation. Deep sedation is
considered a state from which the patient is not easily aroused or in which the
patient does not maintain an adequate airway. Although the distinction is made
in the guidelines, sedation can vary over the course of a procedure to encompass
either state.

The ASA and the accrediting organizations (the Joint Commission [JC] and
the Accreditation Association for Ambulatory Health Care [AAAHC]) no longer
use the term conscious sedation. Instead, they define "moderate sedation" as the
ability to respond *purposefully* to verbal or light tactile stimulation, and "deep
sedation" as the ability to respond *purposefully* to repeated or painful stimulation. Furthermore, "If the patient loses consciousness and the ability to respond
purposefully, the anesthesia care is a general anesthetic, irrespective of whether
airway instrumentation is required" (ASA Position on Monitored Anesthesia
Care, 2003).

Some of the elements of the AAP guidelines should be considered for
all patients. Equipment that *must* be available on-site includes a resuscitation
cart, a source of oxygen, a positive-pressure oxygen delivery system that can
administer at least 90% oxygen for at least 60 minutes, suction, and monitors.
Continuous measurement of oxygen saturation and heart rate by pulse oximetry
as well as intermittent respiratory rate and blood pressure monitoring are
required.

An additional person should monitor the patient, and, for patients receiving
deep sedation, the monitoring personnel should have that monitoring as their

only responsibility. There should be documentation not only of vital signs and medication given, but also of a presedation health evaluation, informed consent, recovery parameters, and instructions at discharge to the person responsible for the patient. These and other guidelines are provided as suggestions for care, not absolute standards.[49,50] They can be used as a framework to guide sedation by nonanesthesiologists. When the anesthesia staff participates in developing parameters of its own institution, the individual needs of that institution should be incorporated.

It is useful for the anesthesia department to consider the circumstances under which it would be best to have an anesthesiologist involved in sedative care. Often, help is requested after efforts at sedation by another service have failed to provide adequate conditions. It may or may not be reasonable to give additional sedation after multiple doses of drug(s) have already been administered. The anesthesiologist must evaluate the current status of the patient and then decide whether to give additional sedation or to recommend that the procedure be rescheduled. Although some departments may have the flexibility to offer assistance in sedation on short notice, this is often not the case with a busy service.

In the latter situation, it is usually possible to help with sedation only when it has been scheduled in advance. By developing close communication between services, it is generally possible to find a mutually acceptable time when an anesthesiologist will be available to assist. Different arrangements that have been adopted by some include regularly scheduled time for services that often request help, involvement of the anesthesia department's acute pain service or intensive care service personnel, provision of a treatment room coverage at a fixed time of the day, or dedication of an otherwise underused operating room to patients needing sedation for procedures. Each anesthesia department's involvement in sedative care will be decided on a variety of factors, including frequency of use, complexity of patients' medical status, need for specialized equipment, and flexibility of staff schedules.

Preparing for emergencies

When preparing to provide anesthesia services outside the operating room environment, most efforts are directed at providing the equipment, policies, and procedures to deliver care for specific procedures. Part of these efforts must focus on what will be done if there are unexpected emergencies. These emergencies fall into several general categories, including patient care emergencies, equipment failure or lack of availability, and personnel emergencies. Because personnel who work outside the operating rooms do not have the training given to the nurses, technicians, and others who help us in the operating rooms, part of the agreement to provide anesthesia services in new venues should include proper training to accompany the adoption of needed policies, procedures, and protocols.

Patient care emergencies encompass problems such as an unexpected difficult airway, bronchospasm, anaphylactic reaction, myocardial ischemia, or combative patient behaviors. Although these problems are part of the many problems routinely addressed by anesthesiologists, they take on a new complexity outside the normal operating room environment. The personnel who will be present outside the operating room do not have the same experience in helping the anesthesiologist in dealing with these problems. To the extent possible, education should be provided to nursing and other personnel about what is expected of them in emergent situations. The anesthesiologists involved in these situations have a responsibility not only to ensure that education is provided, but also to be very specific in emergent situations about what they need in terms of assistance.

There are two parts to preparing staff to assist with emergencies the anesthesiologist will face in these situations. First, the anesthesiologist chosen to work in these environments must have the communication skills, leadership ability, and insight into the capabilities of support personnel to effectively supervise and direct medical therapies. Widespread experience has confirmed that the radiologist, cardiologist, oncologist, or other physician involved in the diagnostic/therapeutic procedure expects the anesthesiologist to be "in charge" and responsible for dealing with all emergencies. Therefore, it is incumbent on the anesthesiologist to be proactive in directing all personnel present to assist (as needed).

The anesthesia leadership should recognize that not all anesthesiologists are well suited to perform in this environment, which requires considerable self-reliance, patience, and willingness to explore new solutions to complex problems. The second part of preparing staff for emergencies is education. The following are some of the questions that should be reviewed with personnel:

- What kind of personnel will be available during procedures?
- Will there be a registered nurse always available to assist?
- Have the personnel had operating room or critical care experience?

Summary

Anesthesiologists are increasingly asked to provide services outside the traditional operating room environment. The outpatients who come to an institution expect the best of care. This is an opportunity for anesthesiologists to deliver efficient, safe, and humane care for a wide variety of procedures and to increase the recognition of our specialty in areas that previously have had little contact with anesthesiologists.

References

1. Ehrenwerth J, Eisenkraft JB. *Anesthesia Equipment: Principles and Applications.* St Louis, MO: Mosby; 1993:521–533.
2. Committee on Drugs. American Academy of Pediatrics. Guidelines for monitoring and management of pediatric patients during and after sedation for diagnostic and therapeutic procedures: addendum. *Pediatrics.* 2002;110:836–838.

3. American Society of Anesthesiologists: Standards for Basic Anesthetic Monitoring, October 25, 2005.

4. Report of the Advisory Committee on the Biological Effects of Ionizing Radiations: The effects on populations of exposure to low levels of ionizing radiation. Division of Medical Sciences, National Academy of Sciences, National Research Council, BEIR III 1980, Washington, D.C.: National Academy Press; 1980.

5. Robertson RL, Robson CD, Zurakowski D, Antiles S, Strauss K, Mulkern RV. CT versus MR in neonatal brain imaging at term. *Pediatr Radiol*. 2003;33:442–449.

6. Upton AC. National Council on Radiation Protection and Measurements Scientific Committee 1–6. The state of the art in the 1990s: NCRP Report No. 136 on the scientific bases for linearity in the dose-response relationship for ionizing radiation. *Health Phys*. 2003;85:15–22.

7. Modan B, Keinan L, Blumstein T, Sadetzki S. Cancer following cardiac catheterization in childhood. *Int J Epidemiol*. 2000;29:424–428.

8. Mason KP, Zgleszewski SE, Holzman RS. Anesthesia and sedation for sedation for procedures outside the operating room. In: Motoyama EK, Davis PJ, eds. *Smith's Anesthesia for Infants and Children*. 7th ed. Philadelphia, PA: Mosby Elsevier; 2006: 839–855.

9. Cohan RH, Dunnick NR, Bashore TM. Treatment of reactions to radiographic contrast material. *AJR Am J Roentgenol*. 1988;151:263–270.

10. Martin LD, Pasternak LR, Pudimat MA. Total intravenous anesthesia with propofol in pediatric patients outside the operating room. *Anesth Analg*. 1992;74:609–612.

11. Fisher DM, Robinson S, Brett CM. Comparison of enflurance, halothane, and isoflurane for diagnostic and therapeutic procedures in children with malignancies. *Anesthesiology*. 1985;63:647–650.

12. Menon DK, Peden CJ, Hall AS, et al. Magnetic resonance for the anaesthetist. Part 1: physical principles, application, safety aspects. *Anaesthesia*. 1992;47:240–255.

13. Tobin JR, Spurrier EA, Wetzel RC. Anaesthesia for critically ill children during magnetic resonance imaging. *Br J Anaesth*. 1992;69:482–486.

14. Peden CJ, Menon DK, Hall AS, et al. Magnetic resonance for the anaesthetist. Part II: anaesthesia and monitoring in MR units. *Anaesthesia*. 1992;47:508–517.

15. Gold JP, Pulsinelli W, Winchester P, et al. Safety of metallic surgical clips in patients undergoing high-field-strength magnetic resonance imaging. *Ann Thorac Surg*. 1989; 48:643–645.

16. Erlebacher JA, Cahill PT, Pannizzo F, et al. Effect of magnetic resonance imaging on DDD pacemakers. *Am J Cardiol*. 1986;57:437–440.

17. Shellock FG, Curtis JS. MR imaging and biomedical implants, materials, and devices: an updated review. *Radiology*. 1991;180:541–550.

18. Patteson SK, Chesney JT. Anesthetic management for magnetic resonance imaging: problems and solutions. *Anesth Analg*. 1992;74:121–128.

19. Shellock FG. Monitoring during MRI: an evaluation of the effect of high-field MRI on various patient monitors. *Med Electron*. 1986;17:93–97.

20. Dimick RN, Hedlund LW, Herfkens RJ, et al. Optimizing electrocardiographic electrode placement for cardiac-rated magnetic resonance imaging. *Invest Radiol*. 1987; 22:17–22.

21. Shellock FG. Monitoring sedated pediatric patients during MR imaging. *Radiology*. 1990;177:586–587.

22. Cote CJ. Anesthesia outside the operating room. In: Cote CJ, Ryan JF, Todres ID, Goudsouzian NG, eds. *A Practice of Anesthesia for Infants and Children*. 3rd ed. Philadelphia, PA: W.B. Saunders; 2001:571–583.

23. Frankville DD, Spear RM, Dyck JB. The dose of propofol required to prevent children from moving during magnetic resonance imaging. *Anesthesiology*. 1993;79:953–958.

24. Shellock FG. Biological effects of MRI: a clean safety record so far. *Diagnostic Imaging*. 1987;9:96–101.

25. Hammer GB, Hall SC, Davis PJ. Anesthesia for general abdominal, thoracic, urologic and bariatric surgery in pediatric patients. In: Motoyama EK, Davis PJ, eds. *Smith's Anesthesia for Infants and Children*. 7th ed. Philadelphia: Mosby Elsevier; 2006: 685–722.

26. Lebovic S, Reich DL, Steinberg LG, et al. Comparison of propofol versus ketamine for anesthesia in pediatric patients undergoing cardiac catheterization. *Anesth Analg*. 1992;74:490–494.

27. Vida VL, Bottio T, Milanesi O, et al. Critical aortic stenosis in early infancy: surgical treatment for residual lesions after balloon dilation. *Ann Thorac Surg*. 2005;79: 47–51.

28. Koenig P, Cao QL, Heitschmidt M, Waight DJ, Hijazi ZM. Role of intracardiac echocardiographic guidance in transcatheter closure of atrial septal defects and patent foramen ovale using the Amplatzer device. *J Interv Cardiol*. 2003;16:51–62.

29. Wagner KJ, Mollenberg O, Rentrop M, Werner C, Kochs EF. Guide to anaesthetic selection for electroconvulsive therapy. *CNS Drugs*. 2005;19:745–758.

30. Patkar AA, Hill KP, Weinstein SP, Schwartz SL. ECT in the presence of brain tumor and increased intracranial pressure: evaluation and reduction of risk. *J ECT*. 2000; 16:189–197.

31. van den Broek WW, Leentjens AF, Mulder PG, Kusuma A, Bruijn JA. Low-dose esmolol bolus reduces seizure duration during electroconvulsive therapy: a double-blind, placebo-controlled study. *Br J Anaesth*. 1999;83:271–274.

32. Mitchell P, Torda T, Hickie I, Burke C. Propofol as an anaesthetic agent for ECT: effect on outcome and length of course. *Aust NZ J Psych*. 1991;25:2255–2261.

33. Simpson KH, Snaith RP. The use of propofol for anaesthesia during ECT. *Br J Psychiatry*. 1989;154:721–722.

34. Boey WK, Lai FO. Comparison of propofol and thiopentone as anesthetic agents for electroconvulsive therapy. *Anaesthesia*. 1990;45:623–628.

35. Hodgson RE, Dawson P, Hold AR, Rout CC, Zuma K. Anaesthesia for electroconvulsive therapy: a comparison of sevoflurane with propofol. *Anaesth Intensive Care*. 2004;32:241–245.

36. Singh A, Shah G, Young J, Sheridan M, Haas G, Upadhyay J. Ureteral access sheath for the management of pediatric renal and ureteral stones: a single center experience. *J Urol*. 2006;175(3 Pt 1):1080–1082.

37. Liou LS, Streem SB. Long-term renal functional effects of shock wave lithotripsy, percutaneous nephrolithotomy and combination therapy: a comparative study of patients with solitary kidney. *J Urol*. 2001;166:36.

38. Aldridge RD, Aldridge RC, Aldridge LM. Anesthesia for pediatric lithotripsy. *Paediatr Anaesth*. 2006;16:236–241.

39. Roth RA, Beckman F. Complications of extracorporeal shock-wave lithotripsy and percutaneous nephrolithotomy. *Urol Clin North Am*. 1988;15:155–166.

40. Pettersson B, Tiselius HG, Andersson A, Eriksson I. Evaluation of extracorporeal shock wave lithotripsy without anesthesia using a Dornier HM3 lithotriptor without technical modifications. *J Urol*. 1989;142:1189–1192.

41. Cicek M, Koroglu A, Demirbilek S, Teksan H, Ersoy MO. Comparison of propofol-alfentanil and propofol-remifentanil anaesthesia in percutaneous nephrolithotripsy. *Eur J Anaesthesiol*. 2005;22:683–688.

42. Aldridge RD, Aldridge RC, Aldridge LM. Anesthesia for pediatric lithotripsy. *Paediatr Anaesth*. 2006;16:236–241.

43. Zeitlin GL, Roth R. Effects of three anesthetic techniques on the success of extracorporeal shock wave lithotripsy in nephrolithiasis. *Anesthesiology*. 1988;68:272–276.

44. Malhotra V, Long CW, Meister MJU. Intercostal blocks with local infiltration anesthesia for extracorporeal shock wave lithotripsy. *Anesth Analg*. 1987;66:85–88.

45. Tritrakarn T, Lertakyamanee J, Koompong P, et al. Both EMLA and placebo cream reduced pain during extracorporeal piezoelectric shock wave lithotripsy with the Piezolith 2300. *Anesthesiology*. 2000;92:1049–1054.

46. Basar H, Yilmaz E, Ozcan S, et al. Four analgesic techniques for shockwave lithotripsy: eutectic mixture local anesthetic is a good alternative. *J Endourol*. 2003; 17:3–6.

47. Fisher DM: Sedation of pediatric patients: an anesthesiologist's perspective. *Radiology*. 1990;175:613–615.

48. Cote CJ. Sedation for the pediatric patient: a review. *Ped Clin North Am*. 1994; 41:31–58.

49. American Society of Anesthesiologists Task Force on Sedation and Analgesia by Non-Anesthesiologists. Practice guidelines for sedation and analgesia by non-anesthesiologists. *Anesthesiology*. 2002;96:1004–1017.

50. Hoffman GM, Nowakowski R, Troshynski TJ, Berens RJ, Weisman SJ. Risk reduction in pediatric procedural sedation by application of an American Academy of Pediatrics/American Society of Anesthesiologists process model. *Pediatrics*. 2002; 109:236–243.

51. American Society of Anesthesiologists' Guidelines for Nonoperating Room Anesthetizing Locations. American Society of Anesthesiologists; October 15, 2003.

11. Office-based anesthesia

Hector Vila, Jr., MD
Meena S. Desai, MD
Rafael V. Miguel, MD

Definition

Office surgery is defined as any surgical or invasive procedure performed in a location outside a hospital, hospital outpatient department, ambulatory surgery center (ASC), or other diagnostic and treatment center which results in a patient stay of less than 24 hours. All perioperative care (i.e., preoperative assessment and preparation, operation, and postoperative recovery) is usually performed in a one-operating room (OR) suite within a physician's office. Generally speaking, office surgical procedures should not result in the loss of more than 10% of estimated blood volume in a patient with normal hemoglobin, should last less than 6 hours, and should not involve major intracranial, intra-thoracic, or intra-abdominal operations. They are non-emergent and not life-threatening in nature. By contrast, hospital-based ambulatory surgery units and ASCs are licensed by the state and frequently contain more than one OR and provide services for multiple surgeons. The advantages of office surgery include the following:

- Lower cost
- Greater privacy and convenience for the patient
- More control over surgical scheduling
- Potential reimbursement advantages to the surgeon

These advantages have led to the proliferation of office surgical procedures since the year 2000.

Safety

Whereas there are a number of outcomes studies for hospitals and ASCs, there are few for office surgery. Morello et al.[1] reported in 1997 on more than 400,000 plastic surgery procedures. They found a mortality of 1 in 57,000 patients. In 2000, Grazer and de Jong[2] reported on nearly 500,000 cosmetic surgery patients and found a mortality rate of 1 in 5,224 patients (or 19 per hundred thousand patients). Both of these studies relied on voluntary reporting, so it is plausible that physicians who had office surgical deaths may not have completed the survey. Hoefflin et al.[3] reported no office deaths in more than 23,000 cases. This data, however, came from a single fully accredited office with board-certified anesthesiologists and board-certified surgeons. Following an emergently imposed temporary requirement of mandatory reporting in response to a rash of office surgery mortalities in Florida, Vila et al.[4] analyzed and compared morbidity and mortality of office surgery to similar procedures performed in ASCs. They found the risk of injury and/or death was increased more than 10-fold in the office. In this study, the office deaths occurred in accredited facilities only 38% of the time and when an anesthesiologist was present in only 15%. In a more recent analysis of patient safety via an internet-based quality improvement and peer-review program, Keyes et al.[5] reported a death rate of 1 in 58,810 in 411,670 procedures performed in accredited offices during a 2-year period. A summary of the available literature on mortality of ASC and office surgery is contained in Table 11-1.[6-10]

These reviews have identified problems unique to the comparatively unregulated office. These include the following:

- Unqualified individuals participating in the surgery and/or administering sedation and anesthesia.
- Inadequate resuscitative airway equipment and medications.
- Emergency protocols were lacking or not followed. Transfer agreements with hospitals for emergency care were inconsistently available and inappropriately used.

Table 11-1. Summary of published mortality rates per 100,000 patients

Ambulatory surgery centers			Office-based surgery		
Source	Patients	Mortality	Source	Patients	Mortality
Natof HE[6] (1980)	13,433	0	Morello et al.[1] (1997)	400,675	1.7
Warner et al.[7] (1993)	35,598	4.4	Grazer and de Jong[2] (2000)	496,245	19
Mezei and Chung[8] (1999)	17,638	0	Hoefflin et al.[3] (2001)	23,000	0
Letts et al.[9] (2001)	4,899	0	Fleisher et al.[10] (2002)	28,199	35
Fleisher et al.[10] (2002)	175,288	25	Vila et al.[4] (2003)	141,404	9.2
Vila et al.[4] (2003)	2,316,249	0.78	Keyes et al.[5] (2004)	411,670	1.7

Regulations and oversight

State regulations

There are several different ways in which state regulatory bodies provide office surgery oversight. These include legislation, statutes, regulations, and rules. In some cases, states may have a combination of these methodologies. Legislation refers to bills that have been introduced in the legislature that have yet to become law. Statutes are bills that have been signed into law by the State House and Senate. Administrative rules and/or regulations are language that has been adopted by a regulatory body (e.g., state Board of Medicine) that also has the force of law for its constituents (i.e., physicians). Rules adopted by the Boards of Medicine may not have some of the powers of state law (e.g., to determine criminal action), and their scope is established and limited by state law. However, rules do establish guidelines for practice that will serve a basis to determine whether standard of care was violated and disciplinary action against a licensee should be considered.

As of 2006, 20 states had regulated office surgery via statute, rules/regulation, and/or guidelines. Those states are Alabama, California, Colorado, Connecticut, Florida, Illinois, Louisiana, Massachusetts, Mississippi, New Jersey, New York, North Carolina, Ohio, Oklahoma, Pennsylvania, Rhode Island, South Carolina, Tennessee, Texas, and Virginia. A number of other states were considering rule formation. Because of the rapidly changing environment of office-based surgery, it is difficult to provide a reliable current resource for each respective state's existing rules and regulations for readers in this chapter. Instead, the reader is referred to the American Society of Anesthesiologists (ASA) Web site, http://www.asahq.org/Washington/rulesregs.htm, which contains an up-to-date and state-by-state summary.

Accrediting organizations

There are several major nationally recognized accrediting bodies (listed in Table 11-2). The most common national organizations that accredit office surgery are the American Association for Accreditation of Ambulatory Surgery Facilities (AAAASF), the American Association of Ambulatory Health Care (AAAHC), and The Joint Commission. The accreditation process in office surgery assesses a physician's office and compares it to nationally recognized standards. The typical areas for comparison include the following:
- Governance
- Facilities (OR, equipment, etc.)
- Surgical services
- Anesthesia services
- Quality improvement program
- Records

Table 11-2. National office surgery accrediting organizations

Organization	Contact information
Accreditation Association for Ambulatory Health Care (AAAHC)	3201 Old Glenview Road, Suite 300, Wilmette, IL 60091-2992 Telephone: (847) 853-6060 (Source for *Accreditation Handbook of Ambulatory Health Care*) http://www.aaaasf.org
American Association for Accreditation of Ambulatory Surgery Facilities, Inc. (AAAASF) (*Manual for Accreditation of Ambulatory Surgery Facilities*, 1998)	5101 Washington St., Suite 2F, P.O. Box 9500, Gurnee, IL 60031 Telephone: (888) 545-5222 http://www.aaaasf.org
The Joint Commission Preriously Known as Joint Commission on Accreditation of Healthcare Organizations (JCAHO)	One Renaissance Boulevard, Oakbrook Terrace, IL 60181 Telephone: (630) 792-5000 http://www.jointcommission.org
American Osteopathic Association—Healthcare Facilities Accreditation Program (AOA-HFAP)	142 E. Ontario Street, Chicago, IL 60611 Telephone: (800) 621-1773, ext. 8258 http://www.aoa-net.org/Accreditation/HFAP/hfapcontact.htm

- Policy and procedures
- Medication management

Each of the nationally recognized accrediting bodies has mechanisms to ensure verifiable quality care but varies in their requirements. To date, only the AAAASF requires mandatory reporting of adverse outcomes. Accreditation is important for several reasons. Accreditation of offices provides consistency and can demonstrate external recognition of quality. Many states now require accreditation of offices performing surgical procedures. Many payers, including Medicare and private insurance companies, require accreditation of the facility in order to be reimbursed for facility fees; however, because most office-based surgery is elective cosmetic surgery, third-party payers are frequently not involved. This results in further isolation of the office surgical setting with a concomitant greater loss of oversight and outside influence. The incentive for accreditation in cosmetic facilities is often driven by market competition.

In some states, the surgeons' desire to self regulate has led to the development of private accrediting organizations. These organizations have received close scrutiny from state regulators. One concern is that they may be too closely involved with the surgical practitioners to objectively evaluate a practice. These local organizations frequently do not possess the ongoing training, quality improvement program, and necessary qualifications that dedicated established national accrediting organizations have. Other nationally recognized groups have provided guidance. The Federation of State Medical Boards (FSMB) proposed three pathways that state medical boards can adopt for oversight of office-based surgery and anesthesia practices in unregulated settings (http://www.fsmb.org/pdf/2002_grpol_Outpatient_Surgery.pdf):

- Adoption of FSMB Model Guidelines
- Requiring accreditation by a recognized national or state accrediting organization
- Development of individual state standards

In addition, the American Medical Association adopted 10 core principles intended to inform and guide legislative and/or regulatory bodies in setting standards to promote safety. These core principles are found in Table 11-3.

Policies and procedures

Most of the accreditation standards in hospitals are in place to verify that the appropriate personnel, policy, and procedures are present for safe medical care. In the office, the importance of qualified personnel and of the appropriate policies and procedures cannot be overstated and must be comparable to those present in hospitals. At a minimum, the office anesthesiology practitioner is advised to follow the relevant ASA guidelines, standards, and statements. The applicable standards for preoperative evaluation, intraoperative monitoring, and postoperative care that apply in the office environment are no different from those in other ambulatory settings and are covered in the relevant chapters in this book. The reader is referred to the following, which the office surgery practice must have available:

- ASA Guidelines for Office-Based Anesthesia (http://www.asahq.org/publicationsAndServices/standards/12.pdf)
- Credentialing Guidelines for Practitioners who are not Anesthesia Professionals to administer anesthetic drugs to establish a level of moderate sedation (http://www.asahq.org/publicationsAndServices/credentialing.pdf)
- Practice guidelines for the management of patients with obstructive sleep apnea. (http://www.asahq.org/publicationsAndServices/sleepapnea103105.pdf)
- Office-Based Anesthesia - Considerations for Anesthesiologists in Setting Up and Maintaining a Safe Office Anesthesia Environment (http://www2.asahq.org/publications/pc-139-7-office-based-anesthesia-considerations-for-anesthesiologists-in-setting-up-and-maintaining-a-safe.aspx)

The office surgery practice should also have an emergency office procedure manual, outlining steps to follow in the event of the following:

- Fire
- Cardiac arrest
- Electrical failure
- Locally appropriate natural emergencies

The manual should include a record of the performance of drills on a monthly or quarterly basis and regular "crash cart" checks.

Table 11-3. American Medical Association (AMA) core principles for office-based surgery

Core principle 1	Guidelines or regulations for office-based surgery should be developed by states according to levels of anesthesia defined by the American Society of Anesthesiologists (ASA) excluding local anesthesia or minimal sedation. (ASA. Continuum of depth of sedation. Available at: http://www.asahq.org/ PublicationsAndServices/standards/20.pdf. Accessed February 27, 2003.)
Core principle 2	Physicians should select patients for office-based surgery using moderate sedation/analgesia, deep sedation/analgesia, or general anesthesia by criteria including the ASA Physical Status Classification System, and so document. (ASA. ASA physical status classification system. Available at: http:// www.asahq.org/clinical/physicalstatus.htm. Accessed February 27, 2003.)
Core principle 3	Physicians who perform office-based surgery with moderate sedation/analgesia, deep sedation/analgesia, or general anesthesia should have their facilities accredited by the Joint Commission on Accreditation of Healthcare Organizations, Accreditation Association for Ambulatory Health Care, American Association for Accreditation of Ambulatory Surgical Facilities, American Osteopathic Association (AOA), or a state-recognized entity, such as the Institute for Medical Quality, or be state-licensed and/or Medicare-certified.
Core principle 4	Physicians performing office-based surgery with moderate sedation/analgesia, deep sedation/analgesia, or general anesthesia must have admitting privileges at a nearby hospital, have a transfer agreement with another physician who has admitting privileges at a nearby hospital, or maintain an emergency transfer agreement with a nearby hospital.
Core principle 5	States should follow the guidelines outlined by the Federation of State Medical Boards (FSMB) regarding informed consent. (Report of the Special Committee on Outpatient [Office-Based] Surgery. *Med Licensure Discipline.* 2002; 88:160–174.)
Core principle 6	For office surgery with moderate sedation/analgesia, deep sedation/analgesia, or general anesthesia, states should consider legally privileged adverse incident reporting requirements as recommended by the

(Continued)

Table 11-3. *Continued*

	FSMB and accompanied by periodic peer review and a program of Continuous Quality Improvement. (Report of the Special Committee on Outpatient [Office-Based] Surgery. *Med Licensure Discipline.* 2002; 88:160–174.)
Core principle 7	Physicians performing office-based surgery using moderate sedation/analgesia, deep sedation/analgesia, or general anesthesia must obtain and maintain board certification by one of the boards recognized by the American Board of Medical Specialties, AOA, or a board with equivalent standards approved by the state medical board within 5 years of completing an approved residency training program. The procedure must be one that is generally recognized by that certifying board as falling within the scope of training and practice of the physician providing the care.
Core principle 8	Physicians performing office-based surgery with moderate sedation/analgesia, deep sedation/analgesia, or general anesthesia may show competency by maintaining core privileges at an accredited or licensed hospital or ambulatory surgical center for the procedures they perform in the office setting. Alternatively, the governing body of the office facility is responsible for a peer-review process for privileging physicians based on nationally recognized credentialing standards.
Core principle 9	For office-based surgery with moderate sedation/ analgesia, deep sedation/analgesia, or general anesthesia, at least one physician who is currently credentialed in advanced resuscitative techniques (e.g., advanced trauma life support, advanced cardiac life support, or pediatric advanced life support) must be present or immediately available with age- and size-appropriate resuscitative equipment until the patient has met the criteria for discharge from the facility. In addition, other medical personnel with direct patient contact should at a minimum be trained in basic life support.
Core principle 10	Physicians administering or supervising moderate sedation/analgesia, deep sedation/analgesia, or general anesthesia should have appropriate education and training.

Amended core principles as presented by the AMA Board of Trustees (BOT) to the AMA House of Delegates at the I-03 Meeting. For additional information, refer to BOT Report 23 (A-03). Source: http://www.ama-assn.org/ama/pub/category/11807.html.

Personnel

All health care practitioners (physicians, dentists, podiatrists, and allied health personnel) participating in the office surgery procedure should hold a valid license or certificate from the state to perform their assigned duties. An increasing number of states are requiring the surgeon and anesthesiologist to have staff privileges at a licensed hospital to perform the same procedure that is to be performed in the office setting. Some physicians, such as dermatologists and some "cosmetic physicians," may not maintain hospital privileges. In this situation, the physician must be able to document comparable training or experience and specialty board certification/eligibility by a board approved by the American Board of Medical Specialties (ABMS) and be performing procedures generally recognized by that board as within the specialty. Although ABMS board certification is the only board recognized by all 50 states, other specialty boards may be recognized by the respective states as evidence of board certification. An alternative is for the oversight board to consider, on a case-by-case basis, the background, training, and experience of the individual surgeon.

Many regulatory bodies classify office surgery facilities by means of a three-level system detailed in Box 11-1.

Surgeons in an office-based setting providing Level III (and probably Level II, although this requirement is inconsistent) should maintain current advanced cardiac life support (ACLS) certification. At least one other assistant should be currently certified in ACLS, and other medical personnel should maintain training in basic cardiopulmonary resuscitation. However, these requirements vary from state to state. In many of the office deaths reported from the state of Florida, lack of readily available resuscitative equipment contributed to the poor outcome. The state of Florida has instituted a requirement for ACLS training for all surgeons participating in Level II and III office surgery procedures along with another assistant certified in basic life support.[11]

Box 11-1. Office surgery facilities classification

Class A	Level I	Minor surgical procedures such as excision of skin lesions performed under topical or local anesthesia and not involving drug-induced alteration of consciousness other than minimal sedation or anxiolysis
Class B	Level II	Surgical procedures that require moderate sedation, usually administered intravenously
Class C	Level III	Surgical procedures which require, or reasonably should require, deep sedation, general anesthesia, or major conduction blockade to achieve loss of consciousness and vital reflexes

Facility requirements

The ASA OR design manual, developed in 1998 by the Committee on Equipment and Facilities, contains a comprehensive and detailed summary of facility requirements and is the basis for the following information on facility design.[12]

Room size

There are no specific minimum size requirements for office-based surgery. However, keeping in mind the numbers of people in the room (in addition to the patient) and the required equipment, an OR should have approximately 300 square feet. If the center will provide Level III anesthesia, there should be a ventilation system capable of providing 15 air exchanges per hour with at least three of these exchanges provided with fresh outdoor air. Relative humidity should be kept at 50%–60%. Each room should have the ability to adjust its temperature. Piped gases, including air and oxygen, as well as vacuum and outlet and scavenging outlet should be available adjacent to the anesthesia machine. If the piped connections are not available, a suitable dedicated cylinder storage area is required. Wide enough egress is needed to wheel the patient in and out of the OR. Although patients undergoing office-based anesthesia (OBA) are often walked into the OR, sometimes preoperative anxiety requires intravenous (IV) anxiolysis. This may make patients unstable to walk and therefore in need of a chair or stretcher for transfer into the OR. Similarly, patients are frequently unsteady after the operation and will need to be transported to the recovery area. Doors, hallways, and corners should all be wide enough to accommodate the stretcher or chair, hanging IV lines, and the required personnel with ease.

Power requirements

There should be adequate lighting, electrical power outlets with ground fault circuit interrupters, and a backup power source. Typical emergency power systems provide for activation within 10 seconds of power failure and will last at least 90 minutes under normal load. There must be sufficient power capacity to complete any procedure and safely remove patients from the facility. Especially if the surgical facility is above the ground floor, there must also be backup power to the entire building in order to have lighted hallways and elevator operation for patient transport if an interruption in power occurs.

Emergency exit strategy

Access to the office surgery center should be unobstructed. This is particularly relevant in those offices above the ground floor. If a patient requires transfer to a hospital and is hemodynamically unstable, the transfer needs to be done on a stretcher. This requires that the building hallways, access doors, elevators, and (if necessary) stairs be sufficiently large to accommodate such a transfer, and ramps should be accessible and convenient for patient transfer. The office staff needs to be aware of the location of emergency exits so they may use them and direct emergency personnel to the appropriate areas. Periodic review must be performed to ensure that all exits are well marked, clear, unobstructed, and unlocked. There must also be adequate lighting, early fire warning, and backup or redundant exit arrangements.

Facility regulatory bodies

In addition to the aforementioned agencies that will evaluate the suitability of the center and physician to practice medicine within the facility, the facility must comply with all appropriate local, state, and national regulatory requirements. Local jurisdictions may include the Building Department, Fire Marshal, Public Works Department, and Planning and Development Departments. State agencies may include the Certificate of Need Program Office, Health Department, Insurance Commissioner, State Department of Environmental Regulation, and Regional Planning Commissions. At a minimum, the practitioner opening a new office surgery facility should contact the state Department of Health for information on relevant regulations. Federal agencies with possible jurisdiction include the Department of Health and Human Services, Department of Justice (Americans with Disabilities Act), the Department of Labor, the Environmental Protection Agency, and the Occupational Safety and Health Administration.

Basic office layout

The office facility must have a preoperative holding area that can receive patients, provide for changing into surgical apparel, and provide a private space for preoperative interview, administration of preoperative medications if indicated, and obtaining of vital signs. There should also be a substerile area with a scrub sink, an autoclave, and storage for sterile supplies. Storage space is one of the most important requirements and is often overlooked. There should be adequate storage space for OR equipment, supplies, and OR waste.

Fire

Because of the ever-present danger of fire in the OR, fire extinguishers and fire alarm boxes should be located in each facility. Additionally, the house shutoff valve for medical gases should be conveniently located. Every OR should have a smoke detector and a sprinkler system. Appropriate fire codes provide for adequate exits that have been designed to accommodate wheelchairs and/or stretchers. (Typically, the hallway should be a minimum of 4 feet in width with 3′–10″ door openings.)

Preoperative assessment

In the office-based practice, it is key to educate our fellow specialists in proper patient selection. The surgeon or proceduralist and their office staff are the first line in patient selection, and once a list of appropriate patients has been developed, it must be reviewed with the surgeon's office staff as they begin to identify appropriate office patients versus those who should be referred to hospital outpatient or inpatient care (Table 11-4). This list should be updated and revised frequently as guidelines change.

The requirement for preoperative patient evaluation for office surgery is identical to all ambulatory surgery and is detailed in Chapter 3. It is often helpful to have the office patients fill out an initial anesthesia questionnaire that is distributed at the surgeon's office and that allows the patient to anticipate the medical evaluation and the nature of the questions asked in the telephone interview (Figure 11-1).

Table 11-4. Patient selection criteria for selecting appropriate office-based patients

Criteria that suggest a patient may be <u>unsuitable</u> for a procedure in an office setting
  1. Unstable angina
  2. Recent myocardial infarction
  3. Severe cardiomyopathy
  4. Uncontrolled hypertension
  5. Patients with internal defibrillators or pacemakers
  6. End-stage renal disease
  7. Sickle cell disease
  8. Patient on major organ transplant list
  9. Uncontrolled diabetes
  10. Active multiple sclerosis
  11. Severe chronic obstructive pulmonary disease
  12. Abnormal airway/Difficult intubation
  13. Malignant hyperthermia by history
  14. Acute illegal substance abusers
  15. Morbid obesity
  16. Dementia with disorientation
  17. Psychologically unstable: rage/anger problems
  18. Myasthenia gravis
  19. Recent stroke
  20. Obstructive sleep apnea

NOVA ANESTHESIA PROFESSIONALS
Patient Pre-Anesthesia Questionnaire

Name: _____ Age: _____ Weight: _____ Height: _____

Date/Time: _____ Procedure: _____ Surgeon: _____

Person to drive you home: _____ Telephone#: _____

1. Please complete this form and have it available for your anesthesia telephone interview, if possible, please fax this form to XXX-XXX-XXXX.
2. If you should have any questions or do not understand some of the items, we will clarify them at the time of your interview.
3. Please use the comment space to explain any "YES" answers and please provide dates if possible.

List all Medications/Herbals you currently take:
_____
_____
_____

List all previous operations: _____
_____
_____
_____

Any drug allergies:	N Y_____	Have you ever had a problem with anesthesia or
Any latex allergies:	N Y_____	with Malignant Hyperthermia? N Y_____
Do you smoke:	N Y_____	Has anyone in your family had a problem with anesthesia
How many packs a day?_____		or malignant hyperthermia? N Y_____
Do you drink alcohol?	N Y_____	Could you be pregnant? N Y_____
How much?_____		Date of last menstrual period:_____
Do you use recreational drugs? N Y		Do you have a history of:
Do you have any of the following?		Irregular heartbeat or arrhythmia? N Y_____
Asthma or Bronchitis?	N Y_____	Heart murmur/Chest pain? N Y_____
Emphysema?	N Y_____	Mitral Valve prolapse? N Y_____
Difficulty Breathing?	N Y_____	High blood pressure? N Y_____
Sleep Apnea?	N Y_____	Heart attack/angina? N Y_____
Diabetes?	N Y_____	Peptic ulcer disease? N Y_____
Kidney problems?	N Y_____	Hiatal hernia? N Y_____
Bladder problems?	N Y_____	Gastric ulcer/acid reflux? N Y_____
Thyroid disease?	N Y_____	Hepatitis/liver disease? N Y_____
Sickle cell disease?	N Y_____	Stroke? N Y_____
Bleeding problems?	N Y_____	Epilepsy? N Y_____
Anemia?	N Y_____	Seizure? N Y_____
Blood transfusion?	N Y_____	Migraines or headaches? N Y_____
Neck pain?	N Y_____	Do you wear contacts or glasses? N Y_____
Back pain?	N Y_____	Do you have a hearing aid? N Y_____
Arthritis?	N Y_____	Do you have any loose/chipped teeth? N Y_____
Muscle weakness?	N Y_____	Do you have dentures, caps, bridgework N Y_____ or braces?

Any additional comments or concerns not mentioned above?
_____
_____
_____

Signature: _____ Date/Time: _____

Figure 11-1. NOVA Anesthesia Professionals, Inc. (Villanova, PA) patient pre-anesthesia questionnaire.

Table 11-5. Preprocedure testing recommendations for office-based anesthesia

(These tests may be needed for administration of anesthesia and are not intended to limit those required by surgeons for issues specific to their surgical management.)

For healthy individuals under the age of 50, with **no** comorbid conditions, undergoing minimally invasive procedures (cataracts, gastrointestinal, dental, diagnostic imaging, minor gynecological, urological procedures): NO specific preoperative tests are indicated.

Testing for asymptomatic patients for moderately invasive surgery (liposuction, face-lifts, breast augmentations, laparoscopy, arthroscopy, and other plastic and cosmetic procedures)

TEST	MALE	FEMALE
Hgb/Hct	50 and older	Age 12 and older
ECG (within 1 year)	50 and older	50 and older
Beta hCG	N/A	Child-bearing age*

*Pregnancy tests are offered to patients if they think they could be pregnant and if LMP shows missed periods.

For patients over the age of 50, a history and physical within the past 6 months by a primary physician are recommended. For patients **with** comorbid conditions (e.g., HTN, CAD, or DM), a recent history and physical are needed to establish that the patient's comorbid conditions are at their maximal medical management for undergoing an elective procedure with anesthesia. Testing would be selected to identify changes in health.

Patients with comorbid conditions (HTN, CAD, DM, or pulmonary disease) may require additional testing within 1 month or interval as indicated, and it will need to be disease-specific.

TEST	DISEASE
ECG	HTN, CAD, cerebrovascular disease, DM, symptomatic mitral valve prolapse, arrhythmias within 1 year
Glucose	Diabetic: can be serum or glucometer reading on day of procedure
Electrolytes	Patients on diuretics
BUN/Cr	Renal disease
Chest x-ray	If indicated by primary M.D. for advanced pulmonary disease

Significantly abnormal test results will need a statement addressing the patient's eligibility to undergo an elective procedure with anesthesia. This statement will be from a medical director or referred to the primary physician if that is determined to be more appropriate.

CAD, coronary artery disease; DM, diabetes mellitus; ECG, electrocardiogram; hCG, human chorionic gonadotropin; HTN, hypertension; LMP, last menstrual period.

Some of the information required may be available in the patient's office medical record, and a telephone interview may be used to verify and obtain additional information. Arrangements for medical consults and preoperative testing such as laboratory tests and electrocardiogram (ECG) should be made in advance of surgery. As has been recommended by many in the ambulatory field, testing should be performed only on an as-needed basis and not as a general medical screening. Testing should be selected to identify changes in health. Patients with comorbid conditions must have a history and physical that ascertains whether patients are medically stabilized and whether there are any new changes in the patient's condition.

A current preoperative testing guideline (Table 11-5) may be helpful for the surgical offices so they can initiate the ordering of any necessary testing as soon as the patient is scheduled.

When the anesthesia provider has not personally performed a physical examination, the patient should arrive at the office facility early enough to allow for proper evaluation prior to the planned surgical procedure. Although the evaluation of the patient's current medical status is paramount, one must also consider "social factors" of postoperative care such as the patient's psychological status and the support system at home (help at home, ability to get to the hospital if a complication occurs at home, distance from the hospital, etc.).

Setup and delivery of care

General considerations

All basic ASA monitoring standards, including monitoring and equipment, should be followed in office surgery settings as they should be in all surgery locations. Qualified anesthesia personnel must be present in the room throughout the anesthetic, and the patient's oxygenation, ventilation, circulation, and temperature must be continually evaluated. To ensure the presence of adequate ventilation during deep sedation and general anesthesia, the exhaled gases should be continually monitored for the presence of carbon dioxide.

The equipment setup at each location should address the standards and guidelines for office-based anesthesia, but the format should be altered for portability. The "anesthesia red cart" has been modified into a portable tackle box and has a "bag" that holds all disposables.

Portable monitors equipped with automatic electronic defibrillators are provided for our infrequently used office locations. At our frequently used office suites, the anesthesia cart and monitors are stationary and dedicated to the location. Every site should have a source for positive-pressure delivery of oxygen. The dental suites' oxygen delivery systems are modified to have a positive-pressure oxygen delivery capability. A portable emergency E tank of oxygen must be full and available should the occasion arise and standard delivery systems fail. Suction must be available at every site.

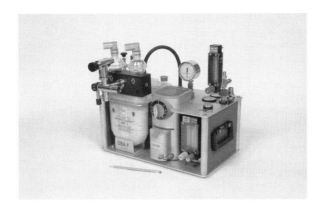

Figure 11-2. The first lightweight, U.S. Food and Drug Administration 510(k)-approved, compact, portable anesthesia machines—the OBA-1® and OBA-1® magnetic resonance imaging units (OBAMED Inc.)—are specifically designed for surgical locations where space or access is limited, such as office-based anesthesia. Reproduced with permission.

An anesthesia machine is required for offices when the use of volatile anesthetic agents is planned. Several new machines have been developed with portability and space limitations in mind (Figure 11-2). Refurbished anesthesia machines are available from numerous companies.

The anesthesia practitioner should confirm that the operative suite can provide adjunctive care for selected procedures as needed (i.e., warming devices, eye protection for laser surgery, foley catheter as needed, and antiembolic stockings). The recovery area must also be equipped with appropriate monitors, oxygen, and suction.

The intraoperative anesthetic record should conform to established ASA standards. The anesthesia record also needs to conform to established guidelines and standards of accrediting organizations, the state, and the ASA.

Anesthetizing locations can be outfitted as the site warrants and as space allows, while at the same time adhering to standards, guidelines, and regulations.

Five different categories of office-based anesthesia practice which outline the challenges faced in each site will be discussed:

1. The one-room plastic or cosmetic surgical suite equipped to provide general anesthesia.
2. The surgeon who equips a large room for periodic IV sedation on an as-needed basis.
3. The dental specialist who sporadically provides IV or inhalational sedation for dental phobics.
4. Pain medicine physicians requiring a suite for interventional pain procedures, typically ultrashort interventions that often require light IV sedation.

5.   The rapid turnover required of a gastrointestinal suite providing IV sedation.

Our anesthesia practice group surveys and documents the layout of each facility prior to starting cases. It is important to document exits, plans for patient flow, and locations of phones, bathrooms, emergency lighting, backup generators, etc. These surveys should be updated as changes occur or at least on an annual basis. One must verify that the facility is in compliance with all local and state regulations. Along with the site survey, collect and verify all the practitioners' state licenses, board specialty status, U.S. Drug Enforcement Agency (DEA) license, and hospital privileges (Table 11-6).

Plastic and cosmetic surgical suite

The general anesthesia operating suite provides the surgeon the greatest flexibility in the numbers and types of plastic and cosmetic procedures performed.[3] The one-room general suite is outfitted much the same way an OR is, with anesthesia machine, monitors, and end-tidal and gas analysis monitoring systems. The recommended calibration of the general anesthesia machine and monitors must be performed to manufacturers' specifications by authorized personnel. The surgical suites must be equipped with all necessary materials for ACLS protocols of resuscitation as well as with the suggested amount of dantrolene for the treatment of malignant hyperthermia. If general anesthesia or triggering agents for malignant hyperthermia, such as volatile anesthetic agents (halothane, enflurane, isoflurane, desflurane, and sevoflurane) or succinylcholine, are used or available in the facility, then a minimum of 12 vials of dantrolene should be immediately available for initial patient rescue. An additional 24 vials of dantrolene must be present or available in a facility in close proximity to the office. A supply of preservative-free sterile water for injection should be kept nearby to mix with dantrolene before injection (60 mL/vial). Malignant Hyperthermia Association of the United States (MHAUS) guidelines recommend that each facility have a full treatment dose (36 vials) on-site. The current cost of maintaining 36 vials in stock is approximately $909 per year (call Procter & Gamble Pharmaceuticals at 800-448-4878 for current pricing, routine ordering, reordering, and emergency orders). In the absence of triggering agents in the facility, dantrolene may not be required; however, verification with state regulations is mandatory. It is also important to note that malignant hyperthermia deaths have occurred in susceptible individuals without the presence of "triggering agents." The reader is advised to stay abreast of current MHAUS recommendations. These can be found at http://www.mhaus.org/index.cfm/fuseaction/Content.Display/PagePK/ProfessionalInfoCenter.cfm. A rapid onset/short acting muscle relaxant must be available for emergency airway management in all office-based practices where deep sedation and general anesthesia are used. To maximize efficiency, there usually is a separate recovery room with the recommended monitors, oxygen, and suction systems. Postanesthesia care unit (PACU) care should be delivered by a registered nurse (RN) with current ACLS certification.

Table 11-6. Office anesthesia checklist

☑ **Facility design:**

	Date completed	Comments
• Sufficient space		
• Recovery area		
• Meets building codes		
• Sufficient electrical outlets		
• Backup power		
• Visual access to patient at all times during surgery/proper lighting		

☑ **Equipment and supplies:**

	Date completed	Comments
• Reliable O_2 source with backup		
• Adequate source of suction and catheters		
• Self-inflating (Ambu) resuscitation bag capable of administering at least 90% O_2 with backup bag		
• Emergency cart/airway equipment/ACLS drugs for population(s) served (i.e., adult, pediatric)		
• Communication device (telephone, intercom within reach)		
• Scavenging system for waste gas		
• Blood pressure, electrocardiogram, stethoscope, pulse oximeter, capnogram		
• Functioning resuscitation equipment and defibrillator		
• Appropriate-sized airways, laryngoscope blade, masks/laryngeal mask airways		
• Dantrolene when using triggering agents		

☑ **General preparedness:**

	Date completed	Comments
• Credentialed and licensed medical doctors		
• ACLS and/or pediatric ALS trained staff on premises until patient discharge		
• Hospital transfer agreement		
• Quality assurance policies/initiatives and peer reviews		

ACLS, advanced cardiac life support; ALS, advanced life support.

Table 11-7. NOVA Anesthesia Professionals, Inc. (Villanova, PA) anesthesiologist bag inventory

Bags: disposable items	Quantity
Endotracheal tubes (6.0, 7.0, 8.0)	1 of each
Yankauer suction	2
Suction hose	1 per patient
Nasal cannulas	3–4 (+1 for each additional patient)
Lactated Ringer or normal saline	3–4 (+1 for each additional patient)
Ambu bag	1
Laryngeal mask airway	1
IV tubing	3 each (minidrip and macrodrip)
Extension IV tubing	3–4 (+1 for each additional patient)
Extension tubing (infusion pump)	3–4 (+1 for each additional patient)
Rubber glove	2 (optional)
Stylettes	2 per bag
Manual sphygnomanometer	1
Stethoscope	1
Oxygen tank with wrench	1 each
Flashlight	1
Scissors	1

Mobile surgical suite for intravenous sedation

IV sedation or monitored anesthesia care techniques are often employed to meet patient and surgeon preferences and when anesthesia gases are not available for a general anesthetic. The surgeon (genitourinary, gynecology, ophthalmology, podiatry, plastic, etc.) who only occasionally uses these services requires all the same elements of care; however, the setup for IV sedation with portable monitors and equipment is provided. Our group uses a three-component portable system:

1. The monitor bag that carries a lightweight monitor for ECG, noninvasive blood pressure and pulse oximetry, and an automatic external defibrillator.
2. The disposables bag that carries fluids, nasal cannula, IV sets, laryngeal mask airway, Yankauer, and additional items (Table 11-7).
3. The medications, resuscitative medications, and controlled substances that are in an organized setup within a tackle box. Opioids are double-locked with the tackle box and assigned to each particular physician as needed (Table 11-8).

Dental suite

The dental specialists who most frequently ask for sedation are oral surgeons, periodontists, prosthodontists, and pedodontists. Each specialty has

Table 11-8. NOVA Anesthesia Professionals, Inc. (Villanova, PA) anesthesiologist tackle box inventory

Tackle box	Quantity
Top drawer items	
Gauze	
Stopcocks	2–3
Oral airways (6.0, 7.0, 8.0)	1 each
Nasal airways 20, 24, 28, 32)	1 each
Electrocardiogram leads	1 bag
Alcohol wipes	
Bandaids	
Tape	1–2 rolls
Laryngoscope (with batteries)	2
C batteries	1 extra set
Mac blade # 4 (laryngoscope)	1
Rusch blade # 3 (laryngoscope)	1
50% Dextrose (injection w/needle)	1
*Ketamine**	*1–2*
*Midazolam**	*1–2*
*Fentanyl**	*1–2*
*Demerol**	*1*
Labels (Fentanyl, Versed, Brevital)	1 roll each
Alupent inhaler	1
Propofol	2
First drawer:	
Sodium bicarb (1 mEg/mL)	1
Epinephrine inj (with needle) (1 mg)	1
1% or 2% Lidocaine (w/needle) (100 mg/mL)	1
Amiordarone	3
Ca chloride 10% (100 mg/mL)	1
Procainamide (1 g/10 mL)	1
Surgilube	1 tube
Tongue blades	10
Second drawer	
IV caths (18, 20, 22 gauge)	10 each
Temp strips	dozen
1% Lidocaine (10 mg/mL)	1 (50 mL vial)
1 cc syringes	8–10 syringes
3 cc syringes	6–8 syringes
5 cc syringes	5–6 syringes
10 cc syringes	5–6 syringes
Needles (18, 22 gauge)	8 each
50% Dextrose	1 (50 mL vial)
Ammonia inhalants	2–4

(Continued)

Table 11-8. *Continued*

Tackle box	Quantity
Third drawer	
Thiopental (Pentothal) (if available)	1 kit
Methohexital (Brevital) (if available)	1 (2.5 g vial)
Dolasetron (Anzemet)	2–4 (1 mL amp)
Metoclopramide (Reglan)	2–4 (1 mL amp)
Glycopyrolate (Robinul)	1 (20 mL vial)
Atropine	1 (20 mL vial)
Cefazolin (Ancef)	1 (1 g vial)
Ampicillin	1 (500 mg vial)
Clindamycin	1 (600 mg vial)
Gentamycin	1–2 (2 mL vial)
Dexamethasone	1 (30 mL vial)
Hydrocortisone (Solu-Cortef)	1 (2 mL act-o-vial)
Furosemide	4 (4 mL vial)
Fourth drawer	
Succinycholine or Rocuronium	1–2 (10 mL vial)
Dopamine	1 (5 mL vial)
Propanolol (Inderal)	1–2 (1 mL amps)
Adenosine (Adenocard)	4 (2 mL amps)
Diphenhydramine (Benadryl)	2–3 (1 mL amps)
Digoxin (Lanoxin)	2–3 (2 mL amps)
Verapamil	1 (2 mL vial)
Nitrostat/Nitropaste	1 (25 sublingual tab vial)
Hydralazine	1 (1 mL vial)
Labetolol (Normodyne)	1 (20 mL vial)
Esmolol (Brevibloc)	1 (10 mL vial)
Phenylephrine	2–4 (1 mL amps)
Ephedrine	2–4 (1 mL amps)
Epinephrine	2–4 (1 mL amps)
Flumazenil (Romazicon)	1 (5 mL vial)
Naloxone (Narcan)	2–3 (1 mL amps)

*These drugs should be kept in a double-lock box.

different needs as the procedures each specialty performs are quite varied. Some dental specialists have had some training and exposure in working with the anesthesia provider and the "sedated" patient. As part of their training, these dental specialists have received education about sedation so they acquire an appreciation of the acuteness of an unprotected airway and its limitations. Everyone must have the same expectations, and patient safety must be the most important factor. Remember that the anesthesiologist's expertise in providing sedation allows the practitioner to accomplish a greater range of procedures, so the training of the specialist is key. Many dentists provide sedation with nitrous oxide and oxygen gases in their office. These gases are delivered via flow systems that are controlled at the wall or with a portable flow meter. A mixture of oxygen and nitrous oxide, between 30% and 50%, is titrated to the patient's comfort. The gas is delivered through a nose mask that sits on the patient's face. The scavenging system is connected to the office's central suction. The nasal mask is not a tight fit and therefore the scavenging system is less efficient. Some practics choose not to use the nitrous oxide gas in sedation cases.

Oral surgeons most commonly require anesthesia for the extraction of impacted molars. These cases are typically 30–35 minutes long and require a deep level of sedation. IV sedation is titrated with bolus administration of midazolam 2–3 mg and fentanyl 50–100 µg at the start. Ketamine may be given in small aliquots (e.g., 5–10 mg) as indicated by patient condition. An IV infusion of propofol or methohexital (Brevital®) may be titrated to 50–150 µg/kg per minute. The drip is titrated to end as the last molars are sutured, and the patient is typically able to walk to recovery within 7–10 minutes.

Periodontists often require anesthesia services for their phobic patients. They use anesthesia for gum surgery, dental implants, and planing and scaling of all mouth quadrants. Close communication with the practitioner, the patient, and the anesthesiologist regarding the details of the patient's phobia and the changing level of anesthesia from lighter to deeper planes of anesthesia is key. The need for patient cooperation during the procedure will necessitate changing levels of anesthesia as the procedure is performed. Continuous IV sedative infusions provide the greatest flexibility with varying levels of anesthesia. Have the dentist select the lowest setting of water spray required with drilling, cleaning, etc., as the airway has decreased protective reflexes and the risk of aspiration increases. Alternatively, the anesthetic level may be lightened so the patient may cooperate with swallowing to avoid aspiration. The use of a mouth prop is invaluable in keeping the mouth open in a sedated patient so that accessibility to the field is ensured. These must be placed before patient cooperation is lost, as mouth opening can be an issue in the sedated patient.

Prosthodontists are the plastic surgeons of dentistry, and the gamut of procedures includes dentures, partial plates, and crowns with post and core preparations. The prosthodontist needs to have many periods of patient cooperation that may involve making of molds, molding articular surfaces, and fitting prosthesis. The technique of continuous infusion of propofol at varying rates and increments of midazolam (Versed®) will provide satisfactory working conditions with effective patient comfort.

Interventional pain

As is true for many other interventional scenarios in the office, sedation may not be required but provides greater patient comfort and compliance. This is the case with interventional pain treatment in which patients with chronic pain often have comorbid conditions such as depression and anxiety. A small amount of IV sedation/anxiolytics can be used to titrate to patient comfort. Opioids should be reserved for those patients with pain at rest who cannot tolerate the position required for performance of the planned intervention.

Use extreme caution in sedating those patients who will receive injections with the potential to harm the spinal neuraxis. Benumof[13] reported on four cases in which interscalene blocks were performed in patients receiving deep sedation or general anesthesia. These patients suffered permanent spinal cord damage by direct needle trauma. Patients who are awake or mildly sedated during blocks are able to communicate and complain of pain on nerve entry and/or compression by injection by the advancing needle. This means that all patients sedated for interventional pain procedures should be responsive to light tactile or verbal stimuli whenever the potential for nerve damage exists, especially when one is advancing a needle in or toward the spinal canal above L3. Furthermore, some procedures (e.g., radiofrequency ablation and spinal cord stimulation) will require significant patient cooperation and feedback, so communication with the operating surgeon beforehand will assist in developing the most appropriate sedation strategy.

Ensuring adequate space in the interventional pain suite is an important consideration. There are frequently a multitude of pieces of equipment with varying power source requirements which occupy large amounts of space. These include the fluoroscopy machine (i.e., "C-Arm") with monitors, ideally placed at the patient's head to facilitate viewing while performing the procedure without the interventionalists having to turn their head. All facilities that use radiologic imaging equipment must comply with basic radiation safety and all applicable regulations. The most basic concept in radiation safety is that the closer an individual is to the source of radiation the higher the level of exposure. Therefore, every attempt should be made to maintain the greatest possible distance away from the radiation beam. Among the other equipment competing for space in the operating suite are the radiofrequency machine and percutaneous disc decompression devices. Radiofrequency machines have been shown to interfere with monitors such as ECG.[14] Therefore, advanced planning is necessary so that the anesthesiologist, with the requisite patient-monitoring equipment, will be in place and ready access to the patient is ensured.

Office gastroenterology procedures

GI endoscopic procedures are among the most common procedures performed in the ambulatory setting. In fact, colonoscopy is the second most frequently performed procedure in ambulatory care, with more than 1.1 million of the almost 1.4 million colonoscopies reported as occurring in the ambulatory setting in 1996 and 9.8 million sigmoidoscopies/colonoscopies ordered or provided in physicians' offices in 2002.[15,16] Colonoscopies are important in detecting colorectal cancer and preventing deaths from this second leading cause of death in the United States. Colorectal cancer screening has been shown to be cost-effective.[17] Colonoscopy allows the endoscopist to remove lesions and polyps at the time of the procedure (unlike a barium enema or virtual colonoscopy) and may detect cancer in patients whose colon cancer would otherwise go undetected.[18] Colonoscopy involves additional cost and risk to patients (such as bowel perforation) and patient discomfort.[19]

The AAAHC recently reported data from 101 ASCs representing more than 378,623 colonoscopy procedures annually.[20] The overall complication rate in their study of 2,416 colonoscopies was found to be 1.4%. The most common complications were abdominal pain, hypotension, difficulty maneuvering scopes, and bleeding requiring treatment. Hypoxemia was reported in two of the patients studied. The type of anesthesia administered was 72% moderate sedation, 24% deep sedation, 3% general, and 1% mild sedation. Midazolam was used in combination with other sedatives/narcotics in 80% of the cases. Opioids (fentanyl or meperidine) were used in approximately 75% of the cases. Propofol was administered either alone or in combination with other medications in approximately 33% of the procedures. In this study, RNs administered nearly half of the sedation anesthetics and certified RN anesthetists administered almost 25% of the anesthetics. Anesthesiologists administered only approximately 15% of the anesthetics; which provider gave which drugs is unknown. The use of propofol by RNs supervised by gastroenterologists has been advocated as safe,[21] but the product prescribing information requires that propofol be administered only by individuals trained in general anesthesia. Because sedation is a continuum and it is not always possible to predict how an individual patient will respond, the ASA has issued a Statement on the Safe Use of Propofol. Due to the potential for rapid, profound changes in sedative/anesthetic depth and the lack of antagonist medications, agents such as propofol require special attention. Even if moderate sedation is intended, patients receiving propofol should receive care consistent with that required for **deep sedation**. All practitioners who administer propofol should be qualified to **rescue** patients whose level of sedation becomes deeper than initially intended and who enter, if briefly, a state of general anesthesia (http://www.asahq.org/publicationsAndServices/standards/37.pdf). In a joint statement by ASA and American Association of Nurse Anesthetists, the societies reinforced that whenever propofol is used for sedation/anesthesia, it should be administered only by persons who are trained in the administration of general anesthesia and who are not simultaneously involved in these surgical or diagnostic procedures.

Propofol's rapid onset and short duration of action make it ideal for endoscopic procedures, and it has been shown to provide more rapid recovery and discharge as well as return to cognitive baseline.[22] However, this study did not show a difference in patient satisfaction.

Anesthesia drugs and techniques

Induction and maintenance of office anesthesia can include IV and inhalation techniques. Short-acting agents are most appropriate and have great versatility of application. More important than agents or techniques is to provide an anesthetic that will give the patient a rapid recovery to normal function, with minimal postoperative pain, nausea, or other side effects. The practice and site dictate the setup at each location.

Opioids

The office practitioner must comply with state rules and requirements regarding controlled medications. Schedule II, III, IV, and V medications are commonly used in providing sedation, analgesia, and anesthesia. Policies and procedures are required to comply with laws and regulations pertaining to controlled drug supply, storage, and administration. In addition, all medications used in anesthesia care need to be secured, and regular inspection and inventory review of the medication supply ensures safety. The office anesthesiologist needs separate U.S. Drug Enforcement Administration (DEA) registration certificates for manufacturing, distributing, dispensing, and administering controlled medications. Also, a separate state-controlled drug registration may be required. The prescribing of any medication in the office setting must be under the direction of state-licensed providers. These individuals should assume administrative responsibility for the use of prescribed medications. It should be clear in the office policies and procedures who is responsible for various medications and how issues such as drug outdating or recall are handled. An anesthesiologist working in the office setting may supply the controlled drugs used for anesthesia care or may use the supply provided by the surgeon's office. If there are multiple office locations where controlled medications may be administered or dispensed, a separate registration number may be needed for each one. These "dispensing entities" must obtain controlled drugs from a medication supplier using DEA form 222 (The DEA Schedule I and II Drug order form). Occasionally, a pharmacy (using a 222 order form) may dispense controlled medications to individual physicians to administer. Records must be maintained that account for the use and wastage of all controlled medications on each patient for each date. DEA regulations should always be followed. Records must be kept for at least 2 years (some states require longer time periods) and are subject to DEA inspection. The recording method and any backup media should be specified.

The choice of narcotics for use in the office setting has also been studied.[23,24] The short-acting remifentanil is clearly more costly, and its very short-acting profile may not leave the homebound postsurgical patient with adequate analgesia. Our choice is to use titrated doses of fentanyl to control moderate to severe postoperative pain sufficiently to transition to oral analgesics and facilitate timely discharge. Changes in clinical practice that are geared toward short-acting agents and titrated well can substantially affect how a patient feels and can shorten the time to discharge.[25]

Sedative hypnotics

Although opioids are an integral part of many anesthetic techniques, there has been a dramatic increase in the use of propofol for moderate sedation and as part of a total IV anesthetic. Propofol has attractive properties (rapid onset/offset, excellent sedation, as well as a potent antinausea effect) that make it particularly useful for ambulatory surgery in general and office surgery in particular.[26]

Ketamine is another general anesthetic that has achieved some popularity in office surgery anesthetics. It also possesses qualities that would appear to make it an excellent choice (i.e., potent analgesia, amnesia, and hemodynamic stability). At least one study found that the coadministration of small-dose ketamine (mean of 3.7 µg/kg per minute) with propofol (33 µg/kg per minute) attenuates propofol-induced hypoventilation, produces positive mood effects without perceptual changes after surgery, and may provide earlier recovery of cognition.[27] However, it is easily overdosed when combined with other sedatives, converting deep sedation into a general anesthetic, with the resultant increase in airway and cardiovascular compromise. In a recent randomized, double-blind study, propofol-ketamine had a postoperative nausea and vomiting (PONV) incidence similar to patients receiving a propofol-fentanyl anesthetic. The ketamine patients manifested increased heart rate, opioid requirements, and dreaming in the PACU compared to patients receiving propofol-fentanyl.[28]

Total intravenous anesthesia

Total intravenous anesthesia (TIVA) techniques are used for deep sedation and general anesthesia, and the level is varied as the procedure dictates.[29] Midazolam and fentanyl can be easily administered by repeated bolus. Therefore, one can try to discontinue their use in the last 90 minutes of the procedure, as residual effects may affect the alertness of the patient, and supplement with propofol as needed. Ketamine is used judiciously, and we typically use it for its dissociative and analgesic properties at the beginning of the case and limit its use to no greater than 25 mg total to avoid its dysphoric effects. It is an especially useful drug during laser procedures in which the use of supplemental oxygen is limited. Additionally, we can supplement this technique with an infusion of propofol or a mixture of methohexital (Brevital®) and propofol in equal concentrations to achieve an appropriate level of sedation. This may be titrated with a pump infusion or a micro drip. Generally, the dose varies between 25 and 150 µg/kg per minute. The addition of methohexital adds a component of sedation that complements propofol, as it provides a deeper sedation with less depression of the respiratory drive. The maximum dose of methohexital used should not exceed 8 mg/kg, as this will bring its undesirable side effects of shivering and masseter muscle spasm movements into play. Methohexital may also be used in bolus increments of 10–20 mg to augment levels of sedation or cover breakthrough alertness during the procedure. As with all cases, the liberal and appropriate use of local anesthetics is invaluable to a successful anesthetic technique. Recently, clinicians are exploring the use of dexmedetomidine infusions as a component of TIVA but cost considerations might limit its widespread use.

Procedures of 30 minutes' duration or less are well managed with bolus techniques without using continuous infusions. In today's cost-conscious environment, we use indicated medications that offer real advantages and we are judicious in the addition of "newer" medications if no real benefit is quantified.

Volatile anesthetics

In the fast-paced, cost-conscious, efficiency-driven environment in the office, it behooves one to use an ideal general anesthetic technique that provides a smooth and rapid induction, optimal operating conditions, and rapid recovery with minimal or no side effects. One would like to tailor the anesthetic technique to allow for safely fast-tracking to facilitate flow.

Several comparisons have been made to allow gauging the selection of the inhalation agent (desflurane versus isoflurane versus sevoflurane) and are addressed in more detail in Chapter 9 (General anesthesia). As further testing amongst these various techniques continues, along with information from bispectral brain function monitor, a clinically significant cost and time saving may possibly be realized.[30] The differences in time can be minor. In the office practice, it is important to remember that inhalational techniques, compared to TIVA, are associated with the increased costs of providing an anesthesia machine and with waste gas scavenging. One option for scavenging in the absence of a central suction is to use a charcoal canister to absorb halogenated anesthetic agents while allowing CO_2, O_2, and water vapor to pass through (Figure 11-3). The ongoing discussion of the use of nitrous oxide in the balanced inhalational anesthetic technique is especially relevant in office-based anesthesia, where

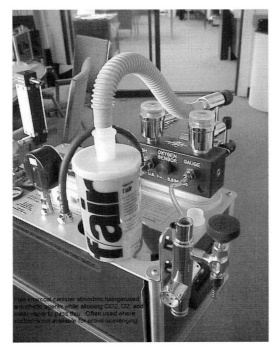

Figure 11-3. OBAMED Inc. F/Air charcoal canister absorbs halogenated anesthetic agents while allowing CO_2, O_2, and water vapor to pass through. Often used where suction is not available for active scavenging. Reproduced with permission.

there is less tolerance for PONV. In our experience, we have eliminated the use of nitrous oxide in our balanced technique as we believe it can increase the incidence of nausea and vomiting in some patients.

Anesthesia considerations for common plastic and cosmetic surgery procedures

Plastic and reconstructive surgery is generally performed on abnormal structures of the body, to improve function, but may also be done to approximate a normal appearance. Cosmetic surgery (also referred to as aesthetic surgery) is performed to reshape normal structures of the body in order to improve the patient's appearance and self-esteem. These surgeries are among the most commonly conducted procedures in offices, and health insurance coverage varies. There is no centralized reporting of the numbers or types of office procedures performed nationally. Some of the more complete data come from Florida, where the Department of Health required reporting of all office procedures. The report is summarized in Table 11-9.[31]

Common plastic and cosmetic surgery procedures include breast augmentations, face-lifts, abdominoplasty, and liposuction. Often, the procedures are combined for patient convenience; however, there have been reports indicating that the combination procedures carry a higher morbidity. Large-volume liposuction, in particular, has also been identified with increased risk. Many states with office surgery regulations restrict the volume of liposuction. The American Society of Plastic Surgery recommends that liposuction be limited to a total aspirant (supernatant fat and fluid) of 5,000 mL.[32] They also recommend that combination procedures such as large-volume liposuction and abdominoplasty be avoided. Abdominoplasty is a procedure that is growing in popularity and has also been identified as carrying a high risk for postoperative fatal pulmonary embolism. Hughes[33] found a mortality of 3.3 per 10,000 procedures. Patients with a history of deep vein thrombosis (DVT) or multiple risk factors for DVT are at a higher risk of developing postoperative DVT. The association of pulmonary embolus and abdominoplasty may be related to the reduction of ease of superficial venous drainage from the pelvis and legs. Adding liposuction to abdominoplasty may not increase the risk of DVT or pulmonary embolus.[34]

Table 11-9. Florida office surgery procedures[31] (n = 144,854)

Procedure	Percentage
Cosmetic/reconstructive	47
Gastroenterology	25
Pain management	17
Ob/gyn	5

Table 11-10. Risk factors for deep venous thrombosis and pulmonary embolism

Virchow's Triad (stasis, hypercoaguability, vascular injury)
Immobilization (such as from surgery or a fracture)
Malignancy
Thrombophlebitis
Pregnancy and for 6 to 12 weeks postpartum
Extremity Trauma
Hormone replacement therapy or oral contraceptives
Smoking
Obesity (body mass index > 30)
Recent myocardial infarction or cerebrovascular accident
Previous history of deep vein thrombosis/pulmonary embolism
History of radiation therapy (especially pelvic)
Antiphospholipid antibody syndrome
Homocystinemia
Polycythemia
Other hypercoaguable states
- Abnormal protein C or S
- Factor V Leiden
- Abnormal factors XIII, IX, and X

Adapted from Most et al.[35]

The American Society of Plastic Surgery has formulated a task force on Deep Venous Thrombosis Prophylaxis and has established guidelines.[35] They recommend that patients be stratified according to their risk of DVT and pulmonary embolus. A list of known risk factors is listed in Table 11-10, and Table 11-11 categorizes the patients according to risk level.

These are the recommended treatments according to risk stratification:

Low-risk patients: Position the patients comfortably on the operating table, with slight knee flexion with a pillow to enhance popliteal venous return. Avoid external pressure on the legs or constricting garments.

Moderate-risk patients: They suggest the same positioning and the use of intermittent pneumatic compression garments worn before, during, and after general anesthesia until the patient is fully awake. If possible, these patients should stop taking thrombogenic medications (such as oral contraceptives) at least 1 week before surgery, although it is unclear (in the literature) whether the risk for DVT and pulmonary embolus normalizes within this time.

High-risk patients: Require the same measures as the other two categories plus a preoperative consultation from hematology and the consideration of low-molecular-weight heparin 2 hours before surgery and until the patient is ambulatory. Prophylactic full anticoagulation, however, is considered optional in procedures with a high risk for hematoma, and the majority of aesthetic procedures fall into this category.

Table 11-11. Deep vein thrombosis (DVT) risk stratification

Level of DVT risk	Age (years)	Number of risk factors	Surgical time (minutes)	Surgical type
Low risk	<40	None	<30	Uncomplicated
Medium risk	>40	Two or more	>30	Uncomplicated
Medium risk	40–60	None	>30	Uncomplicated
Medium risk	>40	None	>30	Major, complicated
High risk	>40	Three or more	>30	Complicated
High risk	>40	One or more	>30	Major, complicated
High risk	>60	None	>30	Uncomplicated or complicated

Intermittent pneumatic compression devices are mechanical devices that increase the pulsatile flow in the veins by preventing stagnation and enhancing endogenous fibrinolytic activity, by reducing levels of tissue plasminogen activator inhibitor. There are two types of devices for use: foot pumps that encircle the ankle and compress the venous plexus in the feet, and sequential compression devices that encircle the leg and compress the veins in the calf and thigh. Most importantly, these devices should be applied and activated prior to the induction of anesthesia and continued until the patient is fully awake. The addition of elastic stockings to intermittent pneumatic compression devices may be considered but is not of proven benefit. Additionally, patients must be aware of the signs and symptoms that may indicate venous stasis and pulmonary embolus as early intervention may decrease morbidity and mortality.

Rhytidectomy

The purpose of the face-lift is to decrease skin wrinkling and rejuvenate the appearance of the face, with the removal of excess skin and suspension of facial fascia and tissues. This is a procedure with many options for anesthetic technique. Some surgeons prefer IV sedation anesthesia and others prefer general endotracheal anesthesia. The choice of anesthesia by the surgeon is dependent on their training and the type of anesthetic that they are comfortable working with. These patients are often elderly and require proper screening and a thorough examination of comorbid conditions to ensure that they are maximally optimized for elective surgery. These procedures are often 4 or more hours and can have a significant impact on the patient. A thorough review of all herbal and other medications also should be noted as many may impact on clotting, and care should be taken to stop all herbals for at least 2 weeks. Premedication with clonidine may be useful for sedation as well as helping with hemodynamic control.

The control of blood pressure during the procedure is key. Aim to maintain it 20%–30% lower during the resection and then bring it back up close to baseline prior to closing. This allows the surgeon to see whether there is additional oozing prior to closing when the patient reaches their normotensive range. Minimize fluid administration as bleeding is minimal and excess fluid administration can contribute significantly to facial edema.

Extubate the patient without coughing and bucking as it increases venous return and bleeding. Most surgeons want complete dressings in place before awakening. Many will apply pressure to minimize postextubation bleeding. Ensure that the head dressing is not too constricting, and elevate the head as soon as is feasible as it helps with postprocedure swelling.

Since local anesthetic is used for face-lifts, there is not much postoperative pain immediately postoperatively. Nausea and vomiting are great concerns and a multiregime plan will have the best results. Some surgeons will "observe" the patient in recovery for some time if they are concerned about potential bleeding; otherwise, the patient may be discharged as discharge criteria are met.

Breast augmentation

Breast augmentation is an extremely popular procedure. According to the American Society of Plastic Surgeons Statistics (http://www.plasticsurgery. org/public_education/loader.cfm?url=/commonspot/security/getfile.cfm& PageID=17870), it is one of the most common cosmetic procedures and the volume has grown 37% from 2000 to 2005. Although many of the patients are in the 40-and-younger age groups, all ages of patients may present themselves. Postprocedure pain management is an important issue, and the preoperative interview is the ideal time to address expectations. The quality of the pain is that of pressure and heaviness. Since a weight has been added to their chest and many will have a firm circumferential pressure dressing, this sensation (of pressure and heaviness) is acutely experienced with each breath. Patients should expect to have pain, but it should be tolerable. The intraoperative stretching of skin is often felt as a deep ache in the shoulders and back. Submuscular dissection and implant placement will also involve postprocedure deep muscular pain.

One of the key factors for a good surgical result is to have total control of the bleeding and oozing in the breast pocket. Bleeding into the pocket is known to increase the incidence of capsule contracture and breast immobility. The placement of the implants also requires the patient's position change intraprocedure from supine to sitting. Consider the lengths of airway circuits and IV ports to enable a smooth and timely change in position.

Arms may be positioned at the patient's side or out on arm boards, at the surgeon's discretion. Check pressure points and abduction angles. Also, ensure that the arms transition safely from supine to sitting as placement of implants is confirmed. Consider the effects of position as it pertains to vascular tone and blood pressure and be prepared to treat it accordingly as one may change supine to sitting positions frequently. Surgical complications include pneumothorax and uncontrolled bleeding from the thoracic vessels. Clearly, a plan for transfer and admission to an acute-care facility must be in place in the event of these complications, which cannot be definitively addressed in the office surgical suite setting.

Postsurgical dressings, as in much of plastic and cosmetic surgery, are the preference of the surgeon. Many will want all dressings on prior to extubation. Dressings will involve wound covering as well as bras and elastic bands or bandages that are positioned to mold the placement of the implant in the pocket. If the surgeon would prefer all dressings in place, one must maintain an adequate level of anesthesia that keeps the patient still as the patient is sat up and circumferential dressings are applied. The ideal awakening would involve extubation without coughing as increases in venous pressures may increase the chance of bleeding and oozing in the pocket. Pain management may be accomplished with continuous local anesthetic infusion pumps (usually primed with bupivacaine), intercostal or incisional blocks.

Liposuction

Contouring lipoplasty is not a weight-loss procedure but is a body-contouring procedure. Almost any area of the body is amenable to liposculpture. Over the years, liposuction has evolved, and today the most common method is the tumescent technique. This technique involves the instillation of saline mixed with dilute (0.05%–0.1%) lidocaine and epinephrine (1:1,000,000) into the areas of lipoplasty. The tumescence mixture is given some time to lipolyse the fat cells and make them more conducive for liposuction. The lidocaine in the mixture provides analgesia, and the epinephrine component is to aid hemostasis. The tumescent technique takes advantage of the tissue-binding capacity of lidocaine; there is the slow uptake of lidocaine into the bloodstream, with serum level peaking as late as 10–14 hours postinfusion. The surgeon keeps a precise tally of the infusion amount of each tumesced site, and specific attention is given to tumescent input and aspirate output.

The most common method of suction is the use of a power suction canister and multiple suction cannulas. These cannula vary in the number and placement of the suction ports and have a varied diameter depending on the effect desired. Fibrous areas of the body are difficult to suction and also are less conducive to the even spread of the tumescent fluid. These difficult fibrous areas may be suctioned using an ultrasonic suction that will first "liquefy" the fat, and then the area will be resuctioned with the standard liposuction machine to remove this liquefied fat. The ultrasonic liposuction adds another element of complexity as one must "time" its use as there is an association of seroma formation with increased time usage. Additionally, heat injury is a concern with this technology and particular care must be taken to watch and protect the skin.

Liposuction is a serious surgery and is of a moderately invasive nature. The most common cause of death is from thromboembolism.[36] Particular attention should be paid to herbal and other medications that may elevate this risk. Oral contraception will increase this risk, and this must be discussed with the patient. Preoperative teaching should include discussions on early ambulation and exercises to ward against venous pooling. The character of liposuction pain is often described as "burning" in the first 12–24 hours, and after 24 hours as a deep ache that is accentuated when the muscles under the suctioned fat are being used. The patient may continue to "ooze" fluid from the suction cannula incisions and may experience some orthostatic symptoms for the first 24 hours. The patient should have immediate home help for that time.

The most immediate anesthetic concern is the fluid management of this patient. It has been shown that much of the tumescent fluid is absorbed by the patient even though it appears that it is aspirated out in the fat elute.[37] With the use of epinephrine, the blood loss is limited and one can visually see the amount of heme staining or "redness" of the aspirate. If the wet technique of liposuction is used, IV fluid administration is kept to a minimum and recommended to be "maintenance" only. Larger amounts of liposuction, greater than 4,000 mL, should be replaced with 0.25 mL IV crystalloid per milliliter of aspirate removed over 4,000 mL. Other intraoperative complications must be considered in the diagnostic differential if difficulties arise. These complications include viscus perforation, pulmonary edema, vascular perforation, fat embolism, local anesthetic toxicity, and hypothermia.[38] Positioning and repositioning the patient from side to side and supine to prone are frequently done as one infuses the tumescence to all the sites and allows it to work and then repositions to suction. This is an intraoperative challenge as one must be careful to position safely and continuously be aware of body alignment and all pressure points. The anesthesiologist must also ensure that all monitoring cables and IV tubing will allow for ease of movement during repositioning. The anesthesiologist must prepare ahead with padding and positioning devices as they are often managing much of the "moves," and it is most helpful to have all the devices handy as one also has to be careful with the instrumented airway. Attention to the patient's temperature is in order as hypothermia is a real risk.[39] The patient has many exposed areas to the loss of convective heat. The infiltration of tumescence is cooling. Often, the skin is "wet" as the surgeon checks for evenness of liposculpture and there is heat loss through evaporation. Methods to increase patient temperature need to involve forced warm air devices and keeping operatory temperatures higher than normal. The procedure ends with "feathering," which involves the suction cannula providing a transition between the suctioned and residual fat to provide a natural contour. This feathering will trespass into less anesthetized areas as the tumescence will not have been infused there. There is often transient pain at the end of procedure and this is best addressed with short-acting hypnotics to manage hemodynamic changes. A snug elastic garment is applied immediately at procedure end to control fluid sequestration, and it is worn for several weeks to ensure smooth skin retraction to the newly sculpted areas.

Despite the use of lidocaine tumescent, there can be pain in the "feathered" areas. One must ensure that the patient is comfortable as they are assessed in the PACU. Our practice uses Nalbuphine in doses of 5 or 7.5 mg up to 10 mg intravenously in the PACU. In doses exceeding 10 mg, there is often an increased element of sedation which will delay discharge. Warming the patient with a forced-air device in the PACU is also essential after liposuction.

Abdominoplasty

Abdominoplasty is designed to remove excess skin and skin laxity and remove fat with the abdominal skin flap. Liposuction does not address the issue of excess skin and this is the definitive procedure to solve this problem. Most abdominoplasty patients are past child-bearing age and many are moderately overweight. The number of men undergoing this procedure is also steadily increasing. The procedure is moderately invasive and patients will need a thorough work-up preoperatively. The procedure is extraperitoneal and often accompanied by liposuction. Liposuction may be done of the hips and flanks; aggressive liposuction of the flap is to be avoided as it compromises the blood supply to the flap and increases the chance of flap necrosis.

As discussed previously, this group of patients is at particularly increased risk for thromboembolic events. The patient must be advised of this particular risk and what their postop role is in the recognition of the symptoms of this complication and their role in decreasing the incidence of this complication. Most abdominoplasties are done using general anesthesia with orotracheal intubation and muscle paralysis. After the imbrication of the muscle diastases is completed, the patient will be positioned in a flex position with the back up and the knees bent. The back is raised and the patient is flexed at approximately 30–40 degrees. This flexion allows the abdominal flap to be closed under tension. The patient is kept in this position throughout the remainder of the procedure and in the PACU. Drains are usually placed and removed in 7–10 days. If pain infusion systems are to be used, they are primed with local anesthetic (usually bupivacaine) and placed at this time. As sutures are closed under tension to stretch the skin for a tighter approximation, one should try and extubate without coughing as the increase in intra-abdominal pressure can impact on the repair.

The greatest immediate concern is to ensure that the patient is comfortable with tolerable pain. Postprocedure, many patients describe a muscular back pain and back muscle spasm and tightness in the first 24 hours. This is best discussed, as it is best addressed with local heat/ice therapy and comfortable positioning. Many practices are now using local pain infusion pumps that will deliver local anesthetic to the site over a number of days. Home instructions need to stress the need of moving about after surgery and leg and feet exercises that can be done to deter venous pooling.

Postoperative care

Care should be handed over in a predetermined and coordinated fashion to the PACU personnel. Immediate postop care may be in the same OR room and then turned over to recovery personnel or may be in an adjacent designated PACU. OBA facilities may have great variability, but one must ensure that the ASA standards for postanesthesia care are followed.[40] The immediate postprocedure (phase 1) care should be provided by an RN with ACLS training. Fast-tracking can be used as is applicable. All patients who receive general anesthesia, regional anesthesia, or monitored anesthesia shall receive appropriate postanesthesia management consistent with the ASA standards for postanesthesia care.

Fast-tracking

Discharge must be an objective and planned process. Several scoring data sheets for objective discharge are available and are discussed in detail in Chapter 13. Fast-tracking patients is the most efficient method of turnover in the office. The goal of the anesthetic technique is to have a patient postprocedure who is awake, alert, and moves from OR bed to PACU bed without assistance. The anesthesiologist typically turns the room over in 10 minutes and begins with the next patient, and most general anesthetic discharges occur within 60 minutes of awakening.

The anesthesia practitioner can only leave the patient in the care of the PACU personnel when the postprocedure condition is stable. After that, the physical presence of the anesthesiologist is not required to address most PACU issues. The proximity of the recovery and operatory suites facilitate this care, and constant and easy communication is key if additional instructions are required. To ensure efficient turnover and continuity of care, the person escorting the patient and aiding in home care should be present in the PACU, so that instructions can be discussed firsthand and follow-up appointments made. All patients should be followed with postprocedure calls, and responses should be documented and evaluated. A postprocedure satisfaction survey is helpful in identifying areas that may require further attention.

Acute pain management

Oftentimes, the office surgical practice has one operatory and one acute recovery bay. The nursing staff, though qualified, is limited and the efficient flow of patients is dependent on no delays in the discharge area. The greatest concerns of patients in the PACU relate to pain management and nausea and vomiting issues.[41,42]

Most plastic and cosmetic surgical procedures involve postprocedure pain. The adequate dosing of an analgesic before awakening is key to prompt discharge in the PACU. The patient who awakens with a tolerable comfort level will fare better with fulfilling the discharge and home-readiness protocols of the center. Our practice largely uses intraoperative fentanyl as it provides cost-effective analgesia and allows for timely discharge with comfort. The patient may resume oral medications at home as soon as they begin to feel pain. Rescue analgesia is provided after the patient is assessed and a pain score value is determined. For pain score values of 7 or less, we will institute treatment with nalbuphine in doses of 5, 7.5, or 10 mg given 5 minutes apart. Nalbuphine, a mixed agonist/antagonist opioid, has a good analgesic profile and has a limited respiratory depression, so we may still monitor the patient after the IV dose and safely discharge the patient. We have found that dosing greater than 10 mg does oftentimes lead to unwanted side effects such as drowsiness that may delay discharge. For pain score values of 8 or greater, we will dose with up to two incremental doses of 25 µg of fentanyl intravenously in the PACU.

Many surgeons are also using continuous infusion pain management techniques that involve local anesthetic pumps that may be patient-controlled as well as continuous infusion via indwelling soaker catheters. They are most commonly used for abdominal surgeries and breast surgeries. The catheters are placed prior to closing, and the initial dosing of local anesthetic is delivered prior to awakening. They are typically kept in place for 3–5 days and then removed at a postprocedure office visit. One such system is the ON-Q System of Post-Op Pain Relief and is distributed by I Flow Corporation. Information is available online at http://www.iflow.com/3_Products/Acute_Pain_Management/onq.html.

Many surgeons may also place local anesthesia in incision sites to decrease postop discomfort. Others may also use intercostal blocks or other local field blocks. Many plastic surgeons are averse to using nonsteroidal anti-inflammatory medications as they do not wish to do anything that may increase the risk of bleeding. Surgeons believe that IV ketorolac has more "bleeding and oozing" and are not open to its use. The recent controversies regarding the COX-2 (cyclooxygenase-2) inhibitors and cardiovascular complications have led some patients and plastic surgeons to avoid their use.

Nausea and vomiting

The other main concern for patients is nausea and vomiting postprocedure. For many in this "white-gloved service," even the feeling of nausea is not acceptable. Many recent analyses have developed a model for predicting high- and low-risk anesthesia groups for nausea and vomiting.[43,44] Our feeling is that at this level of consumerism, one must attend to all aspects of the "surgical experience" and consider everyone as a nausea/vomiting risk. Many patients will consider paying out of pocket for the avoidance of this complication. A simplified PONV Risk Score includes the female gender, history of motion sickness or PONV, nonsmoker, and the use of postoperative opioids as being predictive of risk.[45] Although high-dose narcotics are implicated in increasing nausea, the role of lower doses is more controversial. One study showed that usual narcotic doses used in the course of outpatient surgery do not promote an increased incidence of postoperative nausea or vomiting,[46] whereas others have shown an increased risk with as little as 75 µg of perioperative fentanyl.[47]

Guidelines or consensus statements regarding nausea and vomiting, including indications for multimodal approach, are applicable in office-based surgery and are found in detail in Chapter 12. 5-HT3 blockers, such as ondansteron, may be best administered immediately before the end of surgery for greatest efficacy. The use of a second dose of a 5-HT3 blocker has been shown to have no added efficacy as a rescue drug.[48] Prophylactic IV administration of dexamethasone immediately after induction rather than at the end of anesthesia was most effective in preventing PONV.[49] A single prophylactic dose of dexamethasone has not been shown to have any clinically relevant toxicity in otherwise healthy patients. The combination of dexamethasone and 5-HT3 receptor antagonist may be a more efficacious combination than either one alone. The use of a multidrug regime can reduce the nausea and vomiting propensity of an inhalational general anesthetic. Patients also need to be counseled as to how to deal with the car ride home, especially if they have a propensity toward motion sickness. Specific antimotion sickness medications such as meclizine or scopolamine patch should be considered for the susceptible patient. The ondansetron oral disintegrating tablet (ODT) has been used as part of a multimodal regimen to further reduce postdischarge nausea, particularly following plastic and cosmetic surgery procedures.

Special considerations

Adverse incident reporting and quality improvement activities

A quality improvement policy for the office is important to promote high-quality patient care. Many states require each office to have such a policy, but even where not required by state law it is highly advisable. The anesthesiologist should participate in ongoing continuous quality improvement and risk management activities of each particular office practice. The quality improvement plan should specify the individual who is responsible for performing each element of the plan. An anesthesiologist or an anesthesiology group that provides anesthesia care at multiple facilities may form its own quality improvement unit to evaluate the total anesthesia care it provides. A routine review of anesthesia and surgical morbidity and "adverse" or "sentinel" or outcome events should be integral to the plan. There should be a specific list of quality indicators (see Table 11-12 for examples).

Table 11-12. Ambulatory surgery quality indicators

a. Death, cardiac or respiratory arrest
b. Unplanned reintubation
c. Central nervous system or peripheral nervous system deficit appearing within 2 days of anesthesia
d. Myocardial infarction within 2 days of anesthesia
e. Pulmonary edema within 1 day of anesthesia
f. Aspiration pneumonia
g. Anaphylaxis or adverse drug reactions
h. Postdural puncture headache within 4 days of spinal or epidural anesthesia
i. Dental injury
j. Eye injury
k. Surgical infection rate
l. Excessive blood loss
m. Unplanned admission to a hospital or other acute-care facility
n. Drugs errors
o. Wrong surgical site
p. Incorrect procedure or patient

Additionally, the plan should include an annual review and check of anesthesia equipment to ensure compliance with current safety standards and the standards for the release of waste anesthetic gases.

Emergencies in the office setting

The key to dealing with emergencies in the office-based setting is to be prepared with emergency medications, supplies, and training. All resuscitation medications need to be labeled and organized in a consistent location such as a tackle box. Appoint an individual within the practice to check and update all emergency supplies as ACLS algorithms change. Keep emergency airway rescue items in a disposable bag. Make sure all anesthesia providers are current with ACLS practices and maintain current credentials.

Intraoperative and PACU emergencies need to be dealt with immediately. Understand the limitations of the office and make the decision to transfer to a hospital as necessary. Have emergency plans and policies in place and do not hesitate to activate them, as the appropriate and timely transfer of the patient can be lifesaving. Until 911 ambulance help arrives, administer the appropriate ACLS algorithms. Training for emergencies should be rehearsed well in advance through role-playing.

It is very important to conduct emergency drills every quarter with different scenarios so that role-playing prepares everyone for their role in the event of an emergency. All office personnel, both medical and administrative, should have a clear assigned role.

Anesthesiologists are generally not involved in postdischarge surgical emergencies, such as bleeding after face-lifts or breast implants, etc. These procedures and patients are now higher risk and may involve hemodynamic instability. The potential need for blood administration and invasive monitoring often cannot be addressed in the office setting, should that be required.

Add-ons to the day's schedule are not considered emergencies, and they are done after patients have had the same rigorous medical evaluation and satisfy our NPO (nil per os) and escort policies and other guidelines. Carefully apply all the same policies and procedures to all patients.

Transfer agreements

Transfer agreements must be in place in case hospital admission is needed. Make sure the practitioner or surgeon had a signed transfer agreement to a nearby institution for the admission of a patient. If the client is a dentist or otherwise does not have admitting privileges (such as dermatologic surgeons), make sure they have an agreement with a physician who will admit the patient and care for the patient at a nearby hospital. Children and handicapped patients are best handled by having their local doctor notified that their patient is to undergo a procedure with sedation in the office setting. This communication is useful in the event that the patient needs follow-up care.

Summary

The virtual explosion in office surgery has been a positive experience overall but has been accompanied by avoidable complications. However, well-regulated and prepared offices will likely have better outcomes and should mirror the safety levels achieved at other ambulatory surgery sites if they are to survive. The physician practicing in an office setting should be able to answer the following questions proposed by increasingly well-informed patients:

- Does the surgeon and/or anesthesiologist have privileges to do the same procedure in a nearby hospital or ASC?
- Have the surgeon's or anesthesiologist's privileges to do this procedure ever been denied, withdrawn, or put on probation at any medical facility?
- Is the person who performs sedation or anesthesia fully trained and certified by an appropriate anesthesia organization?
- Will there be a preoperative visit with anesthesia personnel?
- Will the individual administering sedation and/or anesthesia be in constant attendance during surgery?
- Is the anesthesia machine a current model and similar to the machines used in a nearby hospital and ASC? Is the machine serviced and calibrated according to manufacturer's recommendations?
- Will the monitors used during the anesthetic and in the recovery room be the same as would be used if the operation were in a hospital or ASC?
- Who will be with the patient following surgery in the recovery area? Is this person an RN trained and experienced in PACU nursing?
- Is the physician's office fully equipped to handle any type of medical emergency? Is this equipment checked routinely and kept up to date? Are the personnel trained to handle these emergencies?
- How are the instruments sterilized after each surgery, and do all personnel having patient contact wear appropriate surgical attire?
- Are arrangements in place for immediate transfer and admission to a nearby hospital?
- Is this surgeon's office accredited by one of the nationally recognized medical accrediting organizations in the United States?

References

1. Morello DC, Colon GA, Fredricks S, Iverson RE, Singer R. Patient safety in accredited office surgical facilities. *Plast Reconstr Surg*. 1997;99:1496–1499.

2. Grazer FM, de Jong RH. Fatal outcomes from liposuction: census survey of cosmetic surgeons. *Plast Reconstr Surg.* 2000;105:436–446.

3. Hoefflin SM, Bornstein JB, Gordon M. General anesthesia in an office-based plastic surgical facility: a report on more than 23,000 consecutive office-based procedures under general anesthesia with no significant anesthetic complications. *Plast Reconstr Surg.* 2001;107:243–257.

4. Vila H, Soto R, Cantor AB, Mackey D. Comparative outcomes analysis of procedures performed in physician offices and ambulatory surgery centers. *Arch Surg.* 2003; 138:991–995.

5. Keyes GR, Singer R, Iverson RE, et al. Analysis of outpatient surgery center safety using an internet-based quality improvement and peer review program. *Plast Reconstr Surg.* 2004;113:1760–1770.

6. Natof HE. Complications associated with ambulatory surgery. *JAMA.* 1980;244: 1116–1118.

7. Warner MA, Shields SE, Chute CG. Major morbidity and mortality within one month of ambulatory surgery and anesthesia. *JAMA.* 1993;270:1437–1441.

8. Mezei G, Chung F. Return hospital visits and hospital readmissions after ambulatory surgery. *Ann Surg.* 1999;230:721.

9. Letts M, Davidson D, Splinter W, Conway P. Analysis of the efficacy of pediatric day surgery. *Can J Surg.* 2001;44:193–198.

10. Fleisher LA, Pasternak R, Barash PG, Anderson G. Safety of outpatient surgery in the elderly: the importance of the patient, system and location of care. *Anesthesiology.* 2002;96:A1127.

11. Florida Board of Medicine Practice Alert. Available at: http://www.doh.state.fl.us/mqa/medical/info_ACLSrule.pdf. Accessed December 20, 2005.

12. ASA Operating Room Design Manual. Ehrenwerth J, ed. Park Ridge, IL: American Society of Anesthesiologists; 1999.

13. Benumof JL. Permanent loss of cervical spinal cord function associated with interscalene block performed under general anesthesia. *Anesthesiology.* 2000;93: 1541–1544.

14. Tong NY, Ru HJ, Ling HY, Cheung YC, Meng LW, Chung C. Extracardiac radio-frequency ablation interferes with pacemaker function but does not damage the device [correspondence]. *Anesthesiology* 2004;Apr;100(4):1041.

15. Owings MF, Kozak LJ. Ambulatory and inpatient procedures in the United States, 1996. National Center for Health Statistics. *Vital Health Stat.* 1998;13:26.

16. Woodwell DA, Cherry DK. National Ambulatory Medical Care Survey: 2002 Summary. *Vital Health Stat.* 2004;346:328.

17. Hawk ET, Levin B. Colorectal cancer prevention. *J Clin Oncol.* 2005;23:378–391.

18. Inger DB. Colorectal cancer screening. *Prim Care.* 1999;26:179–187.

19. Iqbal CW, Chun YS, Farley DR. Colonoscopic perforations: a retrospective review. *J Gastrointest Surg.* 2005;9:1229–1235.

20. AAAHC Institute for Quality Improvement. Colonoscopy 2005 Report. Wilmette, IL: Accreditation Association for Ambulatory Health Care; 2006.

21. Hansen JJ, Ulmer BJ, Rex DK. Technical performance of colonoscopy in patients sedated with nurse-administered propofol. *Am J Gastroenterol.* 2004;99:52–56.

22. Ulmer BJ, Hansen JJ, Overley CA, et al. Propofol versus midazolam/fentanyl for outpatient colonoscopy: administration by nurses supervised by endoscopists. *Clin Gastroenterol Hepatol.* 2003;1:425–432.

23. Song D, Whitten C, White P. Use of remifentanil during anesthetic induction. *Anesth Analg.* 1999;88:734–628.

24. Joshi GP, Warner DS, Twersky RS, et al. A comparison of remifentanil and fentanyl adverse effect profile. *J Clin Anesth.* 2002;14:494.

25. Apfelbaum JL, Walawander CA, Grascla TH, et al. Eliminating intensive postoperative care in same day surgery patients using short acting anesthetics. *Anesthesiology.* 2002;97:66–74.

26. Bitar G, Mullis W, Jacobs W, et al. Safety and efficacy of office based surgery with monitored anesthesia care/sedation in 4778 consecutive plastic surgery procedures. *Plast Reconstr Surg.* 2003;111:150–156.

27. Mortero RF, Clark LD, Tolan MM, et al. The effects of small-dose ketamine on propofol sedation: respiration, postoperative mood, perception, cognition, and pain. *Anesth Analg.* 2001;92:1465–1469.

28. Vallejo MC, Romeo RC, Davis DJ, et al. Propofol-ketamine versus propofol-fentanyl for outpatient laparoscopy: comparison of postoperative nausea, emesis, analgesia, and recovery. *J Clin Anesth.* 2002;14:426–431.

29. Trytko R, Werschler WP. Total intravenous anesthesia for office-based laser facial resurfacing. *Lasers Surg Med.* 1999;25:126–130.

30. Gan TJ, Glass PS, Windsor A. Bispectral index monitoring allows faster emergence and improved recovery. *Anesthesiology.* 1997;87:808

31. Florida Board of Medicine Surgical Care Committee Report. January 5, 2005.

32. Iverson RE and the ASPS Task Force on Patient Safety in Office-based Surgery Facilities. Patient Safety in Office Based Surgery. I. Procedures in office based surgery. *Plast Reconstr Surg.* 2002;110:1337–1342.

33. Hughes CE. Reduction of lipoplasty risks and mortality: an ASPS survey. *Aesthetic Surg.* 2001;21:161–163.

34. McDevitt NB. Deep vein thrombosis prophylaxis. American Society of Plastic and Reconstructive Surgeons. *Plast Reconstr Surg.* 1999;104:1923–1928.

35. Most D, Koslow J, Heller J. Thromboembolism in plastic surgery. *Plast Reconstr Surg.* 2005;115:20e-30e.

36. De Jong RH, Grazer FM. Perioperative management of cosmetic liposuction. *Plast Reconstr Surg.* 2001;107:1039–1044.

37. Trott SA, Beran SJ, Rohrich RJ, et al. Safety consideration and fluid resuscitation in liposuction: an analysis of 53 patients. *Plast Reconstr Surg.* 1998;102:2220–2229.

38. Kenkel JM, Lipschitz AH, Luby M, et al. Hemodynamic physiology and thermoregulation in liposuction. *Plast Reconstr Surg.* 2004;114:503–513.

39. Iverson RE, Lunch DJ, ASPS Committee on Patient Safety. Practice advisory on liposuction. *Plast Reconstr Surg.* 2004;113:1478–1490.

40. Practice Guidelines for Postanesthetic Care: A report of the ASA Task Force on Post Anesthesia Care. *Anesthesiology.* 2002;96:742–752.

41. McHugh GA, Thoms GM. The management of pain following day case surgery. *Anesthesia.* 2002;57:270–275.

42. Pavlin DJ, Chen C, Penaloza DA. Pain as a complicating recovery and discharge after ambulatory surgery. *Anesth Analg.* 2002;95:627–634.

43. Marcus JR, Few JW, Chao JD, et al. Prevention of emesis in plastic surgery; a randomized prosective study. *Plast Reconstr Surg.* 2002;109:2487–2494.

44. Gan TJ, Meyer T, Apfel CC, et al. Consensus guidelines for managing postoperative nausea and vomiting. *Anesth Analg.* 2003;97:62.

45. Apfel CC. A Simplified risk score for predicting postoperative nausea. *Anesthesiology.* 1999;91:693.

46. Cepeda MS, Gonzalez F, Granados V, et al. Incidence of nausea and vomiting in outpatients undergoing and general anesthesia. *J Clin Anesth.* 1996;8:324–328.

47. Rosenblum M, Weller RS, Conard PL, et al. Ibuprofen provides longer lasting analgesia than fentanyl after laparoscopic surgery. *Anesth Analg.* 1991;73:255–259.

48. Barbosa MV, Nahas FX, Ferreira LM. Ondansetron for the prevention of postoperative nausea and vomiting: which is the best dosage for aesthetic plastic surgery. *Aesthetic Plast Surg.* 2004;28:33–36.

49. Fuji Y, Tanaka H, Toyooka H. The effects of dexamethasone on posantiemetics in female patients. *Anesth Analg.* 1997;85:913–917.

12. Postanesthesia care recovery and management

Johnathan L. Pregler, MD
Patricia A. Kapur, MD

Anesthesia for ambulatory surgical patients is conducted in a variety of clinical settings. The specifics of each facility's environment will determine the characteristics of the setting for postoperative care. Ambulatory patients may be fully integrated with inpatients in the main operating room of a full-service hospital, handled in segregated operating rooms within a hospital, or cared for in a separate hospital-affiliated or freestanding building. These arrangements affect patient selection, the type of surgery offered, and management of the recovery process. The following discussion will focus on generic aspects of postanesthesia care for the ambulatory patient which must be adapted for individual institutional circumstances.

Recovery area design and function

The physical characteristics of the recovery room will play a major role in determining efficiency and function of patient care. Traditionally, a recovery unit for ambulatory anesthesia has consisted of two functions. The first function is an acute-care recovery area (phase 1 recovery or postanesthesia care unit [PACU]) for the initial phase of recovery after anesthesia. The secondary recovery function (PACU phase 2, short-stay recovery unit or predischarge area) handles the care of the patient after discharge from the first-stage recovery and patients who go directly from the operating room to a phase 2 recovery (fast-track) until discharged. It is important to note that "fast-track recovery" is an expedited total recovery process, not just a change in physical location.

Physical arrangement of units

There are multiple models for how to physically arrange the two units. Ideally, the two units should be in close proximity to facilitate the movement of patients. Close proximity also makes it easier to determine when a patient may fast-track past the first phase of recovery. Some facilities have chosen to physically merge PACU phase 1 and phase 2 into a single unit. This is an efficient physical arrangement for patient throughput and staffing. It eliminates the need for patient transfer from one unit to another for all patients, including those who would not meet fast-tracking criteria. The efficiencies of fast-tracking can be applied to all patients, even the ones who require only 10–15 minutes of acute-phase recovery. By combining phases 1 and 2, each patient has only a single nurse caring for them during the entire recovery process. This can streamline clinical care and eliminate the time and effort spent transferring patient care information between staff. Merging the two units eliminates any concerns on the part of the anesthesia provider about fast-tracking a patient who might require slightly more nursing attention in phase 2. Merging the two units does add management complexities, in particular the assignment of patients to nursing staff. The nurse assigning patients as they arrive from the operating room still needs to carefully allocate patients to a virtual phase 1 or phase 2 to avoid overloading any single staff member with patients in the acute phase of recovery. The number of patients to nurses can vary depending on the acuity of each patient.

Other facilities have retained separate phase 1 and phase 2 recovery units. If the units are adjacent, some physical efficiency of the above model is retained. Staff can still flex between units. In this model, the anesthesia and nursing team in the operating room makes the determination of the patient's ability to bypass phase 1 recovery. An advantage of this approach is the efficiency of nurse staffing: the assigned nurses can focus on the similar needs of their assigned patients, and workload can be more easily assigned. In its 2004 guidelines, the American Society of Perianesthesia Nurses recommends a staffing ratio of one nurse for up to three patients in phase 1 recovery.

An ambulatory PACU has equipment and staffing similar to an acute-care hospital PACU but focused toward the lesser acuity of the procedures involved. If the ambulatory unit is not integrated with that of a full-service hospital, options for treating the full range of postoperative complications must be provided. The PACU must be equipped to provide postoperative physiological monitoring for all patients, and backup supplies for invasive hemodynamic monitoring must be available if needed. Because the latter are rare-use items in the ambulatory setting, components can be stored together and in-service training should be conducted at regular intervals so that staff maintain their familiarity and skills. A cardiac arrest cart is mandatory, and cardiac pacemaking capability must be considered. To minimize duplicate stocking of rarely used cardiac medications (e.g., secondary antiarrhythmic drugs), the cart can be considered the principal source for these medications when needed, even in the absence of a cardiac arrest.

The ambulatory PACU also must address the emergency respiratory care of a postoperative patient. Supplies and equipment need to be available for reintubation, oxygen delivery and humidification, and inhaled and nebulized medication delivery. The facility should have a plan for the patient who might need prolonged postoperative mechanical ventilation. The plan could be to use manual ventilation until transfer to a better-equipped facility or a backup anesthesia machine with its ventilator.

Secondary recovery area

The phase 2 unit may share a space with the preoperative preparation area of ambulatory surgical patients or it may be a separate area. By and large, patients are physiologically stable, awake, and oriented in the phase 2 unit. When the patient arrives, a postoperative pain control plan should have already been initiated, and the intravenous (IV) catheter should still be in place. Nurse-to-patient ratios are lower in a phase 2 unit than in phase 1; 1 : 6 nurse-to-patient ratios are often supplemented by nonprofessional caregivers. It is common to allow the family to participate in the secondary recovery process, during which time the patient is usually semirecumbent or sitting. Activities such as ambulation, dressing, and predischarge instruction, as well as nutrition and voiding if indicated, are carried out in the phase 2 unit. Staff should be prepared to treat any nausea and emesis that may occur in this setting and to continue to evaluate patients for late development of postoperative complications.

Overnight observation

Ambulatory surgery is the care of patients who go home on the same day. Additionally, some freestanding facilities expand their services by incorporating space adjacent to or part of the recovery area for an extended observation unit (EOU). The EOU allows patients to stay for a prolonged period, from an overnight stay to several days, in order to offer skilled nursing observation for medically stable patients who may not be able to return home immediately because of postsurgical requirements such as continued parenteral analgesic therapy, unresolved nausea, or additional time for restricted movement to prevent hematoma formation. Extended observation is frequently referred to as a 23-hour stay. Patients who require care for medical conditions that necessitate advanced care such as angina or bronchospasm and patients with postsurgical conditions that require higher levels of care such as airway obstruction or postsurgical bleeding should be admitted to a full-service hospital. Third-party insurance reimbursement for EOU care is variable and may depend on the surgical procedure or other justifiable indication. The allowable duration of an extended care course will depend on the licensure of the particular facility and the local regulations regarding the facility.

Staffing

Management of patient flow through ambulatory recovery will play a key role in the overall efficiency of the facility and in managing costs. Staffing efficiency and effectiveness are key elements in maintaining strong performance in these areas. As a general principle, overall facility designs that allow staff to perform multiple functions in the same physical area are the most cost-efficient from a staffing perspective. A single large unit that accommodates preoperative preparation and the entire recovery process will be the most efficient. Nurses can be cross-trained to handle both admission and recovery and discharge duties. Staffing can be increased in the intake area during the early part of the workday when recovery has few patients. In the afternoon, when recovery is busier and the preoperative area has few patients, staff can shift to assist with recovery and discharge functions. When the facility consists of one large unit, staff can respond to acute changes in workload more efficiently and can even handle tasks in both areas simultaneously. If there is limited space, having the intake area and phase 2 PACU together improves efficiency. Intake and phase 2 share common processes in admission and discharge and have similar patient care acuity so staff can be easily cross-trained. The two units will need similar staffing categories, such as personnel for transport, assisting family members who enter and exit the unit, and storing and recovering patient belongings. Similarly, linking phases 1 and 2 of PACU gains the efficiency of having all the personnel required for the entire recovery process in one place. In addition, the need for complex protocols and decision-making regarding fast-tracking can be eliminated, allowing patients to move efficiently through the recovery process. Separating all three units in a facility should be avoided since it will permanently hinder the effectiveness of the staff and will result in higher costs to the facility.

The phase 1 PACU has the potential to hold up the operating room function when its throughput, staffing, or space cannot support the flow of patients from the operating rooms. Staffing is the single most important variable factor that will determine how effective the PACU is. The faster a patient moves from the operating room to discharge, the more recovery beds will be available to accommodate fresh surgical patients and the less chance there is that the PACU will hold up the start of surgical cases. Ideally, staffing should peak when the need for patient care peaks on the unit. To minimize costs, staffing should also be reduced during hours when there is less patient care activity. Juggling staffing patterns to ideally match this workflow is difficult. The problem is complicated by all of the possible permutations of personnel schedules, shift length, and cross-training that can add variability. Staggered nursing shifts can be an important part of the answer. There are cost-effective computer systems that can assist with developing a staffing strategy that meets the needs of the facility. If the PACU does hinder the flow of patients out of the operating room, several strategies can help remedy the problem. Time-motion studies can be performed to identify where in the recovery process patients are delayed and to determine which type of additional staff will best improve efficiency. If staffing and space are being maximally used, it may be necessary to evaluate the operating room schedule to optimize the flow of patients to the PACU. Ideally, the PACU should receive a steady number of new patients that match the ability of the unit to discharge patients. Changing the sequence of cases in the operating room can help eliminate variability in the number of new arrivals per time interval in the PACU.[1] In addition, if the facility has an EOU, patients who will stay overnight should ideally be scheduled as the last patients of the day in the operating room. A successful PACU not only will provide quality postsurgical care to patients but also will efficiently support the flow of patients through the facility.

Selection of staff with appropriate characteristics is of utmost importance in the ambulatory recovery room. The tasks of a recovery nurse in the ambulatory setting are very different from those of acute-care hospital PACU staff. Patients are awake much sooner and are transitioning back to their normal, nonhospitalized life. The staff needs to have personal qualities that allow them to effectively communicate with awake patients and their families or caregivers. The ambulatory recovery staff will need to provide patient education and discharge readiness tasks that are traditionally handled on the surgical ward in acute-care hospitals. Patients may need emotional support to reassure them that they will be able to return to normal activity, care for dressings, and appropriately use pain medication after discharge. The successful PACU nurse has to enjoy these interactions with patients and family members and needs the ability to effectively communicate in a caring manner in these situations. The attitude and ability to work with patients and their families make a tremendous difference in the efficiency of the unit. The characteristics of each individual nurse have a great influence on the speed with which patients move through the recovery process.[2] It is important to hire individuals who will support the goal of an outpatient recovery room.

Transport for urgent care

All ambulatory surgery facilities must have complete plans in place to be able to transport patients to a location where they may receive an increased level of care. This may involve stabilizing the patient's condition at the ambulatory center before transport or transporting the patient emergently to a higher-level facility. Reasons for transport include the need for urgent additional surgery or a more invasive procedure that is better performed at a full-service facility, newly developed medical instability, or care of a postsurgical sequelae. All staff should be current in their knowledge of transport protocols. Arrangements must be made in advance with a transport service or the local municipal paramedics to facilitate transport. It may also be necessary for a registered nurse or anesthesia provider to travel with the patient in order to ensure the continuation of medical care during transit.

Criteria-based recovery

The registered nursing staff needs to be supported by principles of care and policy and procedures that allow them to function in an efficient manner. It is well established that recovery assessment should be made on outcome-based criteria as opposed to specific time requirements. Patients should progress from the operating room to discharge based upon their physiologic state and the return of normal cognitive functions. Anesthetic techniques and agents have improved significantly enough that patients often are awake, alert, and responsive with stable vital signs very early in the recovery process. With advance planning and the use of regional or local anesthesia, many patients have little to no pain and nausea symptoms. There is no reason that these patients cannot be moved from operating room to discharge as expeditiously as possible.

Criteria-based recovery should be applied across the entire recovery process. A patient who is admitted to phase 1 PACU should not be required to stay a certain length of time. Once the patient has met the criteria for admission to phase 2, the transfer should be done. Also in phase 2, there is no need to have patients spend a specific time interval prior to discharge. If a patient meets the criteria for discharge upon arrival, it is appropriate to immediately begin preparing the patient to go home. Meeting the facility's discharge criteria should be the only barrier for a safe and efficient discharge to home. Specific criteria will be discussed in Chapter 13.

Ambulatory recovery issues

Postoperative pain

The plan for postoperative pain management should be developed and implemented before the patient enters and leaves the operating room. Also, the recovery staff must have a clear understanding of analgesic medications and protocols and be prepared to treat pain early to optimize recovery time. The anesthetic technique should be chosen to minimize the amount of postoperative pain that a patient will experience. Regional anesthetic techniques or local anesthesia applied in the surgical field should be used as much as possible to reduce the patient's postoperative pain. If a general anesthetic is required or desired, it must be recognized that neither propofol nor the inhaled anesthetic agents alone provide good postoperative analgesia. If possible, pain should be controlled prior to the end of the procedure by maximizing the use of local anesthetics and non-narcotic analgesics, supplemented by narcotics as needed.

Narcotics have been the traditional pharmacologic agents used to control intra- and postoperative pain in the conventional surgical setting. They minimize the autonomic responses during surgery, and if administered with appropriate timing near the end of the procedure, they can provide postoperative pain relief. However, narcotics also increase the risk of respiratory depression, nausea and vomiting, and sedation in the postoperative period. Therefore, perioperative narcotics should be used carefully and judiciously in the ambulatory setting. The ultrashort-acting narcotics alfentanil and remifentanil have been promoted as good choices for ambulatory surgery because of their rapid termination of effect postoperatively. This can be an advantage in a surgical procedure with little to no postoperative pain; however, both alfentanil and remifentanil are too short-acting to provide analgesia that lasts in the recovery period. When narcotics are required for analgesia, the intermediate-acting narcotic fentanyl ($1-2\,\mu g/kg$) is the ideal drug for immediate pain control in the PACU. Fentanyl offers the advantage of having long enough duration to allow the patient to transition to the oral medication that they will be taking after discharge. Fentanyl also has a short duration that limits the chances of residual sedation and respiratory depression that might hinder discharge, although nausea persists longer than the other side effects. If necessary, longer-acting narcotics such as dihydromorphone or morphine may be used for pain that is not adequately controlled with oral drugs. These should be used as early as possible, before the end of surgery or early in the postoperative process, because the risk with using longer-acting narcotics is that sedation and emetic symptoms may also last longer.[3] Table 12-1 lists the characteristics of the parenteral opioids. If a patient is discharged during the 3–4 hours when these longer-acting drugs are working, the patient may experience severe pain at home when the analgesic effects wear off. As part of the process of preparing the patient for discharge, it is essential the patient be transitioned to oral medications that will provide adequate analgesia at home. If this is not possible due to ongoing pain, the patient should be considered for overnight admission for parenteral pain medication. Commonly used oral opiates and opioid-nonopioid combinations are listed in Table 12-2.

Alternatives to opioid pain management should be actively sought for every patient and procedure since the opioids can cause nausea and vomiting and sedation that will delay discharge. Analgesic techniques that should be

Table 12-1. Commonly used parenteral opioids

Drug	Dose range	Peak effect (minutes)	Duration (hours)
Fentanyl	$25-100\,\mu g$	5–15	0.5–1
Morphine	2.5–15 mg	5–20	2–7
Hydromorphone	0.2–2 mg	5–20	2–4

Doses should be titrated starting with the lower recommended dose.

Table 12-2. Oral preparations of opioid and nonopioid analgesic combinations

Drug	Duration of action (hours)
Acetaminophen/propoxyphene napsylate (Darvocet)	4–6
Acetaminophen/oxycodone (Percocet)	6
Acetaminophen/codeine (Tylenol with codeine)	4
Acetaminophen/hydrocodone (Vicodin)	4–6

considered include local anesthetic infiltration, intra-articular instillation of local anesthetic and opioids,[4] nonsteroidal anti-inflammatory drugs (NSAIDs), and regional anesthesia.[5]

Whether pre-emptive analgesic interventions are more effective than conventional regimens in managing acute postoperative pain remains controversial. Several reviews have addressed this question and have drawn fundamentally different conclusions. The emphasis of pre-emptive analgesia should be on the pathophysiologic phenomenon of antinociception that should prevent altered sensory processing. Therefore, pre-emptive may not simply mean "before incision." An insufficient afferent blockade cannot be pre-emptive, even if it is administered before the incision.[6]

Whereas the evidence on pre-emptive analgesia in animal studies is very convincing,[7] results from human clinical studies remain inconsistent. Though not specifically focusing on ambulatory patients, a recent meta-analysis of 66 studies of different pre-emptive analgesic interventions reported significant effect with epidural analgesia, local infiltration, and systemic NSAIDs but was equivocal for opioids and NMDA (N-methyl-D-aspartic acid) receptor antagonists.[6]

NSAIDs can function as a parenteral or oral replacement for narcotics for mild to moderate pain. The nonspecific NSAID agents such as ibuprofen, diclofenac, and naproxen and ketorolac have all proven effective for mild to moderate pain provided that they are administered with sufficient time to have an effect postoperatively.[8] Administration of NSAIDs may reduce postoperative nausea but may not reduce the need for opioids in ambulatory procedures.[9] Whereas earlier studies suggest no benefit from the use of NSAIDs with regard to nausea or analgesia requirements,[10] a more recent meta-analysis has demonstrated opioid-sparing effects as well as reduction of opioid-related adverse effects.[11] More detailed studies are needed in ambulatory patients to define whether the achieved effect from NSAIDs is due to the reduced pain per se or strictly to the reduction in opioid use. The use of nonspecific NSAIDs has been limited due to concerns regarding potential gastrointestinal and renal side effects and platelet dysfunction.

The newer cyclooxygenase-2 (COX-2) selective antagonists provide effective postoperative pain relief without the risks of postoperative bleeding associated with the traditional NSAIDs. Their implementation, however, has been hampered by the increased risk of cardiovascular side effects after long-term use that resulted in the removal of rofecoxib (Vioxx) and valdecoxib (Bextra) from the market. Research on the effectiveness of the COX-2 agents has shown that they can be useful in reducing the amount of postop narcotic needed in the recovery room due to a reduction in pain scores and in reducing the number of patients who require narcotic medication after discharge.[12] Use of these drugs has been limited due to the withdrawal of the vast majority of oral compounds and to the absence of a parenteral form that can be administered perioperatively, although the preoperative administration of a variety of oral drugs is gaining acceptance. Parecoxib is an injectable COX-2 agent that has been shown to be superior to other oral NSAIDs in the control of postoperative pain and effective in reducing early postoperative narcotic requirements but is not available in the U.S. at this time. At present, celecoxib is the one remaining COX-2 agent that can be prescribed for postoperative analgesia in the U.S. The 400-mg dose was found to provide superior analgesia to the 200-mg dose, and 400 mg is now the recommended dose.[13] Despite the opioid-sparing effects of the perioperative use of COX-2 drugs, a recent review concluded that the incidence of opioid side effects may not be reduced by the addition of the COX-2 drugs.[14] Finally, the use of COX-2 agents may be limited due to a negative influence on bone growth since COX-2 activity is important for bone healing. Hopefully, with the continued development of more specific NSAIDs, these agents will become more valuable in treating postoperative pain and reducing the side effects of narcotic use in the recovery process. Aspirin and salicylate compounds may be prescribed by the surgeon if there is no significant risk of bleeding. Table 12-3 contains a list of available nonopioid analgesics.

Table 12-3. Selected nonopioid analgesics for adult outpatient postoperative pain management

Drug	Dose range	Onset time (minutes)	Duration (hours)
Nonsteroidal anti-inflammatory drugs			
Ibuprofen	400–800 mg PO	30	2–4
Naproxen sodium	550 mg PO	60	6–8
Naproxen	500 mg PO	60	6–8
Ketorolac	10–20 mg PO	30–60	4–6
	30–60 mg IM/IV	15–45	
Ketoprofen	25–50 mg	30	4–6
Diclofenac	75 mg IM (not available in the U.S.)	30	4–6
Indomethacin	25–50 mg PO	30	4–6
	100 mg PR		
p-Aminophenols			
Acetaminophen	500 mg	30	2–4
Cyclooxygenase-2 antagonists			
Celecoxib	400 mg PO	45–60	4–8

Doses should be titrated starting with the lower recommended dose. This list is not intended to be exhaustive. IM, intramuscular; IV, intravenous; PO, per os; PR, per rectum.

Another drug that is being re-evaluated for its analgesic effectiveness is the unique IV anesthetic, ketamine. Ketamine fell out of use as an anesthetic agent in ambulatory anesthesia practice because of its side effects, which include psychomimetic reactions, nausea and vomiting, dizziness, confusion, and diplopia.[15] A recent study on patients having gynecologic laparoscopy demonstrated that small doses of IV ketamine (0.15 mg/kg) improved analgesia for the first 6 hours after surgery with no increase in side effects.[16] A similar study done on patients having knee arthroscopy and using the same dose of ketamine demonstrated improvement in pain scores for 2 days postoperatively with no increase in side effects or times to discharge.[17] However, there are also other well-controlled studies that have failed to demonstrate that ketamine has pre-emptive effect on postsurgical pain,[18] and the risk of visual disturbances and other less-common psychomimetic reactions remains. Further studies are needed to define ketamine's role as an analgesic in ambulatory anesthesia practice.

Several other agents have been examined recently for outpatient postoperative pain control. Dexmedetomidine is an alpha 2 adrenergic agonist that has anesthetic and analgesic effects. In studies done in an inpatient setting, dexmedetomidine has been shown to significantly reduce the need for postoperative narcotics without adding to recovery time.[19,20] However, limited studies in ambulatory surgery populations have reported excessively prolonged sedation. Gabapentin is an anticonvulsant that has been used to treat neuropathic pain and shows promise in reducing anxiety and postoperative pain. In a study on patients having arthroscopic anterior cruciate ligament repair, premedication with gabapentin provided improved anxiolysis and postoperative analgesia and facilitated early knee mobilization.[21] Further research on the use of dexmedetomidine and gabapentin in the outpatient setting will need to be done before these two drugs become routine analgesics.

Regional anesthesia techniques can completely eliminate pain in the early postoperative period. With the use of longer-acting local anesthetic formulations or postoperative local anesthetic delivery systems, regional anesthesia can provide complete relief of pain from 24 hours to several days.[22] Common regional anesthesia blocks done in the outpatient setting include the following:

- Wound infiltration
- Ilioninguinal-iliohypogastric
- Penile and dorsal
- Upper extremity: Bier (IV regional), axillary, and interscalene
- Lower extremity: femoral, lateral femoral cutaneous, sciatic, popliteal fossa, and ankle
- Central neuraxial: spinal, epidural, and caudal

These blocks are addressed in more detail in Chapter 8. Regional anesthetics have the added benefit of reducing the incidence of postoperative nausea and vomiting (PONV),[23] allowing more patients to fast-track and enabling faster discharge times to home,[24] with fewer hospital admissions and improved patient satisfaction.[25] As a result, studies have demonstrated that regional anesthesia has the potential to significantly reduce hospital costs versus general anesthesia.[26] The most recent development in outpatient regional anesthesia is the use of continuous catheters. Catheters can be placed at the location of the block or in the intra-articular space to provide continuous infusion of local anesthetic by pump for the first 24–48 hours of postoperative care.[27] Catheter techniques have the potential to provide an almost completely pain-free postoperative experience.

Local anesthetic and opioid applied at the surgical site has also been demonstrated to significantly reduce pain and improve discharge times. A nerve block in the surgical field combined with monitored anesthesia care (MAC) anesthesia has been demonstrated to significantly reduce postoperative pain versus general anesthesia, speed time to discharge, and reduce hospital costs.[24] Single-shot intra-articular local anesthetics and opioids have been studied for arthroscopic procedures and have been found to provide good postoperative analgesia during the intermediate recovery period[5,28] and a reduction in the requirements for postoperative opioids.[29]

Patients who require pain control postoperatively in the EOU should be offered pain control by the same modalities offered to inpatients. Patient-controlled analgesia is particularly helpful for the management of patients with challenging postoperative pain problems. The continued development of new alternative techniques of pain management has resulted in fewer patients needing an overnight stay in the EOU. One example is the change in the postoperative care of the patient for anterior cruciate ligament repair which has occurred over the past decade. What was once an inpatient procedure now is usually done with a single-shot or catheter-based regional anesthetic. The majority of these patients return home on the same day as surgery and have little to no pain in the first postoperative day, although they need careful postop instruction to begin oral analgesics before the block goes and to take medications on schedule, so that pain does not become significant.

Nausea and emesis

PONV continues to be the most common overall postoperative complication. Studies done of patients' preferences have demonstrated that nausea and vomiting are the postoperative symptoms that patients most want to avoid. In one study, individuals would choose to have more pain, somnolence, and other side effects if they were not nauseated postoperatively.[30] In another study, patients surveyed were willing to pay up to $100 for treatment that would eliminate PONV.[31] Despite resolution of numerous other surgical and anesthesia sequelae, nausea and emesis can unduly postpone discharge and even result in unanticipated admission.[32]

The causes of PONV are multifactorial. Known risk factors supported by strong evidence include female gender postpuberty, younger age, nonsmoker status, history of previous PONV or motion sickness, postoperative use and administration of opioids, and use of general anesthesia with volatile anesthesia and nitrous oxide[33] (Box 12-1). Although evidence for the type and duration of surgery and anesthesia is less strong, they are nevertheless identified as additional risk factors.[34] The types of surgery that might increase the risk of PONV are plastic, ophthalmologic, orthopedic shoulder surgery, ENT (ear, nose, throat), dental, and gynecologic procedures. A simplified risk factor chart using four independent risk factors by Apfel et al.[35] or five risk factors by Koivuranta

Box 12-1. Risk factors for postoperative nausea and vomiting

Patient factors
    Female
    Younger age
    Nonsmoker status
    History of previous postoperative nausea and vomiting
    Susceptible to motion sickness
Anesthesia factors
    General anesthesia with volatile anesthetics
    Nitrous oxide
    High-dose neostigmine
    Intraoperative and postoperative opioids
Surgical factors
    Duration of surgery

et al.[36] is listed in Box 12-2. These factors can be used to predict the risk that an individual patient has of having PONV (Figure 12-1). Patients with no or one risk factor have a risk of 20% or less of having PONV. Patients with two, three, and four risk factors have a risk of approximately 40%, 60%, and 80%, respectively. Prophylactic treatment of patients should be guided by risk stratification. Scoring systems for adults, while only moderately accurate in predictive ability, have improved the clinician's ability to better tailor antiemetic interventions. The consensus guidelines for managing PONV[37] recommend not treating patients at low risk (less than 10% risk or no risk factors) prophylactically. Patients at moderate risk would receive single-drug therapy or combination therapy. Patients

Box 12-2. Simplified risk factors for postoperative nausea and vomiting (PONV)

Risk factors	Points
Female gender	1
Nonsmoker	1
History of PONV/motion sickness	1
Postoperative opioids	1
Sum	0–4
Female gender	1
Nonsmoker	1
History of PONV	1
History of motion sickness	1
Duration of surgery more than 60 minutes	1
Sum	0–5

Adapted from Apfel et al.[35] and Koivuranta et al.[36]

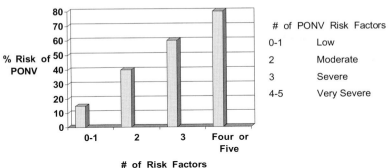

Figure 12-1. Relationship of number of risk factors to level of postoperative nausea and vomiting (PONV) risk.

at high risk would receive prophylaxis with two or three different classes of agents (Figure 12-2). Patients who have nausea or vomiting in the PACU should receive treatment with a drug from a class that they have not received yet in the perioperative period since redosing with the same class is rarely successful.[38] Obtaining an understanding of PONV risk factors and its pathophysiology is complicated by the multifactorial nature of PONV because of the involvement of multiple receptors and stimuli. At least seven neurotransmitter types are documented, or believed to be implicated, in PONV, namely serotonin, dopamine, muscarine, acetylcholine, neurokinin-1, histamine, and opioids. Stimulation of the vestibular-cochlear, glossopharyngeal, or especially vagus nerves is also involved.[33]

In their choice of prophylactic therapy, practitioners should use a rational approach that balances effectiveness and cost against the patient's risk of PONV. A multimodal approach to the prevention of PONV should be applied to each patient, particularly those at high risk. Unless there is a contraindication to infusing IV fluids (as in a patient in renal failure), all patients should receive 20 mL/kg of IV fluids during the surgical procedure. Avoidance of general anesthesia should be considered. There should be a plan to control postoperative pain and, if possible, exclude opiate analgesics. The use of higher inspired concentration of oxygen has not been proven to effectively reduce PONV.[33] Antiemetic drugs are indicated for patients with more than minimal risk. There are many classes of antiemetic agents available for prophylactic use. The use of droperidol at the time of publication is marred by a black box warning issued by the Food and Drug Administration (FDA) because of nine case reports of arrhythmias which have occurred with its use in patients with prolonged QT interval on electrocardiogram (ECG). It should be noted that the FDA black box warning applies to the FDA-approved dose of droperidol, which is greater or equal to 2.5 mg; there currently is no PONV indication or approved dose. The decision

338   J.L. Pregler and P.A. Kapur

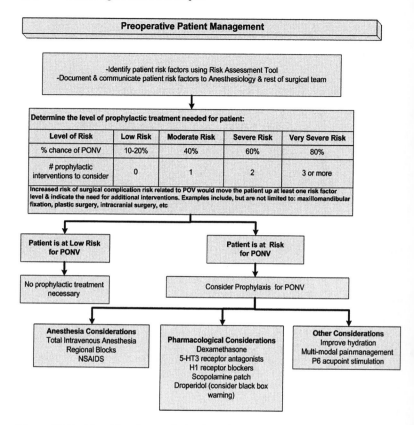

Figure 12-2. Algorithm for prophylactic antiemetic treatment. Adapted with permission from Gan et al.[37] and the American Society of PeriAnesthesia Nurses PONV/PDNV Strategic Work Team.[34] NSAID, nonsteroidal anti-inflammatory drug; PONV, postoperative nausea and vomiting; POV, postoperative vomiting.

to use droperidol is one that each practitioner must make after weighing its antiemetic effectiveness against the potential for complications in each individual patient. With careful screening of the preoperative ECG and monitoring for 2 hours after administration, droperidol can still be an effective option in preventing PONV. Recent studies have shown that droperidol, dexamethasone, and ondansetron are equally effective and reduce the relative risk of PONV by approximately 25%[39] (Figure 12-3). Since the cost of an effective dose of droperidol and dexamethasone is less than a dollar, the most cost-effective option is to use one or two of these drugs as the first round of prophylactic antiemetic therapy. There are also clinical advantages to giving either of these drugs early in the procedure. It has been shown that dexamethasone is more effective when given at the start of the procedure, just after induction, and its effect lasts post-

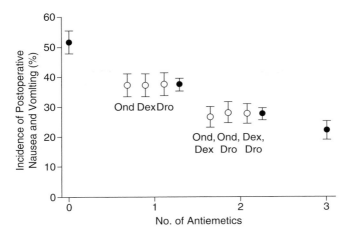

Figure 12-3. Absolute risk reduction in postoperative nausea and vomiting using different combinations of antiemetics. Incidence of postoperative nausea and vomiting associated with the various combinations of antiemetic drugs. The data shown represent outcomes in 5,161 patients. Solid circles represent the average value for each number of prophylactic antiemetics, and open symbols the incidence for each antiemetic or combination of antiemetics. Dex, dexamethasone; Dro, droperidol; Ond, ondansetron. I bars represent 95% confidence intervals. Source: Apfel et al.[39] © 2004 Massachusetts Medical Society. All rights reserved. Used with permission.

discharge for 24 hours.[40] For several reasons, droperidol is also best given immediately after induction. Giving it early allows adequate time for observation of the patient's cardiac rhythm to satisfy the FDA's recommendation on its safe use. Droperidol also has dysphoric and sedative side effects that taper after administration. By administering droperidol early in the case, these side effects can be minimized while the antiemetic effect continues. Haloperidol is currently being considered as an alternative to droperidol, although the minimal fully effective dose is not known and the side effect profile is not well defined.[33] Serotonin antagonists should be added as the third drug for patients at high risk for PONV and should be given near the end of the surgical procedure or for treatment. Dolasetron is a pro-drug and should be administered 30 minutes prior to anesthetic emergence to allow for its metabolism to an active drug. The time to effectiveness for ondansetron is also up to 30 minutes. Other drugs that have similar efficacy, though with fewer studies, are transdermal scopolamine, intramuscular ephedrine, and higher-dose metoclopramide.[37]

If nausea and vomiting occur after surgery and prior to discharge, the number of agents available to treat is more limited (Figure 12-4). It is well established that treatment with a second dose of the same class of antiemetic is much less likely to be effective and the consensus papers recommend using a

Antiemetic Treatment for PONV

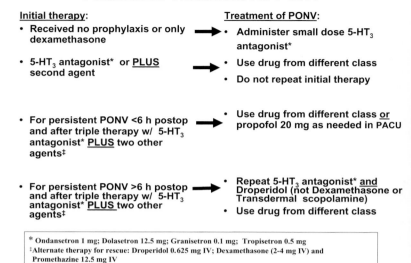

Initial therapy:

Treatment of PONV:

- **Received no prophylaxis or only dexamethasone** ➤ • **Administer small dose 5-HT$_3$ antagonist***

- **5-HT$_3$ antagonist* or PLUS second agent** ➤ • **Use drug from different class**
  - **Do not repeat initial therapy**

- **For persistent PONV <6 h postop and after triple therapy w/ 5-HT$_3$ antagonist* PLUS two other agents‡** ➤ • **Use drug from different class or propofol 20 mg as needed in PACU**

- **For persistent PONV >6 h postop and after triple therapy w/ 5-HT$_3$ antagonist* PLUS two other agents‡** ➤ • **Repeat 5-HT$_3$ antagonist* and Droperidol (not Dexamethasone or Transdermal scopolamine)**
  - **Use drug from different class**

---

* Ondansetron 1 mg; Dolasetron 12.5 mg; Granisetron 0.1 mg; Tropisetron 0.5 mg
‡Alternate therapy for rescue: Droperidol 0.625 mg IV; Dexamethasone (2-4 mg IV) and
  Promethazine 12.5 mg IV

Figure 12-4. Algorithm for treatment of established postoperative nausea and vomiting (PONV).

different class of drug.[33,34,37] As shown in Table 12-4, most agents have significant side effects that can delay the discharge of the patient. Droperidol can cause dysphoria and drowsiness and comes with the recommendation that the ECG be monitored for 2–3 hours after administration. Its use in the PACU can result in a significant delay in discharge. Prochlorperazine (Compazine) and the antihistamines all can cause significant sedation. However, a lower dose of promethazine (Phenergan) (6.25 mg) has efficacy with minimal sedation. Metoclopramide is not particularly effective as a rescue drug and can cause extrapyramidal effects. Scopolamine patch has a delayed onset that makes it ineffective as a rescue modality, although its use should be considered to provide protection for the ride home and postdischarge. None of these drugs is optimally effective, which is why the serotonin antagonists are the first line of drugs for rescue therapy—unless a serotonin antagonist was used for prevention. In that case, a drug of another class must be chosen. Serotonin antagonists can be associated with significant headache, and the treatment dose may be one fourth the prevention dose. Data show that the efficacy of all serotonin antagonists is similar. After 6 hours, the dose of a serotonin antagonist can be repeated.

Alternative therapies have been evaluated for the prevention and treatment of PONV. Full daily volume replacement of IV fluids is effective. Transcutaneous acupoint electrical stimulation has been found to decrease the symptoms of postop nausea and to enhance the effectiveness of droperidol when used in combination.[41] Preoperative acupuncture therapy has also been shown to reduce PONV in patients who undergo abdominal surgery.[42] Supplemental oxygen has

Table 12-4. Postoperative antiemetic therapy-adults

Drug	Dose	Side effects
Serotonin (5HT₃) antagonists		
Ondansetron (Zofran)	4–8 mg IV	Headache, dizziness
Dolasetron (Anzemet)	12.5–25 mg IV	
Granisetron (Kytril)	0.35–1.0 mg IV	
Butyrophenones		
Droperidol	0.625–1.25 mg IV	Extrapyramidal effects, dysphoria, drowsiness, dizziness
Neurokinin (NK-1) antagonists		
Aprepitant (Emend)	40 mg PO	Headache, constipation, pruritis
Steroids		
Dexamethasone	4–10 mg IV	Rare with single dose
Phenothiazines		
Prochlorperazine (Compazine)	5–10 mg IV, IM, PO 25 mg PR suppository	Sedation, drowsiness, hypotension
Antihistamines (H-1) antagonists		
Promethazine (Phenergan)	6.25–12.5 mg IV 12.5–50 mg PR suppository	Sedation
Hydroxyzine (Vistaril)	12.5–25 mg IV, IM	
Benzamides		
Trimethobenzamide (Tigan)	100–200 mg IV, IM 200 mg PR suppository	Extrapyramidal effects, dysphoria, drowsiness, anxiety, dizziness
Anticholinergics		
Scopolamine patch (Transderm Scop)	1.5 mg transdermal	Dry mouth, blurred visions, hallucinations

IM, intramuscular; IV, intravenous; PO, per os; PR, per rectum.

been shown to reduce PONV in some studies[43] and has been ineffective in others,[44] and overall is probably not effective. No alternative therapy has yet become as important as pharmacologic therapy for the prevention and treatment of PONV. A patient-controlled regimen of propofol administration in the PACU has been demonstrated to reduce the number of episodes of vomiting in the PACU and the need for rescue antiemetics.[45] The effectiveness of propofol diminishes as the serum concentration falls, so this method does not provide long-term relief of PONV and is not a practical solution for the problem. Future therapies might be directed toward neurokinin 1 (NK1) receptors that are highly concentrated in the brainstem vomiting center. Pharmacological therapy using NK1 receptor antagonists is being evaluated to augment other multimodal treatments for prophylaxis. No alternative therapy has yet become as important as pharmacologic therapy for the prevention and treatment of PONV. Further PONV research examining patient genetic characteristics and underinvestigated potential clinical risk factors in outpatients and children should lead to predictive systems with improved discriminating power and applicability.

Postdischarge nausea and vomiting

Nausea and vomiting is an under-recognized problem in the postdischarge period, affecting approximately one third of ambulatory surgery patients.[46] Even so, very little research has been conducted regarding the incidence, prediction, or pharmacologic and nonpharmacologic treatment of this problem. No guidelines to this point have included recommendations for patients past the point of discharge. Based on the limited research, a similar algorithm to PONV has been suggested (Figure 12-5).

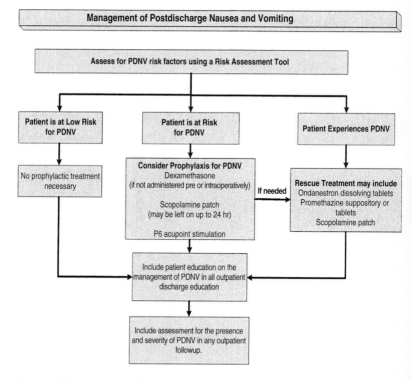

Figure 12-5. Algorithm for management of postdischarge nausea and vomiting (PDNV). Adapted with permission from Gupta et al.[46] and the American Society of PeriAnesthesia Nurses PONV/PDNV Strategic Work Team.[34]

Cardiovascular alterations

Hypertension

Elevated blood pressure is frequently encountered during the recovery from anesthesia and surgery in patients with good myocardial function. A search should be made for obvious etiologies (Box 12-3) such as pain, bladder distention, hypoxemia, hypercarbia, agitation, or abrupt preoperative cessation of chronic antihypertensive medications. In patients with prior good health, in the absence of an identified cause, treatment should be approached cautiously because of wide variability among patients in their response to antihypertensive medications. Patients with a history of chronic hypertension, with or without discernable end-organ damage, need to be treated promptly, taking into account possible pharmacologic interactions of acutely administered drugs with chronic medications. The concern is that, for the at-risk cardiac patient, increased blood pressure may reflect an increased afterload that may cause an imbalance in myocardial oxygen supply and demand. Unless remedied, a spiraling course of cardiac compromise may result.

Treatment of hypertension in the recovering surgical patient consists of either vasodilator or myocardial depressant drugs (Table 12-5). The former category includes the vasodilating calcium channel blocking drugs and longer-acting direct vasodilators as well as the short-acting agents that can be given by IV bolus or infusion, such as nitroglycerin or nitroprusside. Beta-adrenergic antagonists may be employed to lower blood pressure by reducing cardiac output. Esmolol, propranolol, and metoprolol are all available for IV administration, though with differences in pharmacokinetic properties and relative cardiac selectivity. Labetalol, a mixed alpha- and beta-adrenergic antagonist with predominant nonselective beta-adrenergic antagonist properties, can be used to treat postoperative hypertension[47] but also causes a lowered cardiac output. All of the beta-adrenergic antagonists have the potential to exacerbate bronchoconstriction in a dose-dependent manner in individual patients. All beta-adrenergic antagonists should be used with extreme caution in patients with poor ventricular function.

Hypotension

Systemic hypotension is another cause for concern during the recovery period. For the appropriate intervention to be undertaken, the etiology of

Box 12-3. Etiology of postoperative hypertension

Pain
Bladder distention
Hypoxemia
Hypercarbia
Agitation
Cessation of chronic antihypertensive medications

Table 12-5. Treatment modalities for postoperative hypertension

Drug	Dose range	Half-life
Beta blockers		
Propranolol (Inderal)	0.5–1.0 mg IV	2–4 hours
Labetalol (mixed alpha and beta) (Trandate, Normodyne)	5–10 mg bolus IV	4–6 hours
Esmolol (beta 1-selective) (Brevibloc)	0.25–0.5 mg/kg bolus IV 50–200 µg/kg per minute infusion	9 minutes
Metoprolol (beta 1-selective) (Lopressor)	5–25 mg IV increments	2.5–4.5 hours
Vasodilators		
Hydralazine (Apresoline)	2.5–5.0 mg IV increments	4–6 hours
Nitroglycerin	50–100 µg IV bolus 0.1 µg/kg per minute	4–6 hours
Calcium channel blockers		
Nicardipene (Cardene)	2.5 mg IV	6 hours
ACE Inhibitors		
Enalapril (Vasotec)	2.5 mg IV	4–6 hours

IV, intravenous.

hypotension must be sought among the broad general categories of reduced myocardial preload, decreased systemic vascular resistance, or decreased cardiac output (Box 12-4).

Decreased cardiac filling results from insufficient perioperative fluid administration to replace maintenance fluid requirements and surgical losses. Ongoing postoperative blood loss must be one of the considerations when assessing the recovering patient. Specific treatment includes using the head-down position,

Box 12-4. Causes of postoperative hypotension

Reduced myocardial preload
    Hypovolemia
    Venodilation
Decreased systemic vascular resistance
    Venodilating medications
    Sympathectomy from regional anesthesia
    Arterio-venous shunts
    Hyperthermia
    Sepsis
Decreased cardiac output
    Myocardial ischemia
    Dysrhythmias

administering volume resuscitation with appropriate fluids, and making a diligent search for and consideration of possible reoperation to remedy sources of continuing blood loss.

Causes of decreased afterload are summarized in Box 12-4. Vasoconstricting medications may be needed to counter the effect of vasodilators or until the effects of a spinal or epidural anesthetic wane. In the case of severe hypotension in the absence of ongoing myocardial ischemia, myocardial stimulating medications, such as direct- and indirect-acting sympathomimetics, may serve to temporize until the proximate cause of the hypotension can be diagnosed and treated.

Hypotension associated with poor myocardial performance results from inadequate pump function or from arrhythmias that result in impaired chamber filling and/or ejection. Inadequate pump function of the heart may be chronic or acute. Chronically depressed myocardial function would presumably be detected during the prescreening process before anesthesia, and inappropriate patients should have their procedures done in an acute-care facility. Acute myocardial pump decompensation during the recovery period typically indicates ongoing myocardial ischemia. In this situation, treatment requires improving the imbalance between myocardial oxygen supply and demand by administering a coronary vasodilator such as nitroglycerin or by reducing myocardial oxygen demand. Decreasing afterload with a vasodilator or heart rate with a beta-adrenergic antagonist can reduce myocardial oxygen demand.

Myocardial ischemia

As a result of intrinsic changes in coronary artery vascular tone, myocardial ischemia may also develop in the absence of measurable hemodynamic alterations. Coronary vasoconstriction may occur with or without concomitant obstructive coronary artery disease. The occurrence of unexpected chest pain or unexpected symptoms of congestive heart failure in the postoperative period must be thoroughly evaluated, the former to rule out chest wall or gastrointestinal etiologies of parasternal pain, the latter to rule out noncardiogenic causes of pulmonary edema. If a cardiac diagnosis is made, treatment is similar to that for myocardial ischemia. Vasodilating calcium channel blockers are the treatment of choice for the specific diagnosis of coronary vasospasm.

Patients who have experienced a postoperative episode of significant hypertension or hypotension or possible ischemic event may need to be admitted to a full-service hospital. If a discernible cause for the cardiovascular alteration has been identified, and the patient has responded predictably and promptly to the treatment, discharge to home may be the most appropriate measure. Patients not meeting these criteria merit hospital admission for observation and further treatment.

Rhythm disturbances

Rhythm disturbances in the postoperative period may be the cause or result of impaired cardiac performance (Box 12-5). In all cases of rhythm disturbance, adequacy of ventilation must be assessed to rule out hypoxia and hypercarbia. Dysrhythmias associated with myocardial ischemia are treated by resolving the ischemic condition. Treatment of dysrhythmias that are secondary to another

Box 12-5. Etiology of dysrhythmias

Hypoxia or hypercarbia
Myocardial ischemia
Electrolyte imbalance
Drug toxicity
Excessive catecholamine activity
Breakthrough of chronic dysrhythmia upon cessation of chronic antiarrhythmic medications

abnormality, such as an electrolyte imbalance, requires treatment of the underlying cause. Bradyarrhythmias, in the absence of hypoxia, hypercarbia, or other treatable causes, should be corrected with an anticholinergic drug, such as atropine, a beta-1 agonist, or by cardiac pacing in order to prevent potential compromise of vital organ perfusion. Resurgence of chronic arrhythmias that recur when medication levels fall requires acute treatment and re-establishment of therapeutic drug levels by resumption of the chronic medication regimen.

Management of chronic cardiac medications

Patients should continue taking their cardiac medications until the time of surgery and then reinstitute the medications following surgery. Since many perioperative pharmacy areas do not carry a wide array of oral medications, patients should be instructed to bring their daily chronic medications with them so the doses can be administered as closely on schedule as possible after surgery. If nausea and vomiting are a problem postoperatively, other plans must be made to provide the patient uninterrupted pharmacologic control of the cardiovascular problem. Topical preparations are available for some medications, such as nitrates and clonidine. With other drugs, IV substitutions may be administered if oral intake is temporarily precluded postoperatively.

Airway and pulmonary complications

Pulmonary sequelae of anesthesia and surgery may include atelectasis, bronchospasm, croup, or aspiration. Fortunately, many ambulatory procedures are of reasonably short duration such that atelectasis is rarely an ambulatory surgery complication. Reduced functional residual capacity, however, may compromise respiratory sufficiency during recovery in patients such as the supine obese patient, the advanced pregnant patient, or the patient nursed in the head-down position.

Bronchospasm

Selected patients with prior known history of stable, well-controlled bronchospastic disease can be safely cared for on an ambulatory basis. Such patients should be carefully evaluated preoperatively regarding the severity, predictability, and degree of control of their symptoms. Those judged suitable for ambulatory anesthesia and surgery should continue taking their medication up until surgery and bring their inhalers with them to the ambulatory center. In the recovery area, these patients should be carefully assessed for the degree of bronchospasm. Preoperative medication regimes should be reinstituted as soon as practicable. Center personnel should be able to deliver aerosolized bronchodilators by nebulizer, if required, and beta-adrenergic agonists should be available. Persistent postoperative bronchospasm requiring repeated treatments or continuous IV therapy might indicate the need for hospital admission for additional observation and treatment.

Postintubation stridor

The prevention of postoperative stridor requires careful screening for predisposing factors (e.g., prior intubation difficulties and recent upper respiratory infection). Treatment of stridor should include humidified oxygen, dexamethasone, and/or aerosolized racemic epinephrine treatments. An airway at risk of obstruction may need to be resecured, and additional postanesthetic observation is indicated. Careful assessment should be made regarding discharge. See Chapter 4 for further discussion of postintubation stridor in pediatrics.

Pulmonary aspiration

With careful patient selection, preoperative preparation, and modern intraoperative precautions, the incidence of pulmonary aspiration is quite low. Aspiration in the presence of oropharyngeal gastric contents or blood may occur at any time during the perioperative period, including at the time of tracheal extubation or in the recovery suite. In the latter environment, special attention should be paid to patients with compromised airway reflexes caused by residual anesthetics, sedatives, or narcotics or in patients with neurologic compromise of the airway for any reason. Some patients at higher risk during the perioperative period include those with hiatal hernia, obesity, pregnancy, upper abdominal surgery, compromised gastroesophageal sphincter function, or recent ingestion of solid foods.[48]

Symptoms and sequelae of pulmonary aspiration are related to the volume, type of fluid, and acid content of the aspirate. The airway should be cleared and oxygenation of the patient ensured. Assessment includes chest x-ray, which may or may not show changes early on, and arterial blood gas measurement. If severe aspiration is indicated by a low PaO_2 (partial pressure of oxygen, arterial) value, possibly with pulmonary edema, vigorous therapy including mechanical ventilation may be required. If the patient is experiencing no respiratory distress and oxygenation is adequate, the aspiration may have been mild and careful observation to rule out development of a worsening clinical presentation may be all that is required.[49]

Surgical complications

Surgical complications include postoperative bleeding, more extensive surgery than originally anticipated, or a surgical mishap that requires additional postoperative care (e.g., perforated viscus). Prompt recognition and appropriate supportive measures can contribute to an optimized outcome. Several procedures common to the ambulatory arena have their own unique complications.

Abdominal insufflation associated with laparoscopy can cause subcutaneous emphysema that may dissect into the mediastinum or pericardium, or pulmonary gas embolism. The main concern during the recovery period for either of these complications is the appropriate ongoing management of any severe cardiopulmonary sequelae, including continued ventilatory and/or inotropic support while awaiting transport to an acute-care facility.

Hemodilution syndrome is another complication, which can result from visceral irrigation during transurethral prostate surgery or hysteroscopy. Intravascular absorption of irrigation fluid occurs via prostatic sinuses or severed uterine venous channels or possibly from peritoneal absorption of irrigation fluid that has passed out of the fallopian tubes.[50] If dilutional hyponatremia is symptomatic, treatment to restore normal serum sodium levels is based on the patient's central nervous system status and/or current serum sodium level and may require diuresis or IV administration of hypertonic saline solutions. Air embolus has also been reported as a complication of hysteroscopy.

Temperature abnormalities

Hypothermia

Wide changes in patient core temperature are less common with brief ambulatory surgeries, but hypothermia can occur. Modern methods to preserve body heat should be used in longer outpatient cases.[51] Complications of hypothermia include excessive metabolic oxygen consumption with the potential to cause increased cardiac output, prolonged time in the PACU, and patient discomfort from thermoregulatory shivering. Patients undergoing surgery under MAC with sedation, or regional anesthesia techniques, are very appreciative of efforts to keep them warm in the cold operating room environment. If lowered core temperature is detected postoperatively (particularly in the presence of shivering), warming lights and forced-air warming blankets should be used. Small doses of IV meperidine are helpful in reducing the severity of shivering,[52] but it is important to note that this treatment is only masking symptoms.

Malignant hyperthermia

As in any center in which anesthetics are administered, ambulatory centers must be able to differentiate causes of elevated core temperature, including malignant hyperthermia. Patients at risk for malignant hyperthermia have been safely anesthetized in ambulatory centers, taking the precautions in anesthetic technique recommended for such patients, with an adequate postoperative observation period.[53] Prompt access to dantrolene sodium should be available. Consideration can be given to accessibility of blood gas and/or serum electrolyte determinations for the treatment of this condition if it arises unexpectedly.[54]

Box 12-6. Minor complications after ambulatory surgery

Postdischarge nausea
Headache
Myalgias
Sore throat/hoarseness
Dizziness/light-headedness
General malaise

Adapted from Philip BK.[55]

Minor complications

In general, ambulatory anesthesia patients and their families expect very little morbidity from their perioperative experience. Nevertheless, ambulatory patients may experience one or more of a host of minor complications, including postdischarge nausea, sore throat, hoarseness, myalgias, dizziness/light headedness, and general malaise, related to the physiologic trespass of the surgery and related maneuvers[55] (Box 12-6). Laparoscopy patients may not recover their general sense of well-being for 3 to 5 days postoperatively. Care must be taken throughout the entire perioperative period to prevent other minor complications such as corneal abrasion, dental damage, tape irritation, and multiple needle puncture marks.

Influence of anesthetics and anesthesia techniques on recovery

Anesthetic techniques currently being used for ambulatory anesthesia include MAC, regional anesthesia with or without IV sedation, and general anesthesia. The ambulatory anesthesia setting is certainly one area where justification for the use of newer, albeit more expensive, shorter-acting sedative/hypnotic anesthetics and muscle-relaxant drugs can rationally be supported if offsetting savings can be achieved. Cost savings from better patient flow can occur because of reduced consumption of recovery room supplies and staff time when patients have shortened time to return to baseline faculties and from reduced need for observation and treatment of anesthetic sequelae such as persistent sedation or nausea.

In considering anesthetic drugs, the modern anesthetic agents all provide rapid awakening with variation only on the scale of minutes. Whereas minor differences may be apparent in measures of immediate recovery on the operating table, very little difference if any can be shown in overall recovery times.[56] Length of stay is determined more by type and length of surgery, adverse events, pain, PONV, dizziness, drowsiness, and cardiovascular events.[57] As already discussed in this chapter, anesthetic choices that focus on minimizing these sequelae will have the greatest effect on improving patient care and time to discharge in the recovery area and on the ability of the patient to resume their normal activities. Significant improvement in care can be gained from maximizing the use of peripheral regional anesthetics and sedation techniques and avoiding the use of general anesthetics.

Summary

The design, staffing, and medical treatment rendered in the recovery areas of an ambulatory surgery center are integrally related to achieving the goal of safe, high-quality, efficient, cost-effective, patient-oriented perioperative care that incorporates the most up-to-date concepts in ambulatory surgery and anesthesia. In contrast to inpatients and their families, who may remember or know little of operating room events, the generally alert recovering ambulatory anesthesia patient is able to fully appreciate the care and concern shown during the recovery process. A center that is prepared to prospectively and proactively address the range of potential postoperative events, from prevention of discomfort and possible complications to preparation for postrecovery discharge, is appreciated by patients, their surgeons, and referring physicians and ultimately by third-party payers, who ever more frequently determine to which ambulatory facilities patients will be directed.

References

1. Dexter F, Epstein R, Marcon E, de Matta R. Strategies to reduce delays in admission into a postanesthesia care unit from operating rooms. *J Perianesth Nurs.* 2005;20: 92–102.
2. Pavlin DJ, Rapp SE, Polissar NL, et al. Factors affecting discharge time in adult outpatients. *Anesth Analg.* 1998;87:816–26.
3. Claxton AR, McGuire G, Chung F, Cruise C. Evaluation of morphine versus fentanyl for postoperative analgesia after ambulatory surgical procedures. *Anesth Analg.* 1997;84:509–514.
4. Joshi G, McCarroll S, O'Brien T, et al. Intraarticular analgesia following knee arthroscopy. *Anesth Analg.* 1993;76:333–336.
5. Bridenbaugh L. Regional anaesthesia for outpatient surgery—a summary of 12 years' experience. *Can Anaesth Soc J.* 1983;30:548–552.
6. Ong CK, Lirk P, Seymour RA, Jenkins BJ. The efficacy of preemptive analgesia for acute postoperative pain management: a meta-analysis. *Anesth Analg.* 2005;100: 757–773.
7. Woolf CJ, Chong MS. Pre-emptive analgesia: treating postoperative pain by preventing the establishment of central sensitization. *Anesth Analg.* 1993;77:362–379.
8. Wong H, Carpenter R, Kpacz D, et al. A randomized double-blind evaluation of ketorolac tromethamine for post-operative analgesia in ambulatory surgery patients. *Anesthesiology.* 1993;78:6–14.

9. Sukhani R, Vasquez J, Pappas AL, et al. Recovery after propofol with and without intraoperative fentanyl in patients undergoing ambulatory gynecologic laparoscopy. *Anesth Analg.* 1996;83:975–981.

10. Ding Y, White P. Comparative effects of ketorolac, dezocine and fentanyl as adjuvants during outpatient anesthesia. *Anesth Analg.* 1992;75:566–571.

11. Marret E, Kurdi O, Zufferey P, Bonnet F. Effects of nonsteroidal antiinflamatory drugs on patient-controlled analgesia morphine side effects: meta-analysis of randomized controlled trials. *Anesthesiology.* 2005;102:1249–1260.

12. Joshi G, Viscusi E, Gan T, et al. Effective treatment of laparoscopic cholecystectomy pain with intravenous followed by oral COX-2 specific inhibitor. *Anesth Analg.* 2004;98:336–342.

13. Recart A, Issioui T, White P. The efficacy of celecoxib premedication on postoperative pain and recovery times after ambulatory surgery: a dose-ranging study. *Anesth Analg.* 2003;96:1631–1635.

14. Romsing J, Moiniche S, Mathiesen O, et al. Reduction of opioid-related adverse events using opioid-sparing analgesia with COX-2 inhibitors lacks documentation: a systematic review. *Acta Anaesthesiol Scand.* 2005;49:133–142.

15. White P. The changing role of non-opioid analgesic techniques in the management of postoperative pain. *Anesth Analg.* 2005;101:S5–S22.

16. Kwok R, Lim J, Chan M, et al. Preoperative ketamine improves postoperative analgesia after gynecologic laparoscopic surgery. *Anesth Analg.* 2004;98:1044–1049.

17. Menigaux C, Guignard B, Fletcher D, et al. Intraoperative small-dose ketamine enhances analgesia after outpatient knee arthroscopy. *Anesth Analg.* 2001;93:606–612.

18. Adam F, Libier M, Oszustowicz T, et al. Preoperative small-dose ketamine has no preemptive analgesic effect in patients undergoing total mastectomy. *Anesth Analg.* 1999;89:444–447.

19. Arain SR, Ruehlow RM, Uhrich TD, Ebert TJ. The efficacy of dexmedetomidine versus morphine for postoperative analgesia after major inpatient surgery. *Anesth Analg.* 2004;98:153–158.

20. Unlugenc H, Gunduz M, Guler T, Yagmur O, Isik G. The effect of pre-anaesthetic administration of intravenous dexmedetomidine on postoperative pain in patients receiving patient-controlled morphine. *Eur J Anaesthesiol.* 2005;22:386–391.

21. Menigaux C, Adam F, Guignard, et al. Preoperative gabapentin decreased anxiety and improves early functional recovery from knee surgery. *Anesth Analg.* 2005;100:1394–1399.

22. Lu L, Fine N. The efficacy of continuous local anesthetic infiltration in breast surgery: Reduction Mammoplasty and reconstruction. *Plast Reconstr Surg.* 2005;115:1927–1934.

23. Kairaluoma P, Bachmann M, Korpinen A, et al. Single-injection paravertebral block before general anesthesia enhances analgesia after breast cancer surgery with and without associated lymph node biopsy. *Anesth Analg.* 2004;99:1837–1843.

24. Hadzic A, Karaca P, Hobeika P, et al. Peripheral nerve blocks result in superior recovery profile compared with general anesthesia in outpatient knee arthroscopy. *Anesth Analg.* 2005;100:976–981.

352   J.L. Pregler and P.A. Kapur

25. Terheggen M, Sille F, Rinkes I, et al. Paravertebral blockade for minor breast surgery. *Anesth Analg.* 2002;94:355–359.
26. Williams B, Kentor M, Vogt M, et al. Economics of nerve block pain management after anterior cruciate ligament reconstruction. *Anesthesiology.* 2004;100:697–706.
27. Mulroy M. Advances in regional anesthesia for outpatients. *Curr Opin Anaesthesiol.* 2002;15:641–645.
28. Khoury G, Chen A, Garland D, et al. Intraarticular morphine, bupivacaine, and morphine/bupivacaine for pain control after knee videoarthroscopy. *Anesthesiology.* 1992;77:263–266.
29. Goodwin R, Amjadi F, Parker R. Short-term analgesic effects of intra-articular injections after knee arthroscopy. *Arthroscopy.* 2005;21:307–312.
30. Orkin F. What do patients want? Preferences for immediate postoperative recovery. *Anesth Analg.* 1992;74:S225.
31. Gan TJ, Sloan F, Dear G, et al. How much are patients willing to pay to avoid postoperative nausea and vomiting? *Anesth Analg.* 2001;92:393–400.
32. Gold BS, Kitz DS, Lecky JH, et al. Unanticipated admission to the hospital following ambulatory surgery. *JAMA.* 1989;262:3008–3010.
33. Gan TJ. Risk factors for postoperative nausea and vomiting. *Anesth Analg.* 2006; 102:1884–1898.
34. American Society of PeriAnesthesia Nurses PONV/PDNV Strategic Work Team. ASPAN'S Evidence-Based Clinical Practice Guideline for the Prevention and/or Management of PONV/PDNV. *J Perianesth Nurs.* 2006;21:230–250. Available at: http://www.aspan.org/ponv_pdnv_guidelines.htm. Accessed July 13, 2007.
35. Apfel C, Laara E, Koivuranta M, et al. A simplified risk score for predicting postoperative nausea and vomiting. *Anesthesiology.* 1999;91:693–700.
36. Koivuranta M, Laara E, Snare L, et al. A survey of postoperative nausea and vomiting. *Anaesthesia.* 1997;52:443–449.
37. Gan T, Meyer T, Apfel C, et al. Society for ambulatory anesthesia guidelines for the Management of postoperative nausea and vomiting. *Anesth Analg.* 2007;105: 1615–28.
38. White P, Watcha M. Postoperative nausea and vomiting: prophylaxis versus treatment. *Anesth Analg.* 1999;89:1337–1339.
39. Apfel C, Korttila K, Abdalla M, et al. A factorial trial of six interventions for the prevention of postoperative nausea and vomiting. *N Engl J Med.* 2004;350:2441–2451.
40. Wang J, Ho S, Tzeng J, et al. The effect of timing of dexamethasone administration on its efficacy as a prophylactic antiemetic for postoperative nausea and vomiting. *Anesth Analg.* 2000;91:136–139.
41. White P, Issioui T, Hu J, et al. Comparative efficacy of acustimulation versus ondansetron in combination with droperidol for preventing nausea and vomiting. *Anesthesiology.* 2002;97:1075–1081.
42. Kotani N, Hashimoto H, Sato Y, et al. Preoperative intradermal acupuncture reduces postoperative pain, nausea and vomiting, analgesic requirement and sympathoadrenal responses. *Anesthesiology.* 2001;95:349–356.

43. Greif R, Laciny S, Rapf B, et al. Supplemental oxygen reduces the incidence of post-operative nausea and vomiting. *Anesthesiology*. 1999;91:1246–1252.

44. Purhonen S, Turunen M, Ruohoaho U, et al. Supplemental oxygen does not reduce the incidence of postoperative nausea and vomiting after ambulatory gynecologic surgery. *Anesth Analg*. 2003;96:91–96.

45. Gan T, El-Molem H, Ray J, et al. Patient-controlled antiemesis: a randomized, double-blind comparison of two doses of propofol versus placebo. *Anesthesiology*. 1999: 90;1564–1570.

46. Gupta A, Wu CL, Elkassabany N, et al. Does the routine prophylactic use of antiemetics affect the incidence of postdischarge nausea and vomiting following ambulatory surgery? A systematic review of randomized controlled trials. *Anesthesiology*. 2003;99:488–495.

47. Dimich I, Lingham R, Gabrielson G, et al. Comparative hemodynamic effects of labetalol and hydralazine in the treatment of postoperative hypertension. *J Clin Anesth*. 1989;1:201–206.

48. Kallar SK, Jones GW. Postoperative complications. In: White PF, ed. *Outpatient Anesthesia*. New York, NY: Churchill Livingstone; 1990:397–415.

49. Warner MA, Warner ME, Weber JG. Clinical significance of pulmonary aspiration during the perioperative period. *Anesthesiology*. 1993;78:56–62.

50. Isaacson KB. Complications of hysteroscopy. *Obstet Gynecol Clin North Am*. 1999; 26:39–51.

51. Slotman GJ, Jed EH, Burchard KW. Adverse effects of hypothermia in postoperative patients. *Am J Surg*. 1985;149:495–501.

52. Macintyre PE, Pavlin EG, Dwersteg JF. Effect of meperidine on oxygen consumption, carbon dioxide production, and respiratory gas exchange in postanesthesia shivering. *Anesth Analg*. 1987;66:751–755.

53. Yentis SM, Levine MF, Hartley EJ. Should all children with suspected or confirmed malignant hyperthermia susceptibility be admitted after surgery? A 10-year review. *Anesth Analg*. 1992;75:345–350.

54. Strazis KP, Fox AW. Malignant hyperthermia: a review of published cases. *Anesth Analg*. 1993;77:297–304.

55. Philip BK. Patients' assessment of ambulatory anesthesia and surgery. *J Clin Anesth*. 1992;4:355–358.

56. Ashworth J, Smith I. Comparison of desflurane with isoflurane or propofol in spontaneously breathing ambulatory patients. *Anesth Analg*. 1998;87:312–318.

57. Chung F, Mezei G. Factors contributing to a prolonged stay after ambulatory surgery. *Anesth Analg*. 1999;89:1352–1359.

13. Discharge process

Frances Chung, MD, FRCPC
Jeremy Lermitte, BM, FRCA

Ambulatory surgery is continually evolving, with more complex procedures being performed on patients with increasing comorbidities. Recently, more emphasis has been placed on patient recovery and discharge to ensure patient safety and an efficient running of the service.

This chapter will examine the various criteria used to pass through the discharge process, review the fast-track concept, and provide an overview on the factors that delay discharge. We will also review some discharge controversies, including whether oral intake or voiding is required prior to discharge, driving postanesthesia, and the need for escorts. Lastly, the various tests to assess recovery and satisfaction will be examined.

Definition of recovery

Recovery is an ongoing process that begins when the intraoperative period has ended and continues until the patient returns to their preoperative physiological state.[1] This process is divided into three phases:

- Early recovery (phase 1) occurs from the discontinuation of anesthetic agents until the recovery of the protective reflexes and motor function.
- Intermediate recovery (phase 2) is the period during which the criteria for discharge from the ambulatory surgical unit (ASU) are obtained.
- Late recovery (phase 3) lasts for several days and continues until the patient is back to their preoperative functional status and is able to resume their daily activities.

Discharge from the postanesthesia care unit

Phase 1 recovery occurs in the postanesthesia care unit (PACU). Various criteria have been devised to safely discharge patients from the PACU to the step-down unit or ASU. The Aldrete scoring system assesses motor function, respiration, circulation, consciousness, and color, grading each 0, 1, or 2.[2] Pulse oximetry has replaced the color assessment component that was considered subjective (Table 13-1).[3] With this scoring system, each patient requires a score of more than or equal to 9 to be discharged from the PACU.

Table 13-1. The modified Aldrete scoring system for determining when patients are ready for discharge from the postanesthesia care unit

Discharge criteria from PACU	Score
Activity: Able to move voluntarily or on command	
Four extremities	2
Two extremities	1
Zero extremities	0
Respiration	
Able to deep breathe and cough freely	2
Dyspnea, shallow or limited breathing	1
Apneic	0
Circulation	
Blood pressure ±20% of preanesthetic level	2
Blood pressure ±20%–49% of preanesthetic level	1
Blood pressure ±50% of preanesthetic level	0

(Continued)

Table 13-1. *Continued*

Discharge criteria from PACU	Score
Consciousness	
Fully awake	2
Arousable on calling	1
Not responding	0
O_2 saturation	
Able to maintain O_2 saturation >92% on room air	2
Needs O_2 inhalation to maintain O_2 saturation >90%	1
O_2 saturation <90% even with O_2 supplementation	0

A score of greater than or equal to 9 was required for discharge. Reprinted from Aldrete JA[3] © 1995 with permission from Elsevier.

Fast-tracking

Fast-tracking is a clinical pathway that involves transferring the patient from the operating room to ASU directly without entering the PACU. Historically, achieving an Aldrete score of 9 or 10 in the operating room has been used to bypass the PACU. However, the Aldrete scoring system does not address pain, nausea, and vomiting, which are common side effects in the PACU. White and Song[4] have devised a scoring system that includes pain and emetic symptoms within the Aldrete scoring system (Table 13-2). Under the new fast-tracking scoring system, a score of 12 with no score less than 1 in any category provides criteria for bypassing the PACU.

The fast-track concept has been devised to set a higher standard for patient care and to reduce nursing workload and cost. Nursing and personnel costs account for the majority of PACU expenditure as opposed to only 2% related to medication and supplies.[5] In a large multicenter study by Apfelbaum et al.,[6] the recovery times of patients who were fast-tracked were significantly shorter compared to patients who were not fast-tracked (85 ± 62 versus 175 ± 99 minutes, $P < 0.001$, with no change in patient outcome).

Patients who have had regional anesthesia are less likely to have adverse events, including pain and nausea, but are more likely to have a degree of immobility. In view of these differences, Williams et al.[7] devised the RAPBC (regional anesthesia PACU bypass criteria) (Table 13-3). By means of these criteria, patients were discharged home earlier and had a lower incidence of unplanned hospital admissions. However, they needed more nursing intervention in ASU when compared with patients who did not bypass the PACU.[8]

A recent prospective study randomly assigned 207 patients undergoing standardized general anesthesia (GA) into two groups: fast-track and PACU.[9] The fast-track criteria were met by 97% undergoing arthroscopy surgery but by only 72% undergoing gynecological laparoscopy. In this study, the time to discharge was shorter in the fast-track group. However, the total numbers of nursing

Table 13-2. White and Song[4] scoring system to determine whether outpatients can be transferred directly from the operating room to the step-down (phase 2) unit

Parameters	Score
Level of consciousness	
Awake and oriented	2
Arousable with minimal stimulation	1
Responsive only to tactile stimulation	0
Physical activity	
Able to move all extremities on command	2
Some weakness in movement of extremities	1
Unable to voluntarily move extremities	0
Hemodynamic stability	
Blood pressure <15% of baseline MAP value	2
Blood pressure 15%–30% of baseline MAP value	1
Blood pressure >30% below baseline MAP value	0
Respiratory stability	
Able to breathe deeply	2
Tachypnea with good cough	1
Dyspneic with weak cough	0
Oxygen saturation status	
Maintains value >90% on room air	2
Requires supplemental oxygen (nasal prongs)	1
Saturation <90% with supplemental oxygen	0
Postoperative pain assessment	
None or mild discomfort	2
Moderate to severe pain controlled with intravenous analgesics	1
Persistent severe pain	0
Postoperative emetic symptoms	
None or mild nausea with no active vomiting	2
Transient vomiting or retching	1
Persistent moderate-to-severe nausea and vomiting	0
Total possible score	14

A minimal score of 12 (with no score below 1 in any individual category) would be required for a patient to be fast-tracked (i.e., bypass the postanesthesia care unit) after general anesthesia. MAP, mean arterial pressure. Source: White and Song.[4] Used with permission from Lippincott Williams & Wilkins.

interventions and nursing hours were not different between the two recovery groups.

The early phase of recovery represents only a tiny proportion of the overall nursing input. Therefore, it is not surprising that no cost savings were made using the fast-track approach. From the above studies, fast-tracking patients might not be justified on the basis of cost saving only, as there may be no improvement in outcome and cost savings.[10]

Table 13-3. Postanesthesia care unit (PACU) bypass score following regional anesthesia from the University of Pittsburgh Medical Center-Montefiore Surgicenter

Parameters	Score
Movement	
Purposeful movement of (at least) one lower and one upper extremity	2
Purposeful movement of at least one upper extremity but neither lower extremity	1
No purposeful movement	0
Blood pressure	
Within 20% of baseline, without orthostatic changes	2
Between 20% and 40% of baseline, without orthostatic changes	1
Less than 40% of baseline, or orthostatic changes	0
Level of consciousness	
Awake, follows commands	2
Arousable, follows commands	1
Obtunded or persistently somnolent	0
Respiratory efforts	
Able to cough involuntary on command	2
Only able to cough involuntary but not on command	1
Dyspnea or apnea	0
Pulse oximeter score	
$SpO_2 \geq 95\%$ on room air	2
$SpO_2 \geq 95\%$ with face mask or nasal cannula	1
$SpO_2 < 95\%$	0
Total possible score	10

The minimum score to qualify for PACU bypass is 8. Patients considered for PACU bypass should not require interventions for pain, postoperative nausea and vomiting, or shivering. SpO_2, oxygen saturation as measured by pulse oximetry. Source: Williams et al.[7] Used with permission from Lippincott Williams & Wilkins.

Discharge criteria from the ambulatory surgical unit

Discharge of patients home from ASU requires strict adherence to validated criteria to ensure patient safety and to prevent unnecessary litigation. This is ultimately a physician responsibility (American Society of Anesthesiologists [ASA] Guidelines for Ambulatory Anesthesia and Surgery, 2003) but may be delegated to qualified nurses in the ASU unit who adhere to written protocols for patient discharge.

Criteria for the safe discharge home following ambulatory surgery have been developed by both Kortilla,[11] an outcome-based system, and Chung et al.,[12] the postanesthesia discharge score (PADS) system. The latter has been subsequently

Table 13-4. Revised postanesthesia discharge scoring system (PADS) for determining home readiness

Parameters	Score
Vital signs	
Within 20% of preoperative baseline	2
20%–40% of preoperative baseline	1
40% of preoperative baseline	0
Activity level	
Steady gait, no dizziness, consistent with preoperative level	2
Requires assistance	1
Unable to ambulate/assess	0
Nausea and vomiting	
Minimal: mild, no treatment needed	2
Moderate: treatment effective	1
Severe: treatment not effective	0
Pain	
VAS = 0–3 the patient has minimal or no pain prior to discharge	2
VAS = 4–6 the patient has moderate pain	1
VAS = 7–10 the patient has severe pain	0
Surgical bleeding	
Minimal: does not require dressing change	2
Moderate: required up to two dressing changes with no further bleeding	1
Severe: required three or more dressing changes and continues bleeding	0

Maximum score is 10. Patients scoring greater than or equal to 9 are fit for discharge. VAS, visual analog scale. Source: Awad and Chung.[14] Used with permission from the *Canadian Journal of Anesthesia.*

modified to eliminate the fluid intake and output parameters, permitting discharge of an additional 20% of patients.[13] The PADS measures patients' home-readiness by using five major criteria: vital signs, activity level, pain, postoperative nausea and vomiting (PONV), and surgical bleeding.

The pain criterion has been further refined and scores pain with a visual analog scale of 1–10 (Table 13-4). Patients who achieve a score of 9 or greater and who have an adult escort are considered fit for discharge. The PADS permits evaluation of all patients who have had various surgical procedures and anesthesia. Also, this system permits the early discharge of patients by not keeping them longer than necessary.[14]

Patients are often discharged in 1–2 hours or less following ambulatory surgery. It has been adopted in many ambulatory facilities. Also, many ambulatory surgery facilities use outcome-based criteria for discharge instead of numerical scoring like the PADS. All the parameters of an outcome-based system need to be met prior to discharge and typically include the following:

- Alert and orientated to time and place
- Stable vital signs
- Pain controlled by oral analgesics
- Nausea or emesis controlled
- Able to walk without dizziness
- Regional anesthesia: block appropriately resolved
- No unexpected bleeding from the operative site
- Given discharge instructions (from surgeon and anesthesiologist) and prescriptions
- Patient accepts readiness for discharge
- Adult present to accompany patient home

Psychomotor tests of recovery

Psychomotor tests of recovery include paper-and-pencil tests and nonpaper tests. The use of these tests is frequently adapted from other settings for evaluating the recovery period. The Trieger dot test is an example of a paper-and-pencil test. The nonpaper tests include the Maddox wing (a device to test extraocular muscle balance), driving simulators, reaction time tests, pegboard tests, the flicker fusion threshold (which measures the frequency at which the patient perceives a flashing light to be continuous), perceptual speed tests, and the digit symbol substitution test.

The multiple sleep latency test measuring sleepiness and assessment of patients' balance by standing them on a dual-force plate has been suggested.[15] Many of these tests are complex and impractical in the clinical setting, and none has been specifically validated by follow-up studies providing adequate criteria to guide discharge in the ambulatory setting.

Discharge controversies

Is oral fluid intake necessary before discharge?

Schreiner et al.[16] demonstrated that children mandated to drink prior to leaving the ASU experienced a higher incidence of vomiting and a prolonged hospital stay. In addition, Kearney et al.[17] showed that children having oral fluids withheld for 4 to 6 hours postoperatively had a lower incidence of vomiting.

The greatest effect of withholding oral fluids was seen in patients receiving opioids; vomiting was reduced from 73% to 36%. However, for adults, drinking did not influence the incidence of PONV or duration of hospital stay.[18] Drinking oral fluids is not a requirement prior to discharge from the ASU and this has now been incorporated into the practice guidelines produced by the ASA.[19]

Taking oral intake is necessary only for selected patients on a case-by-case basis.

Is voiding necessary before discharge?

Both general and spinal anesthesia affect the detrusor muscle function. However, the main risk factors for postoperative urinary retention are anorectal surgery, old age, male gender, spinal anesthesia, and hernia surgery.[20] Distension beyond the volume associated with voluntary emptying causes bladder atony, impaired voiding after return of function, and subsequently retention of urine.

In current practice, voiding is not a requirement before discharge from the ASU, as it could delay the discharge of 5%–11% of patients who have no risk factors of urinary retention after ambulatory surgery.[21] The incidence of urinary retention in low-risk patients is less than 1% using inability to void at a bladder volume of 600 ml as criteria for defining urinary retention.[22] Low-risk patients can be discharged but should be given written instructions to seek medical help if they are unable to void within 6 to 8 hours of discharge.

In high-risk patients, ultrasound monitoring of bladder volume is better than clinical judgment for determining the need for catheterization.[23] However, the routine use of ultrasound may not be practical for man-power and logistical reasons. Using short-acting spinal anesthetics in low-risk procedures is associated with minimal risk of retention, and patients can be discharged home without the need to void prior to discharge.[24]

Is an escort needed following ambulatory surgery?

The ASA recommends having an adult escort to accompany patients home after ambulatory surgical procedures.[25] Various studies have shown that there is a significant psychomotor and cognitive impairment after anesthesia and therefore a responsible adult escort is required to accompany patients undergoing ambulatory surgery home.[26–28] A prospective case-controlled study conducted over the span of 38 months demonstrated an incidence of 0.2% (60/28,391) of patients without an escort.[29]

In this study, two groups of patients without an escort were identified: patients known not to have an escort preoperatively ($n = 24$) and patients whose escort did not show ($n = 36$). A separate question is the need for a companion for the first postoperative night. Even if patients have an escort, it does not guarantee that they have someone to stay with them overnight. In one telephone survey, 4% of patients had no one to stay with them overnight following ambulatory surgery.[30] In the same study, 4.1% of patients drove and a further 2% consumed alcohol in the first 24 hours after surgery.

When can you drive following ambulatory surgery?

Historically, general anesthetic agents have been shown to impair psychomotor function and skills related to driving for up to 8 hours postoperatively.[31,32] Newer short-acting agents commonly used in ambulatory surgery provide a faster recovery and an earlier return to normal daily activity. In volunteers, general anesthetic agents have been shown to permit prompt return of driving skills at 2, 3, and 4 hours postanesthesia when compared to controls.[33]

However, healthy volunteers (unlike patients) do not experience perioperative anxiety, sleep deprivation, and postoperative pain. Furthermore, patients (unlike volunteers) may receive sedative medication, analgesics, and antiemetics. Recently, a prospective study involving ambulatory surgery demonstrated that patients have lower alertness levels and impaired driving skills preoperatively and 2 hours postoperatively.[34] These parameters returned to normal at 24 hours. Therefore, it is safe for patients to drive 24 hours after a general anesthetic.

However, even after the effects of an anesthetic have abated, certain types of surgery may impair the ability to drive.[35] Also, there is evidence that cognitive impairment may persist 3 days after ambulatory surgery when assessed using a questionnaire specifically designed to assess cognitive function.[36] The authors suggest that some patients are able to perform satisfactorily for short periods of objective psychometric or cognitive testing despite residual cognitive impairment. A study demonstrated that 3.5% of elderly patients have cognitive impairment 1 week after minor surgery.[37]

Discharge following regional anesthesia

Patients having regional anesthesia for upper-limb surgery can achieve PACU bypass criteria more quickly, have reduced rates of pain and nausea, are discharged home faster, and have a lower incidence of unplanned hospital admission when compared with GA.[38,39] Even when combined with GA, a suprascapular block can improve recovery profiles and facilitate early discharge after arthroscopic shoulder surgery.[40]

A recent meta-analysis has compared the recovery profiles of regional anesthesia and GA.[41] In this study, peripheral nerve blocks improved the ability to bypass the PACU and reduced the incidence of nausea, unlike central neuraxial blocks. Pain scores and analgesic requirements were reduced by both techniques of regional anesthesia. However, the ASU discharge time was not reduced relative to GA.

Spinal anesthesia is a simple and reliable technique that has been widely used for ambulatory anesthesia, and its use is more extensively discussed in Chapter 8. Currently, the use of lidocaine has declined because of the neurotoxic effects of the 5% hyperbaric solution, with numerous reports of transient neurological symptoms after its use in spinal anesthesia.

Other alternatives include combining a smaller dose of lidocaine with an opiate, using procaine 5%, or using a low-dose regime of bupivacaine.[42] One factor limiting the popularity of outpatient spinal anesthesia among anesthesiologists is the incidence of postdural puncture headaches (PDPHs). However, 25-gauge pencil-point needles produce an incidence of PDPHs of less than 1%, and the headaches that do occur are mild and self-limiting. In a prospective study involving 676 patients assigned to 27G whitacre or 27G Quincke, the incidences of PDPH were 0.37% and 1.51%, respectively.[43]

Factors delaying discharge

The unanticipated postoperative admission rate from the ASU is an important outcome measurement; in most centers, it averages 1%–2%. In practice, the most common causes for admission in adults and children are surgical factors, such as pain, bleeding, and extensive surgery.[44,45]

Extended recovery facilities

To allow the expansion of ambulatory surgery, many logistical changes have occurred in addition to advances in anesthesia and surgery. By having a 23-hour discharge policy, some institutions have undertaken more complicated surgery in the ambulatory setting. This has reduced cancellation rates for surgery and achieved cost savings. An alternative way to obtain these benefits is the hotel bed.

This accommodation is provided in or near the hospital and is staffed by non-nursing personnel. Patients who have no telephone or escort or who live a great distance from the hospital can be operated on with increased safety. Also, this kind of facility encourages surgeons to do more procedures in the ambulatory setting. It is, however, debatable whether this is indeed ambulatory/1-day surgery in the classic definition.

Assessment of recovery following discharge

Recovery following ambulatory surgery can be measured using numerous outcome measures. However, many of the clinically orientated outcomes, including mortality and morbidity, are exceedingly rare. Postoperative minor symptoms, including nausea and vomiting, are more frequent and can be easily quantified. Recent evidence demonstrates that, even on day 7 postdischarge, 24% of patients experienced symptoms.[46]

The commonest symptom in adults was pain, and in the pediatric population it was drowsiness. However, a great deal of anesthetic research has already focused on the area of postoperative symptoms. Also, despite having no adverse events, a large proportion of patients will subjectively feel that their ability to perform normal activities is impaired for a significant period of time following ambulatory surgery. Focusing on patient-related, rather than traditional, outcomes will allow assessment and improvements to patient satisfaction, quality of life, and quality of recovery outcomes. Future research should examine the quality of recovery rather than just measure physiological endpoints or the incidence of minor adverse events.

Psychometric questionnaires have been used to assess the quality of recovery.[47] Unfortunately, there is no gold standard to assess these tools against. Because recovery is subjective, it should be measured from the patient's perspective. To achieve this, patients should be involved in the questionnaire-generation process and the items generated grouped into dimensions of care. The tool should then be piloted to allow refinement.

How do we determine whether the questionnaire is good? First, it should have a high validity, which is a measure of the appropriateness of the test. Second, it should demonstrate high reliability referring to the reproducibility of the results. Third, the questionnaire must be responsive to be able to detect changes over time. Last, to be useful in clinical practice, it must be interpretable. The questionnaire used by Myles et al.[47] has been well developed and has good validity and reliability. Researchers need to explore how clinical outcomes influence psychometric questionnaire outcomes to improve interpretability.

Postoperative instructions

The success and safety of an ambulatory surgery program depend on patients' understanding and compliance. A lot of responsibility has been placed on patients to adhere to the information and instruction given to them before their surgery. Patients often forget verbal instructions or ignore them.[48] Instructional video presentations shown to patients preoperatively have not been demonstrated to improve patients' knowledge about the perioperative period.[49]

Most institutions provide written instructions to improve patient compliance. However, a recent study suggests that failure to adhere to written instructions could be related to low health literacy and increasing age.[50] Despite these limitations, written postoperative instructions improve patient satisfaction, can give links to further sources of quality information, and provide advice, including emergency telephone numbers for problem-solving.

Patient satisfaction

Patient satisfaction can be defined as "a healthcare recipient's reaction to their care, a reaction that is composed of both cognitive evaluation and an emotional response." The theory behind the process of arriving at a satisfaction level can be divided into three stages:[51]
- First, the patient must have a standard or expectation level regarding their potential care. The expectation may vary depending upon patient background, education, past experience, and their ideals.
- Second, the patient receives a level of care.

- Third, the patient makes a judgment to determine the difference between the expected care and the actual care. Therefore, the level of care provided is only one factor determining a particular satisfaction level. Also, we do not know how a patient determines their expectation level or judges the discrepancy between expected care and actual care.

Because satisfaction is multidimensional, it is difficult to measure. A satisfaction questionnaire must evaluate a number of components of care to be effective. The Patient Satisfaction Questionnaire examines eight dimensions of ambulatory care.[52] An alternative, the Patient Judgments of Hospital Quality Questionnaire, is divided into hospital services or phases of hospital care.[53] In addition, multi-item scales should be used to allow greater discrimination between differing levels of satisfaction. This can be achieved by using a well-constructed psychometric questionnaire. The questionnaire will be more relevant if it has been generated using patients and pilot-tested allowing refinement.

Patients differentiate poorly between the technical and interpersonal dimensions of care. Also, they are often reticent to criticize health care providers and put disproportionate weight on positive impressions unless directly questioned about specific problems.

Many surveys using single-item scales demonstrate high levels of satisfaction but do not show that changes in care alter patient satisfaction levels.[54] This reinforces the need for questionnaires with multi-item scales that are broad, encompassing many aspects of care. For a number of reasons, the nature of anesthesia supports the use of psychometric questionnaires to assess patient satisfaction:

- Many patients are naïve about the role of an anesthesiologist and their qualifications.
- Many surveys to date are biased toward the anesthesiologists who constructed them.
- With poorly constructed surveys, the effect of anesthetic care may be indistinguishable from perioperative care in general. Psychometric tests of good construction include the Iowa Satisfaction with Anesthesia Scale[55] for monitored anesthesia care and the scale of Whitty et al.[56] for patients undergoing ophthalmologic and maxillofacial surgery under GA.

Numerous factors influence the results of a satisfaction survey, including the manner of sampling, patient characteristics, preoperative expectations, the case mix of the institution, the characteristics of nonrespondents, and timing of questionnaire administration. These factors must be considered if the results are to be extrapolated to other settings.

Postoperative follow-up

Follow-up of patients is an important part of ambulatory surgery. This process can increase patient satisfaction, give advice to patients, allow audit to improve practice, and can set new standards through research. The Toronto Western Hospital achieves many of these aims with the aid of a postoperative telephone questionnaire (Table 13-5).

Table 13-5. Ambulatory surgery postoperative telephone interview

Patient details:

Surgeon:

Date of surgery:

Procedure:

Do you wish to be called?
(Yes/No)

Timing of telephone call:

How have you been since your surgery?

Have you experienced any pain in the last 24 hours?
(Yes/No)

Average pain score during last 24 hours
(scale 0–10)

Did you feel prepared to manage your pain at home?
(Yes/No)

How clear were your instructions regarding your analgesic schedule?
(None/Unclear or forgot/Somewhat unclear/Absolutely clear)

How clear were your instructions to alter your analgesic medication schedule?
(None given/Unclear or forgot/Somewhat unclear/Absolutely clear)

Symptom history?
(Nausea and vomiting/Bleeding/Sore throat/Voiding/Bowels/No voiced problems)

Follow-up telephone advice:

Medical help?
(Phone call/Unplanned M.D. office visit/Emergency room visit/Hospital admission)

Did you receive enough information to take care of yourself after surgery?
(Yes/No)

Did you find the instruction sheet you received in the day surgery unit helpful?
(Yes/No)

Did the day surgery staff listen to and answer your questions?
(Yes/No)

How would you rate the care you received in the day surgery unit?
(Excellent/Good/Fair/Poor)

Do you have suggestions on how we could improve your care?

Date completed:

Person conducting interview:

Adapted from Toronto Western Hospital telephone interview record.

Summary

Ambulatory surgery will continue to grow and expand in the future. It is our responsibility to use validated criteria or discharge scoring systems to discharge patients safely home. Regional anesthesia for limb surgery is growing in popularity and plays a significant role in eliminating postoperative symptoms that can delay discharge.

Fast-tracking needs further evaluation to optimize cost and time saving without compromising patient care. Future research needs to be undertaken to assess recovery from the patient's perspective. Psychometric questionnaires need to be well constructed to assess patient satisfaction and recovery. Evaluating the effect of clinical outcomes upon these tools will make them increasingly practical and interpretable.

References

1. Marshall SI, Chung F. Discharge criteria and complications after ambulatory surgery. *Anesth Analg.* 1999;88:508–517.
2. Aldrete JA, Kroulik DA. Postanesthetic recovery score. *Anesth Analg.* 1970;49: 924–934.
3. Aldrete JA. The post anesthesia recovery score revisited [letter]. *J Clin Anesth.* 1995;7:89–91.
4. White PF, Song D. New criteria for fast-tracking after outpatient anesthesia: a comparison with the modified Aldrete's scoring system. *Anesth Analg.* 1999;88: 1069–1072.
5. Dexter F, Tinker J. Analysis of strategies to decrease postanesthesia care unit costs. *Anesthesiology.* 1995;82:94–101.
6. Apfelbaum JL, Walawander CA, Grasela TH, et al. Eliminating intensive postoperative care in same-day surgery patients using short-acting anesthetics. *Anesthesiology.* 2002;97:66–74.
7. Williams BA, Kentor ML, Williams JP, et al. Process analysis in outpatient knee surgery: Effects of regional and general anesthesia on anesthesia-controlled time. *Anesthesiology.* 2000;93:529–538.
8. Williams BA, Kentor ML, Williams JP, et al. PACU bypass after outpatient knee surgery is associated with fewer unplanned hospital admissions but more phase II nursing interventions. *Anesthesiology.* 2002;97:981–988.
9. Song D, Chung F, Ronayne M, et al. Fast-tracking (bypassing the PACU) does not reduce nursing workload after ambulatory surgery. *Br J Anaesth.* 2004;93: 968–974.
10. Millar J. Fast-tracking in day surgery. Is your journey to the recovery room really necessary? *Br J Anaesth.* 2004;93:756–758.
11. Kortilla KT. Post-anaesthesia psychomotor and cognitive function. *Eur J Anaesthesiol Suppl.* 1995;12:43–46.

12. Chung F, Chan V, Ong D. A post-anesthetic discharge scoring system for home-readiness after ambulatory surgery. *J Clin Anesth*. 1995;7:500–506.

13. Chung F. Discharge criteria–a new trend. *Can J Anaesth*. 1995;42:1056–1058.

14. Awad IT, Chung F. Factors affecting recovery and discharge following ambulatory surgery. *Can J Anesth*. 2006;53:858–872.

15. Lichtor JL, Alessi R, Lane BS. Sleep tendency as a measure of recovery after drugs used for ambulatory surgery. *Anesthesiology*. 2002;96:878–883.

16. Schreiner MS, Nicholson SC, Martin T, et al. Should children drink before discharge from day surgery? *Anesthesiology*. 1992;76:528–533.

17. Kearney R, Mack C, Entwistle L. Withholding oral fluids from children undergoing day surgery reduces vomiting. *Paediatr Anaesth*. 1998;8:331–336.

18. Jin FL, Norris A, Chung F. Should adult patients drink fluids before discharge from ambulatory surgery? *Can J Anaesth*. 1998;87:306–311.

19. Practice Guidelines for Postanesthetic Care. A report by the American Society of Anesthesiologists Task Force on Postanesthetic Care. *Anesthesiology*. 2002;96:742–752.

20. Lau H, Lam B. Management of postoperative urinary retention: a randomized trial of in-out versus overnight catheterization. *ANZ J Surg*. 2004;74:658–661.

21. Pavlin DJ, Rapp SE, Polissar NL, et al. Factors affecting discharge time in adult outpatients. *Anesth Analg*. 1998;87:816–826.

22. Pavlin DJ, Pavlin EG, Gunn HC, et al. Voiding in patients managed with or without ultrasound monitoring of bladder volume after outpatient surgery. *Anesth Analg*. 1999;89:90–97.

23. Rosseland LA, Stubhaug A, Breivik H. Detecting postoperative urinary retention with an ultrasound scanner. *Acta Anaesthesiol Scand*. 2002;46:279–282.

24. Mulroy MF, Salinas FV, Larkin KL, et al. Ambulatory surgery patients may be discharged before voiding after short-acting spinal and epidural anesthesia. *Anesthesiology*. 2002;97:315–319.

25. ASA Guidelines for Ambulatory Anesthesia and Surgery, last affirmed Oct. 25, 2003. Available at: http://www.asahq.org/publicationsAndServices/standards/04.pdf. Accessed July 9, 2007.

26. Apfelbaum JL, Lichtor JL, Lane BS, et al. Awakening, clinical recovery and psychomotor effects after desflurane and propofol anesthesia. *Anesth Analg*. 1996;83:721–725.

27. Grant SA, Murdoch J, Millar K, et al. Blood propofol concentration and psychomotor effects on driving skills. *Br J Anaesth*. 2000;85:396–400.

28. Sinclair D, Chung F, Smiley A. Recovery and simulated driving after ambulatory anesthesia. *Can J Anesth*. 2003;50:238–245.

29. Chung F, Imasogie N, Prahbu A, et al. A follow up of ambulatory surgical patients with no escorts. *Can J Anesth*. 2005;52:1022–1026.

30. Correa R, Menzes RB, Wong J, et al. Compliance with postoperative instructions: a telephone survey of 750 day surgery patients. *Anaesthesia*. 2001;56:481–484.

31. Korttila K, Tammisito T, Ertama P, et al. Recovery, psychomotor skills, and simulated driving after brief inhalational anesthesia with halothane, or enflurane combined with nitrous oxide and oxygen. *Anesthesiology*. 1977;46:20–27.

32. Korttila K, Linnoila M, Ertama P, et al. Recovery and simulated driving after intravenous anesthesia with thiopental, methohexital, propanidid, or alphadione. *Anesthesiology*. 1975;43:291–299.

33. Sinclair DR, Chung F, Smiley A. General anesthesia does not impair simulator driving skills in volunteers in the immediate recovery period—a pilot study. *Can J Anaesth*. 2003;50:238–245.

34. Chung F, Kayumov L, Sinclair DR, et al. What is the driving performance of ambulatory surgical patients after general anesthesia? *Anesthesiology*. 2005;103:951–956.

35. Amid PK. Driving after repair of groin hernia. *BMJ*. 2000;321:1033–1034.

36. Tzabar Y, Asbury AJ, Millar K. Cognitive failures after general anaesthesia for day-case surgery. *Br J Anaesth*. 1996;76:194–197.

37. Canet J, Raeder J, Rasmussen LS, et al. Cognitive dysfunction after minor surgery in the elderly. *Acta Anaesth Sand*. 2003;47:1204–1210.

38. Hadzic A, Arliss J, Kerimoglu B, et al. A comparison of infraclavicular nerve block versus general anesthesia for hand and wrist day-case surgeries. *Anesthesiology*. 2004;101:127–132.

39. Hadzic A, Karaca PE, Hobeika P, et al. Peripheral nerve blocks result in superior recovery profile compared with general anesthesia in outpatient knee arthroscopy. *Anesth Analg*. 2005;100:976–981.

40. Ritchie ED, Tong D, Chung F, et al. Suprascapular nerve block for pain relief after arthroscopic shoulder surgery: is it effective? *Anesth Analg*. 1997;84:1306–1312.

41. Liu SS, Strodtbeck WM, Richman JM, et al. A comparison of regional versus general anesthesia for ambulatory anesthesia: a meta-analysis of randomized controlled trials. *Anesth Analg*. 2005;101:1634–1642.

42. Ben-David B, Levin H, Solomon E, et al. Spinal bupivacaine in ambulatory surgery: the effect of saline dilution. *Anesth Analg*. 1996;83:716–720.

43. Santanen U, Rautoma P, Luurila H, et al. Comparison of 27-gauge (0.41-mm) Whitacre and Quincke spinal needles with respect to post-dural puncture headache and nondural puncture headache. *Acta Anaesthesiol Scand*. 2004;48:474–479.

44. Gold BS, Kitz DS, Lecky JH, et al. Unanticipated admission to the hospital following ambulatory surgery. *JAMA*. 1989;262:3008–3010.

45. Fortier J, Chung F, Su J. Unanticipated admission after ambulatory surgery–a prospective study. *Can J Anaesth*. 1998;45:612–619.

46. Mattila K, Toivonen J, Janhunen L, et al. Postdischarge symptoms after ambulatory surgery: first week incidence, intensity, and risk factors. *Anesth Analg*. 2005;101:1643–1650.

47. Myles PS, Weitkamp B, Jones K, et al. Validity and reliability of a postoperative quality of recovery score: the QoR-40. *Br J Anaesth*. 2000;84:11–15.

48. Laffey JG, Carroll M, Donnelly N, et al. Instructions for ambulatory surgery–patient comprehension and compliance. *Ir J Med Sci*. 1998;167:160–163.

49. Zvara DA, Mathes DD, Brooker RF, et al. Video as a patient teaching tool: does it add to the preoperative anesthetic visit? *Anesth Analg*. 1996;82:1065–1068.

50. Chew LD, Bradley KA, Flum DR, et al. The impact of low health literacy on surgical practice. *Am J Surg*. 2004;188:250–253.

51. Fung D, Cohen MM. Measuring patient satisfaction with anesthesia care: a review of current methodology. *Anesth Analg*. 1998;87:1089–1098.
52. Ware JEJ, Snyder MK, Wright WR. Defining and measuring patient satisfaction with medical care. *Eval Program Plan*. 1983;6:247–263.
53. Meterko M, Rubin H, Ware JE Jr. Patient judgements of hospital quality questionnaire. *Med Care*. 1990;9(suppl):S1–44. As cited in Ref 51.
54. Klock PA, Roizen M. More or better: educating patients about the anesthesiologist's role as perioperative physician. *Anesth Analg*. 1996;83:671–672.
55. Dexter F, Aker J, Wright J. Development of a measure of patient satisfaction with monitored anesthesia care. *Anesthesiology*. 1997;87:865–873.
56. Whitty PM, Shaw IH, Goodwin DR. Patient satisfaction with general anesthesia. *Anaesthesia*. 1996;51:327–332.

14. Quality management, regulation, and accreditation

Jerry A. Cohen, MS, MD
Sorin J. Brull, MD
Walter G. Maurer, MD

Objectives of regulation and regulators of medical practice

A brief review of the nomenclature may be helpful to start: *accreditation* is the act of granting credit or recognition, especially with respect to an institution that maintains suitable standards; *certification* (or *credentialing* or *qualification*) is a designation earned by a person that indicates that the individual has a specific knowledge, set of skills, or abilities in the view of a certifying body; *privileging* is a special advantage, qualification, permission, right, or benefit that is granted to an individual by an institution, usually based on the individual's specific knowledge or set of skills (credentials). Regulation of medical practice (where *regulation* is defined as "a rule created by an administrative agency or body that interprets the statute(s) defining an agency's purpose and powers, or the circumstances of applying the statute") may take various forms. The objective of regulation in medical practice is to control cost and improve services rendered, by laying down ground rules for the structures, processes, and acceptable outcomes of care while at the same time establishing a fair and consistent, legally defensible basis for credentialing and privileging.

Standards appeal to regulators because they establish minimal levels of performance that their constituents will accept, delineate which services should be reimbursed, and limit the number of services rendered to an economically manageable set. In the U.S., regulation of ambulatory surgical centers (ASCs) is generally accomplished through accreditation standards. The primary accrediting bodies are the Accreditation Association for Ambulatory Health Care (AAAHC) (http://www.aaahc.org), the Joint Commission (JC) (http://www.jointcommission.org), formerly JCAHO, and the American Association for Accreditation of Ambulatory Surgery Facilities (AAAASF) (http://www.aaaasf.org). Because standards must apply to broad groups of beneficiaries and providers, they are written to apply broadly and be audited easily. This is both practical and severely limiting; what applies to all, to an extent applies to none, and is the nexus of tension between the standards survey process and the interpretation of what constitutes compliance with it, classically with the JC.

Compliance with standards does not necessarily by itself improve quality. Standards tend to decrease the variability of the bell curve that describes quality; however, they do so by raising the height of the bell curve (increasing the number of occupants at the middle) while reducing the number of occupants on the tails (outliers). Optimally, a good standard should have the effect of shifting the curve's mean and the left/low tail toward the right but will not shift the right/high tail toward the center. Minimally acceptable practices are most effective in making standards broadly applicable. Standards rarely stimulate improvement for the most creative entities. When ASC managers unfamiliar with day-to-day practice enact overly obsessive rules to guarantee compliance, the results can stultify improvement. The resulting frustrations borne by local practitioners are also felt by accreditation leadership, who sometimes cannot recognize in the accredited facility's policies the accreditor's own goals and standards they thought they were promulgating.

Is it possible, therefore, to integrate quality management and compliance with standards to improve performance? Do accrediting organizations taint performance improvement by making it just another regulatory requirement rather than a strategic planning tool? The accrediting organizations would say, "Absolutely not." They have been roundly criticized for their failures to connect increasingly detailed regulation with meaningful improvements in practice. These organizations have worked to address these criticisms. For example, the JC has undergone a major change in direction over the last few years and has now set out to prove that it is a strategic partner with health care organizations in shaping better (health) care, not just Medicare and insurance reimbursement. Will it work? As Thomas Paine said, "Time makes more converts than reason."[1]

History of the Joint Commission accreditation program

Emergence of continuous quality improvement

The goal of most of the JC standards is to promote the improvement of performance through continuous quality improvement (CQI). In this chapter, the principal aim is to address compliance and interaction with the JC's regulatory requirements rather than the details of CQI methodology. Some additional discussion of quality and performance improvement is essential to that task, although the details appear in other sections of this chapter.

The effect of the concepts of CQI on the JC was fully manifest in the late 1980s as the JC initiative known as "The Agenda for Change."[2,3] This replaced episodic procedure- and diagnosis-based audits with a continuous approach, based on concurrent monitoring of important points along the care pathway.[4] This approach requires ongoing data-gathering to monitor the stability of processes, support improvement strategies, and measures of success. In the JC model, CQI is highly dependent on measured indicators of care that are related to structure and process and outcome. The indicators are used to quantify the presence or absence of processes (preoperative evaluation, patient consent, and use of sterile technique), outcomes (hemodynamic stability, airway control, and use of regional anesthesia), or structures (equipment performance, logistical support, and medication availability). The specific data to be collected are based on the services offered that are high-volume, high-risk, and problem-prone—what the JC refers to as the "service-risk profile."[2] Examples for an ambulatory anesthesia department appear below:

High-risk indicators	High-volume indicators	Problem-prone indicators
Full stomach	General/Regional anesthesia	Pain blocks
Contagious disease	Intravenous access	Rapid sequence
Cardiac instability	Intubation	Obesity
Metabolic derangement/	Preop evaluation	Airway operations
Malignant hyperthermia	Postop recovery/disposition	Surgery on infants
Airway compromise		

The JC fell short of a well-developed quality management process because of its changing visions, the arcane language of the accreditation manual, the lack of explanations for the rationale for standards, and the inconsistencies in the survey process. This failure made it difficult for facilities to build on past experience with accreditation, compromised their ability to use the standards for total quality management due to constantly changing theories and standards, eroded the credibility of the JC, and drove an expensive pre-survey consultation market. To compound the problem, these consultations did not always deliver the correct JC standards interpretation to the institutions that hired them.

"Shared visions-new pathways"

Responding to criticism about the JC's lack of standardization in the quality management process and to the increasingly successful competition by the AAAHC and AAAASF as alternative accrediting organizations, the JC embarked on its current paradigm, known as "Shared visions-new pathways."[5] This process builds on the previous approaches to CQI but is more continuous and more collaborative and introduces major changes to the survey processes. The proffered benefits of the "Shared visions" program are that it requires less survey preparation, is oriented toward useful systems improvement, is organization-wide in scope, and is care-path-oriented. Furthermore, the accreditation manual was rewritten to improve its clarity. Standards are now broad goals that are not surveyed for compliance (e.g., the first standard in the performance improvement chapter, "The facility collects data to monitor its performance"). After each standard, there is a "rationale" section that explains why the goal is essential, as well as the steps to be taken, in the words of the JC "elements of performance" (EPs) needed to achieve the goal. The EPs are highly specific, but the methods that the facility elects to implement in order to achieve the goals are not prescribed.

The survey process uses the so-called "tracer methodology" that follows problems of actual patients rather than reviewing policies. The new emphasis is on system analysis, safety, self-evaluation, and periodic reporting, the aim of which is to make CQI a strategic management tool. The basic elements of the "Shared visions" processes are defined below:

- Periodic performance review (PPR)—yearly self-assessment via the Web with collaborative corrective action planning between the ASC and the JC; serves as a presurvey tool.
- Priority focus process (PFP)—converts a variety of presurvey data into information that focuses the survey on specific existing problems. PFP consistently focuses surveys on critical patient-care processes based on presurvey data related to:
  - Common significant outcomes: sentinel events, serious adverse events, complaints, medication errors, etc.
  - Critical systems that are at risk of causing adverse outcomes

Additionally, the PFP:
  - Uses data that are known predictors of adverse outcomes
  - Supports customized surveys—based on presurvey data

- ▪ Focuses on self-reporting of issues
- ▪ Uses "tracer" methods—it follows actual patient's care along the care pathway throughout the organization while questioning the caregivers about EPs
- • Priority focus tool—statistical methods for converting a variety of data to information that supports the PFP
- • Priority focus areas—critical systems, structures, and processes that most affect quality or produce negative outcomes if they fail; correspond closely to the standards' chapter headings (e.g., Performance Improvement and Leadership)

The "Shared visions" process is aimed at making accreditation a continuous, ongoing process through periodic self-assessment that provides the focal point for periodic unannounced surveys. The JC believes that this approach reduces the triennial presurvey panic period, although the unannounced nature of the process could produce a smoldering low level of anxiety or gradual relaxation of attention to the details of accreditation. Thus, ambulatory facilities are able to take more initiative for improvement and compliance because standards are reviewed internally, with continual electronic reporting to the JC on a yearly basis (begun in 2006). Between institutional surveys, the JC will work with organizations to approve proposed problem resolution action plans, so that problems are resolved before the survey occurs. This PPR does not affect an organization's current accreditation status. The physical survey is expected to be more consultative and less punitive by focusing on validating resolution of system problems.

The Joint Commission performance improvement model

In the eyes of the JC, performance improvement begins with the organization's collection of data to monitor its performance. Data are used to monitor the stability of processes and to support improvement strategies. Data must be collected for processes that are high-risk (e.g., medication management and operative and invasive procedures), high-volume, and problem-prone. Data may also be collected to determine the satisfaction of patients and staff and to assess the perceptions of staff regarding patient safety. Generally, data must be objective and related to measurable outcomes, not just a collection of anecdotal recollections. The organization then aggregates and analyzes the data to determine how performance levels compare with internal and external benchmarks (Box 14-1).

Statistically valid analysis converts data into information that is useful for strategic and quality improvement (QI) initiatives. The JC expects the information obtained from this analysis be used to support improvements that reduce the risk of sentinel events, improve performance, and enhance patient safety. The improvements must be in the form of well-defined changes that are expected to lead to measurable improvement. Ultimately, the organization must be able to demonstrate that the changes have resulted in sustainable improvement. In addition, the organization must annually identify a high-risk process that might

Box 14-1. Analysis of performance data

Joint Commission: Analysis of performance data is essential when data show the following:
- Trends toward uncontrolled variability in processes
- Variation from expected patterns
- For specific priority issues deemed by leadership to be critical to the facility
- For all substantive high-risk processes (e.g., medication errors, serious adverse reactions, and patterns of adverse events during sedation or anesthesia)
- For sentinel events

fail, the resultant consequences, and potential modes of failure and must delineate steps to prevent failure before a sentinel event occurs. Sentinel events are defined by the JC as "any unanticipated event in a health care setting resulting in death or serious physical or psychological injury to a person or persons, not related to the natural course of the patient's illness."

Root cause analysis

When individual or organization-related performance problems are detected or when a sentinel event does occur, accredited facilities are expected to conduct a root cause analysis (RCA) to determine the factors causing variation from the expected outcome. RCA concentrates on analysis of both special causes (unpredictable or occasional spikes in variability not related to the expected variability in a process) or common causes (variation inherent in the process that could be reduced by improving the process) to determine exactly why the event occurred. The facility must evaluate both human and system factors. The RCA determines potential changes that will improve performance and safety, while reducing risk. It may also determine that there is no reasonable opportunity for improvement, but if this occurs, the findings must be validated. In general, improvement results predominantly from changes to systems, not by replacing individuals. Structured peer-review models in anesthesiology can be applied to RCA when they look at system errors as critically as human errors. Such models demonstrate that adverse outcomes in health care, like other industries, are primarily due to faults in the system.[6] RCA must include participation by both leadership as well as those individuals closest to the process being reviewed.

The characteristics of RCA, above, are detailed in the "Sentinel event and performance improvement" chapters of the JC accreditation manual,[5] but the exact model for RCA is not prescribed. Numerous models exist. Most have the same elements, but often with different names. Below are the essential elements of the "FADE" process described by Organizational Dynamics, Inc. (ODI).[7] The methodologies put forth by ODI preceded and greatly influenced the structure of the JC QI model. The process was conceived as a general approach to systematic QI, but it can also support RCA. The FADE process consists of the following:

Focus on a statement of the problem—derived from preliminary data, reports of individuals, sentinel events, and priority issues determined by leadership
- Brainstorm for problems/issues
- Prioritize issues
- Reach consensus on issue(s)
- Define/verify issue(s)

Analysis of the problem and collection of essential data—delves deeper into the potential causes and determines the data that will accurately characterize the problem on which solutions can be based
- Determine what you know/don't know/need to know
- Collect/analyze data to set baselines, verify problems
- Determine influential factors
- Prioritize most influential factors to determine key factor(s) and cause(s)
- Collect/analyze data to verify key factor(s)

Develop solutions and recommendations that will improve outcome
- Brainstorm for solutions
- Determine optimal solution
- Develop plan for implementing solution

Execute the plan—implement the changes
- Gain commitment for plan
- Implement plan and measurements
- Measure results
- Continue to monitor results
- Plan for "Holding the gain"

Sentinel event reporting and alerts

The key element in all JC standards for QI is the identification and analysis of trends that identify undesirable patterns of performance. Routine tracking of outcomes requires analysis when trends exceed acceptable performance limits, performance or outcome varies excessively, and for certain events mandated by the JC. These mandated events include adverse drug reactions, staffing effectiveness, adverse events related to anesthesia and sedation, and (as of 1996) sentinel events.[5]

The potential for harm rather than the uniqueness of the circumstances characterizes the JC's definition of a sentinel event. Systems engineers define a sentinel event as a failure resulting from the confluence of factors previously not thought to occur together. For the JC, it is "an unexpected occurrence involving death or serious physical or psychological injury, or the risk thereof." Kaiser Permanente goes somewhat further and includes near misses and other events that threaten the well-being, performance, assets, and reputation

Box 14-2. Identifying and managing sentinel events
- Review of all events causing death or loss of function not related to disease
- Reporting of sentinel events as required by law
- Root cause analysis within 45 days

of the organization (http://xnet.kp.org/permanentejournal/spring00pj/event.html).

Reviewable sentinel events

To reduce the frequency of catastrophic failures, institutions must have a process that has defined EPs (Box 14-2) for identifying and managing sentinel events.

Examples of JC sentinel events related to the surgical process which require review include wrong-site or wrong-patient surgery, hemolytic transfusion reactions due to major blood group incompatibility, and awareness under anesthesia if it results in substantial psychological harm. The RCA (see the JC performance improvement model, above) must be done within 45 days of reporting to or notification from the JC. Reporting events to the JC is voluntary, but RCA is mandatory if the JC determines through external means that an organization has had a reviewable sentinel event. Failure of the organization to conduct an RCA can result in the organization being placed on accreditation watch, which does not change accreditation status but will result in a higher level of surveillance.

Sentinel event alerts

Since 1998, the JC has been publishing important alerts about sentinel events in its database that have reached a sufficient level of concern to warrant wide dissemination. From time to time, alerts may also come from outside experts and organizations. The alerts include a description of the event, its causes, and outline steps to prevent or reduce its recurrence. One of the latest topics, sentinel event alert (SEA) 32, pertained to awareness during anesthesia. The entire list of alerts can be found at the JC Web site, http://www.jointcommission.org/SentinelEvents/SentinelEventAlert/, and further discussion of SEA 32 (unintended intraoperative awareness) can be found on the American Society of Anesthesiologists (ASA) Web site, http://www.asahq.org/clinical/toolkit/sea32.htm.

Alerts are recommendations, not scored standards, but they are to be implemented and considered in QI planning, which is surveyable. Many ASCs, therefore, have produced plans for dealing with awareness during anesthesia. These plans can serve as a model for how to include SEAs in the facility's QI plan.

National patient safety goals

The national patient safety goals (NPSGs) have been issued yearly by the JC Sentinel Event Advisory Group since 2002. The JC recognizes that these goals are important processes that affect patient care. The NPSGs are based on a review of the literature, the Sentinel Event Database, as well as input from the public and professional organizations. Although they are considered goals, and not standards, accredited organizations must demonstrate consistent compliance with the goals applicable to their program. The goals are program-specific (ambulatory surgery centers must comply with those for ambulatory health care, offices with those for office-based surgery). Over time, goals may be incorporated into the accreditation standards when they are determined to be more appropriately surveyed as part of a standard. Organizations can apply for a waiver from compliance with the specific requirements to meet a particular JC NPSG if their approach meets or exceeds those of the JC.

For 2005, twelve goals were proposed, eight of which are relevant to anesthesiologists:

- Improve the accuracy of patient identification (two forms of patient identification, prior marking of surgical site, and time out to establish correct patient procedure and surgical site)
- Improve the effectiveness of communication among caregivers (timely reporting of critical tests, read-back of laboratory data and orders, and standardized abbreviations)
- Improve the safety of using medications (remove concentrated electrolytes, review sound-alike drugs, and standardize concentrations)
- Eliminate wrong-site, wrong-patient, and wrong-procedure surgery
- Improve the safety of using infusion pumps (by introducing free-flow protection)
- Reduce the risk of health care-associated infections
- Reconcile medications across the continuum of care (accurate documentation listing all medications prescribed to a patient)
- Reduce the risk of surgical fires (ambulatory centers only)

The relevant 2006 NPSGs[8] include those listed above and the following additional goals:

- Implement a standardized approach to "hand off" communications, including an opportunity for the involved clinicians to ask and respond to questions about the patient
- Label all medications, medication containers (e.g., syringes, medicine cups, and basins), or other solutions on and off the sterile field in perioperative and other procedural settings

The relevant 2007 NPSGs as applied to ambulatory care and office-based surgery continued to highlight patient identification, caregiver communication, medication safety, and reducing the risk of surgical fires while providing more detail and emphasis on the following:

- Reducing infections through compliance with the Centers for Disease Control hand-washing guidelines

- Listing all patient medications at the time of discharge or transfer from the ASC
- Encouraging patients and families to report safety concerns

"Proposed" 2008 NPSGs intend to add the following:

- Planning for the use of technology to assist in correct patient identification
- Reducing the risks associated with anticoagulation therapy
- Use of special teams (generally called "rapid response teams") to assess critical changes in a patient's condition
- Reduce the risk of obstructive sleep apnea
- Assessing the effect of health care worker fatigue on patient care

Although the intent of most of the goals seems clear, occasionally anesthesiologists find some of the goals to be difficult to apply in the clinical arena. Implementing the medication labeling goal, for instance, required that "All labels are verified both verbally and visually by two qualified individuals. No more than one medication or solution is labeled at one time." The goal is derived from the JC's attempt to improve safety on the operative field. However, literal application to anesthesia practice (especially in a busy ASC) would require the circulator to be constantly available to check labeling with the anesthesiologist. This would affect timely administration of these drugs, while ignoring the issue of misreading the label. Anesthesiologists certainly are committed to the overarching concepts of improving safety and reducing medication errors; however, when this goal is applied to the anesthesia setting, it is more an example of a problem than a solution to a known problem. It is important to understand the JC's requirements for implementing an NPSG. The implementation expectations can be found on the JC Web site. There may be disagreements between the organization and the surveyor or consultant, and what to do if this happens is discussed at the end of this chapter (see "Avoiding problems at the time of survey" in the subheading "What to do when there is a disagreement regarding compliance with a standard").

Other accreditation organizations: Accreditation Association for Ambulatory Health Care and American Association for Accreditation of Ambulatory Surgery Facilities

AAAHC quality management and improvement

The AAAHC is the largest accreditor of ambulatory surgery centers and office surgery facilities. The AAAHC has delineated a list of organizational characteristics that serve as the basis for the development and implementation of a high-quality CQI program. The stated goal of the AAAHC program is to promote effective and efficient use of facilities and services; in order to accomplish these goals, the accreditable organization must maintain an active, integrated, organized, peer-based program of quality management and improvement that links peer review, QI activities, and risk management.[9] The AAAHC model includes three subchapters:

1. Peer review, in which:
   a. Health care professionals understand and participate in a peer-review program
   b. A minimum of two physicians or dentists provide the peer-based review
   c. All health care professionals participate in the development of the criteria used to assess the care they provide
   d. Data are collected continually and are evaluated periodically to identify trends
   e. The results of peer review are reported to the governing body
   f. The results of peer review are used in the process of granting clinical privileges
   g. The data are readily available and encourage health care professionals' participation in continuing educational programs
2. QI program, which has the following characteristics:
   a. The QI program is broad in scope and addresses clinical, administrative, cost-of-care performance, and patient outcomes and patient safety issues
   b. The organization conducts specific QI activities that support the goals of the QI program
   c. The organization's QI program must participate in performance benchmarking activities that will allow for comparison of key performance measures with other similar organizations
3. Risk management, in which:
   a. The organization's governing body is responsible for the oversight of the risk management program
   b. The organization must designate a person or committee responsible for the risk management program
   c. The risk management program addresses safety of patients
   d. The risk management program conducts a periodic review of clinical records and policies
   e. Education in risk management activities is provided to all staff and affiliated personnel

AAAASF quality assessment and improvement

The AAAASF is a voluntary program of inspection and accreditation of surgical facilities with the goal of improving patient safety and quality care (http://www.aaaasf.org). The AAAASF standards are designed to ensure verifiable quality care, and all AAAASF-accredited facilities are regularly monitored and improved through an analysis of individual facility performance compared to established standards. The AAAASF quality assessment/QI standards include requirements in five areas:

- A written QI program, with QI surveys that monitor and evaluate quality of patient care, evaluate methods to improve patient care, and identify and correct deficiencies, involving the medical director to resolve current problems.
- Peer review performed at least every 6 months, including both random cases and unanticipated operative sequelae, using a required AAAASF format with online reporting. Peer review must be done by a recognized peer-review organization or an M.D. other than the operating room (OR) surgeon.
- Random case review, assessing specific components of the case record.
- Review of all unanticipated operative sequelae that occur within 30 days of surgery. Specific sequelae must be addressed. The chart review of each unanticipated operative sequela must include identification and analysis of the problem and its cause and treatment.
- Adherence to a Patient's Bill of Rights.

Under other standards, the AAAASF accreditation inspection process also reviews additional quality-related aspects of the surgery center, including patient charts, personnel records and qualifications, safety procedures, and patient selection criteria. The inspection also assesses the scope of procedures performed in the ambulatory center to ensure that the operating surgeon has comparable core hospital privileges covering the procedures performed.

Peer review: relating performance guidelines to performance using outcome measurements of quality

One of the more difficult issues the accrediting organizations and ASCs have had to address is the linkage between the review of performance, quality measurement, and privileging. Quality management requires leveraging change in both individuals and processes based on measured outcome at important points in the care pathway. Improved outcome is a consequence of performing processes optimally and performing optimal processes. If the processes and their structural supports (equipment, pharmaceuticals, and staffing levels) are inadequate, quality suffers, but it may not be the result of performance and consequently may not be improved by modifying peer behavior. When a health care professional's patient outcomes compare poorly to his peers, that professional's performance is in question. In brief, performance improvement requires that groups adopt valid processes and that individuals use them. Outcome is predicated on individual performance but will be poor if the processes and structures are deficient.

All evaluation of performance begins with accurate measurements of the outcomes of defined critical processes. The hours invested in clearly defining what is to be measured, how it will be measured, exclusions and exceptions, and where the data are to be found will save months of wasted time down the line, when the facility is deciding what actions to take based on the data. The outcome indicators contemplated by the ASA and others are a good starting set. Some outcome-related indicators appear in Table 14-1 and in the ASA's "Outcome Indicators for Office-Based and Ambulatory Surgery."[10] Performance measures (e.g., glucose control or intraoperative hypothermia) are valid measures of individual performance only if the variables controlling them are under

Table 14-1. Quality indicators and report form for ambulatory surgery facilities

Date _____

OR# _____
Operation _____
ASA class _____
Age _____

Anesthetic [ ] General   [ ] Regional
Anesthesiologist 1 _____
Surgeon 1 _____
PACU nurse _____

[□] NO UNTOWARD EVENTS

Preoperative evaluation:
[ ] Complete
[ ] Completed in OR
[ ] Incomplete (explain)
[ ] Made by another anesthetist
[ ] Plan changed (explain)

[ ] Monitored anesthesia care
Anesthesiologist 2 _____
Surgeon 2 _____
Discharge [ ] Home
          [ ] Hospital admission

[□] UNTOWARD EVENTS
(enter below)

Airway
☐ Dental trauma
☐ Stridor, laryngospasm, obstruction
☐ Failed rapid sequence induction
☐ Hypoxemia/hypercapnia
☐ Nose bleed or other trauma of airway
☐ Inability to intubate by route originally planned
☐ Esophageal intubation
☐ Accidental extubation
☐ Other

Regional
☐ Pain unresponsive to block
☐ Failed block, inadequate block
☐ Adverse reaction to anesthetic
☐ Excessive block (high spinal)
☐ Wet tap (epidural)
☐ Other

Cardiovascular
☐ Death
☐ Cardiac arrest
☐ Hypertension (sustained>30% above preoperative systolic)
☐ Hypotension (sustained>30% below preoperative diastolic)
☐ Bradycardia (30% below preoperative or that associated with hypotension)
☐ Tachycardia (30% above preoperative or that associated with hypertension)
☐ Myocardial ischemia/myocardial infarction suspected
☐ Congestive failure/pulmonary edema
☐ Dysrhythmia associated with one or more of above
☐ Other

(Continued)

Table 14-1. *Continued*

Miscellaneous
- ☐ Other (describe below)
- ☐ Hyperpyrexia>38°C
- ☐ Hypothermia<34°C (uninduced)
- ☐ Wrong medication/dose given (describe below)
- ☐ Drug reaction (allergic/adverse)
- ☐ Intravascular line problem
- ☐ Nausea and vomiting
- ☐ Equipment failure
- ☐ Equipment not available
- ☐ Pain control problem
- ☐ Other

Discharge planning
- ☐ Unplanned hospital admission
- ☐ Unplanned return to OR
- ☐ Delayed>3-hour stay in recovery room
- ☐ Delayed waiting for M.D. to evaluate
- ☐ Delay due to lack of caregiver
- ☐ Other delay (explain below)

Respiratory
- ☐ Post op ventilatory assistance
- ☐ Significant hypoxemia
- ☐ Pneumothorax
- ☐ Inappropriate bronchial intubation
- ☐ Ventilatory arrest
- ☐ Aspiration-respiratory distress syndrome
- ☐ Reintubation (other than accidental extubation)
- ☐ Bronchospasm
- ☐ Other

Neurological
- ☐ Prolonged neuromuscular block
- ☐ Prolonged sedation/change in neurological status
- ☐ Peripheral nerve injury
- ☐ Recall
- ☐ Seizure
- ☐ Change in vision
- ☐ Other

Describe each event on back, including event (number each, above), location (OR, PACU), cause, treatment, and outcome

ASA, American Society of Anesthesiologists; OR, operating room; PACU, postanesthesia care unit. Modified from QA/PDX Manual and used with permission of Quality Assurance Research, Inc. © 2000. A similar form and the entire manual can be obtained by ASA members free of charge at the ASA member Web site, http://www.asahq.org/members.

the control of that individual. For example, if the practitioner follows appropriate warming techniques intraoperatively in an attempt to maintain normothermia, measurement of the patient's temperature at the end of the operation would not be a good measure of peer performance, because hypothermia might occur despite appropriate intraoperative management. Rather, the outcome indicator of patient's postoperative temperature might better reflect the validity of the guidelines that may need to be changed (for instance, the intraoperative OR temperature setting) before outcome is likely to improve. If, on the other hand, effective guidelines are not followed, a change in peer behavior is indicated.

To be useful in evaluating relative performance, outcome data must be aggregated and compared to benchmarks. When this is done, large volumes of data dilute the effect of any one case, the influence of measurement methods, accuracy of measurement, and actual outcome. The difference observed between individuals is likely then to be the result of their actions. High degrees of variability reflect problems with structures and processes. Individually, we are responsible for observing basic standards; corporately, we are responsible for improving them. So, two things emerge from tracking the data: compliance with peer standards and pointers to improving outcome.

It is easier to measure outcomes than complex processes, and for that reason outcomes are practical starting points for evaluating individual and corporate performance. However, outcomes alone are not a substitute for evaluating compliance with processes or the adoption of effective processes. An ASC might find that it has a critical problem with resuscitation of excessively large numbers of overly sedated patients or possibly an unexplained increase in nausea and vomiting causing excessively prolonged postanesthesia care unit (PACU) stays. These problems raise the possibility of inappropriate privileging, inadequate staffing, lack of compliance with guidelines, a change in case mix, or inappropriate application of anesthetic techniques. The performance improvement chapters of the manuals of accreditation organizations provide a guide to measuring performance, but actual success in fostering improvement requires a serious commitment to differentiating problems with peer performance and institutional failures.

Granting, renewal, and changes to privileges

The AAAHC has a well-described process for credentialing and privileging. In the handbook,[9] the Governance chapter deals specifically with the characteristics of the accredited organization in Subchapter II: Credentialing and Privileging. In this subchapter, credentialing is described as a three-phase process of assessing and validating the qualifications of an individual to provide services. The accreditable organization must, at a minimum:

1. Establish the minimum training, experience, and requirements for physicians and other health care professionals
2. Establish a process to review, assess, and validate an individual's qualifications (education, training, experience, certification, licensure, and other educational activities)
3. Carry out the review, assessment, and validation of credentials according to the institutional process.

In the AAAHC standards, privileging is also a three-phase process, with the objective of determining the specific procedures and treatments that a health care professional may perform. The accreditable organization must, at a minimum:

1. Determine the clinical procedures and treatments that are offered to patients
2. Determine the qualifications related to training and experience that are required for obtaining each privilege
3. Establish a process for evaluating the applicant's qualifications using appropriate criteria and approving, modifying, or denying the requested privileges in a nonarbitrary manner.

Occasionally, in addition to the criteria listed above, ASCs may set a minimum number of procedures a physician must perform in order to obtain or retain a particular clinical privilege. The accrediting organizations do not require specific numbers for clinical privileges; they require that a facility establish and follow a privileging policy. Setting minimum numbers of procedures could mean that the ASC requires enumeration of each activity for which one is requesting privileges and an assessment of associated outcomes. For example, if one has privileges for central line placement, the number and complication rate would need to be known to determine the appropriateness of privileges. Instead, it would be reasonable to grant the privilege if the rate of reported complications is within acceptable institutional limits. In short, an assessment is required, but the exact extent to which it is quantitative is not. Neither the AAAHC nor the JC has established any minimum numbers that an institution could rely on in so doing.

The JC or AAAHC has never required separate review of various skills that are bundled into an anesthetic. Instead, the facility has to look critically at their scope of services to accurately determine the competencies required of their anesthesia services. Using a "standardized" anesthesia privileging form that includes procedures appropriate to an inpatient anesthetic practice would be inappropriate for an ASC. However, competency in fiber-optic intubation or advanced cardiac life support certification may be appropriate for an ASC. Furthermore, the JC requires evidence of continued competence based on information collected by the ASC but does not require self-reporting or practitioner-maintained logs. The requirement for excessive numbers of procedures or requirements applied to selective individuals are beyond the pale of regulatory requirements and suggest a hidden agenda within the facility and the need for a skilled negotiator to uncover and resolve the real problem.

Hot-button issues of importance to ambulatory surgical centers

Intraoperative awareness with recall, and brain monitoring

In October 2004, the JC issued SEA 32[11] on Unintended Intraoperative Awareness. Sebel et al.[12] have reported a suspected incidence of awareness with recall of 0.2%. It is not known whether all of these events occurred with general anesthesia rather than sedation or whether the periods of awareness occurred during induction or emergence of anesthesia. From this report, the JC estimated that 10,000 to 40,000 patients experience some form of awareness during anesthesia; the numbers are of inescapable concern. Awareness is more frequent in patients who are unable to tolerate conventional levels of general anesthesia but is not limited to them. A number of patients who have experienced intraoperative awareness later have nightmares and post-traumatic stress syndrome.[13] It is controversial whether brain monitoring is needed for all patients. Although the U.S. Food and Drug Administration has concluded that the use of the bispectral index (BIS) brain monitor may reduce the incidence of awareness in high-risk populations, the JC believes that the role of brain monitors, such as BIS, is not yet sufficiently defined to require their routine use. As part of SEA 32, the JC asked the ASA to investigate the role of various modes of monitoring in preventing intraoperative awareness.

The points addressed in SEA 32 to reduce intraoperative awareness are the following:

- Consider the use of preoperative amnestics
- Sufficient depth of anesthesia during intubation
- Appropriate use of narcotics to prevent pain
- Avoidance of excessive muscle relaxation or beta blockade
- Appropriate opioid therapy considerations for substance-tolerant patients
- Maintaining accuracy of anesthesia delivery systems
- Consideration of brain function monitoring
- Better OR decorum—less talking and loud music at times of expected light anesthesia
- Postoperative review and counseling for patients reporting symptoms or explicit recall
- Informed consent, at least to explain that awareness does occur and that sedation does not prevent awareness

As with other SEAs, the facility must develop a mechanism for addressing the issues raised in the alert. Key elements to be included in a policy for suspected or known incidence of awareness or recall are the following:

- Assure the patient of the credibility of his or her account and sympathize with the patient's experience
- Explain what happened and why, if a reason can be given (e.g., the need for lighter anesthesia because of cardiovascular instability)
- Offer support to the patient, including referral to a psychiatrist or psychologist, if appropriate
- Document any referrals or treatment provided to the patient
- Notify the patient's surgeon and the facility manager about the incident if part of the ASC's risk management protocol
- Complete an occurrence report concerning the event for the purpose of quality management

The ASA has been very active in addressing the issue of unanticipated intraoperative recall, which is a more practical term for what is actually being reported by patients. ASA has continued to develop model facility policies for dealing with reports of awareness with recall and for educating patients and professionals about the situations in which recall is normal (induction, emergence, and during sedation without general anesthesia). In addition, the ASA actively works with regulators such as the JC to ensure that they promote standards based on sufficient scientific evidence.

The ASA has also produced a Practice Advisory for Intraoperative Awareness and Brain Function Monitoring, which was approved by the 2005 ASA House of Delegates.[14] The advisory surveyed more than 150 peer-reviewed articles and recommends a multimodal approach to monitoring depth of anesthesia to minimize awareness, including use of vital signs, lid reflex, response to commands, and movement. A single physiological parameter may not correlate with a specific depth of anesthesia. Brain monitoring by any of the available devices was not routinely recommended, due to a variety of confounding variables, including inconsistent sensitivity with different drugs and patients, and artifacts due to various devices used in the OR. The topic of brain monitoring remains an important issue with the public, but is to some extent driven by the sensationalism in the media and by the influence of the monitor manufacturers on the public and the JC. It is therefore important to have a multimodal plan for addressing the concerns raised in SEA 32 based on current science.

Sedation by nonanesthesiologists

In the late 1980s, the ASA became increasingly concerned about complications from sedation given by nonanesthesiologists. Guidelines for the administration of analgesia and sedation by nonanesthesiologists were approved by the ASA House of Delegates in 1995 and updated in 2001.[15] The recommendations of these guidelines have been incorporated largely verbatim into various documents of the JC and statute, including the concept of the continuum of depth of sedation and anesthesia, preoperative evaluation, monitoring, postoperative care, and skill sets necessary to conduct sedation and rescue from levels of anesthesia that had become deeper than planned. Sedation Standards and their EPs require that sedation planning include sufficient staff to monitor the patient in addition to the individual performing the procedure, presence of resuscitation equipment, perioperative nursing care, and appropriate monitoring equipment. The standard applies to anesthesia as well as sedation. Currently, one of the individuals involved in patient care must be a qualified licensed independent practitioner with appropriate credentials, who also "plans or concurs with the planned anesthesia." The ASA has described the requirements for privileging of nonanesthesia professionals to give moderate sedation in a document approved by the 2005 House of Delegates.[16]

In the past, anesthesiology departments had been required by the JC to oversee all sedation in their facilities. No such requirement now exists, although anesthesiologists are often called upon to assist in the formulation of policy and to serve on sedation and analgesia committees. The published sedation guidelines of the ASA are useful in formulating safe policies.[15]

Effectiveness of clinical alarm systems

The JC issued a frequently asked question for this NPSG that clarified its intent. An alarm is required to alert staff when the patient is at increased risk and requires immediate attention. The JC requires that facility policy dictate at what ranges alarms are set and when alarms may be disabled. Surveyors will then look at the institutional policies and procedures for the setup of alarms (especially with respect to appropriate settings of high and low limits on physiologic monitoring alarm systems) and will check the alarms to see that they are set appropriately. Recently, the ASA Standards for Basic Anesthesia were amended to require audible alarms for both oximetry and capnography.

Immediate availability of anesthesiologists

The ASA Guidelines for the Ethical Practice of Anesthesiology[17] require that anesthesiologists remain continuously available to those they supervise and be present during the most demanding aspects of anesthesia care. The ASA Guidelines for Patient Care in Anesthesia require "On-site medical direction of any nonphysician who participates in the delivery of anesthesia care to the patient." The words are simple and consistent with Centers for Medicare and Medicaid Services (CMS) requirements, which require that an anesthesiologist supervising a nurse anesthetist be immediately available and directly supervise anesthesia given by a physician's assistant. The JC is obligated to enforce the CMS requirements, as part of JC's deeming status for Medicare certification.[18] Problems arise from excessively detailed efforts to locally apply certain words and phrases such as "continuously," "immediately available," and "directly supervise." Some "safe harbor" exceptions appear to be acceptable (attending short emergencies, receiving a patient in the OR for the next surgery, checking and discharging patients from the recovery room, or handling scheduling issues). However, these current "safe harbors" are always at risk of being reinterpreted by the CMS and its intermediaries. Local solutions vary considerably, from the ill-advised "don't ask, don't tell" to obsessive accounting of all concurrent activity. We need a simpler, clearer model. Unfortunately, the CMS moves slowly to adopt change, and currently we are left in a state of some ambiguity. So, what can be said? Anesthesiologists should avoid any activities that involve direct patient care inconsistent with their Medicare carrier's interpretations. If anesthesiologists supervise widely dispersed locations, they should estimate the immediacy of availability as conservatively as would any Medicare auditor walking between those locations. It should be emphasized that the CMS is most concerned with anesthesiologists' billing for multiple concurrent services.

Informed consent

Consent for anesthesia has long been required by the accrediting organizations. More recently, most anesthesiologists document consent separately from the surgeon/proceduralist, in order to demonstrate that the patient has been informed of the relative risks and benefits of the anticipated anesthetic plan and of the options for care. The standards do not prescribe how the practitioner is to document consent, but it is uncommon today to have a combined surgical and anesthesia consent form, as was the routine in the past. A signed form is an acceptable way of documenting consent, but other methods of documentation may also be acceptable, such as documentation on the anesthesia preoperative assessment form or elsewhere in the medical record. The accrediting organizations do not specifically mandate that the patient sign the consent, but they do mandate that the anesthesiologist have a discussion with the patient and/or the patient's family (if the patient is a minor, incompetent, or so desires) about options and risks. It is important for the anesthesia practice, in consultation with the facility's legal counsel, to specifically approve (preferably, by policy) the method by which consent will be obtained. Because methods of compliance vary from facility to facility and may be affected by requirement of state law, it is important to be able to show the surveyor the informed consent policy, how it is being observed, and how this policy is consistently reflected in the medical record.

The addition of specific risks to the informed consent form is done often. When this list is concise and based on actual outcomes as supported by the anesthesia literature, it is helpful. But sometimes a listed risk is suggested by the institutional risk management in response to a catastrophic event that cannot be addressed by a clear preventive measure. It is important to know that consent is not so much a matter of documentation as it is patient education and that while a proper discussion of the risk of the catastrophic event is appropriate in selected patients, the decision to add it to a form is not always appropriate. Frequent updating of anesthesia consent forms by grafting new risks onto an endlessly expandable consent form is neither practical nor advisable. Institutions that place a laundry list of remote and likely risks together on an anesthesia consent form may fall into the trap of thinking that an all-inclusive list is a substitute for conversation with the patient, thereby increasing risk, rather than minimizing it.[19] Instead, to complement the patient discussion, what is probably needed is a basic anesthesia consent form that includes only the potential risks of common/minor complications (such as postoperative nausea and vomiting, pain) as well as rare, but potentially significant, complications (such as dental damage, awareness, brain damage, and death).

Medication security

The JC[5] requires that medications be safely stored according to the facilities' policy and applicable state law, so that they are not accessible by unauthorized individuals. Drugs that are left out in the open and unattended would violate the standard. Secured OR areas with limited access and constant supervision should not need the drug carts to be locked. However, as the JC noted, the then-current CMS definition of "secured" stated that "all medications including nonprescription medications are in locked containers in a room or are under constant surveillance" as stated in rule 42 C.F.R. § 482.25(3)(b)(2). In October 2003, the ASA advocated a change to CMS policy that would ensure that drugs are properly secured but would remain available, if needed, on top of the anesthesia cart, immediately before, during, and after an anesthetic. The drugs would be available as long as there are authorized OR personnel in the OR suite, not necessarily a specific OR. New proposed regulations that would change the applicable regulation to read "All drugs and biologicals must be kept in a secure area, and locked when appropriate" was published March 24, 2005, in the *Federal Register*,[18] and the comment period ended May 24, 2005. The CMS indicated that its intent was consistent with the ASA policy to designate the operating suite, rather than individual ORs, a securable area.[20] The change was expected to apply by late 2006. The final rule was published November 27, 2006.[21] No changes were made to the proposed regulations quoted above. Public comment reinforced the ASA position. Although the JC clearly intended to implement the change, final wording of the CMS Interpretive Guidelines will need to be published in order for the JC to amend the wording of the JC requirements. It is reasonable to expect that the interpretive guidelines will reflect the comments published with the final rule in the *Federal Register*. In particular, the ASA Position Statement approved by the ASA Executive Committee, October 2003, entitled "Security of Medications in the Operating Room" (http://www.asahq.org/clinical), was cited. Also cited were two specific concerns regarding what needs to be locked versus secure and which personnel can have access to secure areas. The final rule specifically comments that hospitals have the flexibility to determine which noncontrolled drugs and biologicals need to be locked versus those that need only be kept in a secured area, and it also "provides hospitals with the flexibility to define which personnel have access to locked areas based on their own needs as well as state and local law. The definition of 'authorized personnel' should be addressed in hospital policies and procedures." The interpretive guidelines will need to be consistent with the simple statement in the rule that, "A medication is considered secure if unauthorized persons are prevented from obtaining access."

What to do when there is a disagreement regarding compliance with a standard

Resolving problems that arise between surveys

Written policies can often effectively address differences between local interpretation and the apparent message in an accreditation manual. By crafting a policy that specifically addresses how an ASC will fulfill the requirements of a standard and the ways in which it will ensure patient safety, potential problems with accreditation may be resolved. Spelling out how a facility's internal policies protect the patient has a great value in helping the surveyor understand the justification for the ASC's approach. Reference in the policy to how it is consistent with external standards (e.g., those of the ASA or the American College of Surgeons) further demonstrates the validity of the institutional policy.

In the past, questions about interpretation of standards have been prompted by preparation for an impending survey. This is appropriate for the AAAASF and AAAHC, but for JC, surveys are now all unannounced. In the final analysis, referring questions of compliance to the ASA head office may be the most expeditious way to get an answer, but other approaches can also be effective.

First, consult with the local on-site individual whom the institution has designated to be in charge of the facility's compliance with the survey and standards process. Sometimes, this person has approached the anesthesiology department first and presented a conflicting view of the regulation's intent which cannot be resolved. If this results from a question about an accreditation standard, it is useful for all parties to arrange for a phone conference with the accrediting agency after clearly characterizing the questions to be answered. If the issue involves a legal interpretation, the facility's attorney should be involved. In all cases, conversations with the accreditation organization should be attended by the department chair or a department member skilled in the interpretation of the accrediting organization's standards. If disagreement still exists after consultation with the accrediting organization, the details of the attempts to resolve the issue may be forwarded to the appropriate professional organizations. Various organizations have committees that function to resolve issues related to accreditation. One example is the ASA's Committee on Quality Management and Departmental Administration (QMDA). QMDA may engage the ASA's representatives to the accrediting organizations or experts in the ASA Division of Legislative and Governmental Affairs, as appropriate. Examples include the ASA's collaboration with the JC and CMS to resolve the interpretation of medication security with respect to the locking of anesthesia medication carts, and with the JC to reword the NPSG for medication labeling by omitting the requirement for two-person verification of the label when the person drawing up the medication is the one giving it.

The need to prepare for surveys has led facilities to hire other outside consultants. These "mock surveys" are a cottage industry of inconsistent value. Mock surveys often provide a means of highlighting likely problems with the real survey, but it is not uncommon for the mock surveyor to be more critical and suggest changes only to justify their employment. Using a reputable consultant is therefore important. In the case of the JC, Joint Commission Resources, Inc. (JCR) (http://www.jcrinc.com) is high quality, for-profit affiliate of, but independent from, the JC that offers publications and consultation to help ". . . health care organizations world-wide to improve the quality of patient care and achieve peak performance." The JCR newsletter is an excellent source of information about the JC, and JCR does not share any of its findings with the JCAHO. AAAHC also has a for-profit, independent subsidiary, Healthcare Consultants International, Inc. (HCI) (http://www.hciconsultants.com). HCI's primary focus is on assisting ambulatory health care organizations prepare for and maintain accreditation, licensure, and certification through broad-based medical and surgical consulting.

Avoiding problems at the time of survey

Most problems with adoption of standards by a facility need to be resolved before the survey. The JC uses tracer methodology that follows a patient's path of care throughout the ASC, and therefore many staff members will need to be knowledgeable about a variety of standards and issues,[22] especially the following:

- Procedures that are routinely performed, have high risk, or are suspected or known to be problem-prone, including identification of patients, operation, and surgical site
- The selection of the appropriate procedure, preoperative evaluation of patients for the procedure, standards relating to performance of the procedure, monitoring of patients during the procedure, and postprocedure care

- Medication use—appropriateness of medications prescribed, preparation, labeling, dispensing, and security of medication
- Blood and blood component administration and monitoring (if applicable to the ASC)
- How the quality of care is monitored, including the identification of problems and their resolution through performance improvement activities
- Preanesthetic evaluation
- Re-evaluation of patients and equipment immediately before induction of anesthesia
- Evaluation of a patient's postoperative status on admission to and from the PACU, including discharge protocols, documentation, and handoffs
- For hospital-based ambulatory surgery units: how comparable levels of quality of surgery and anesthesia care throughout the hospital are maintained, including the need for uniformity between different areas of the ASC, such as the ORs, gastrointestinal, or radiology suites

Inevitably, surveyors will find problems and staff will be tempted to argue. Avoid this. It is better to defer to one's supervisor or chairman than to persist. With the JC, if a surveyor appears to be clearly wrong on a substantial issue, the ASC's survey coordinator may consult with the JC headquarters for clarification. One should not offer opinions about care processes that cannot be substantiated.

The AAAHC handbook[9] contains a detailed section on the policies and procedures used for accreditation and reaccreditation surveys. Additionally, the handbook details the procedures for revoking the accreditation of an organization, including these criteria: (a) the organization no longer satisfies the AAAHC Survey Eligibility Criteria; (b) is no longer in compliance with its policies, procedures, or standards; (c) has significantly compromised patient care; (d) has failed to act in good faith in providing data to the AAAHC; (e) failed to notify the AAAHC within 30 days of any significant organizational, operational, or financial change; (f) failed to notify the AAAHC within 30 days of any imposition of sanctions, changes in license, criminal indictment, or any violation of state or federal law. The chapter on policies and procedures of the handbook also details the process for Appeal of Accreditation Decision, which should help the nonaccredited facility address the reaccreditation process.

Summary

Without a systematic way of collecting performance and outcome indicators and turning them into meaningful information that drives improvement, controlling quality and outcome tends to be haphazard, like flying without instruments. Quality management is becoming an increasingly important strategic tool for effectively managing health care in ASCs and not just as a way of achieving accreditation. The analysis of meaningful metrics is needed to drive performance improvement, respond to regulatory requirements, thrive economically, reduce the potential for malpractice litigation, and achieve accreditation.

Inevitably, accreditation standards must be met, even if they are not the end-all of quality management. Standards are written to apply broadly and be audited easily, which is both practical and severely limiting; what applies to all, to an extent applies to none, and is the nexus of tension between the interpretation of standards and the determination of compliance with them during the accreditation survey. This chapter addresses the information needed to effectively deal with both the details of quality management and critical issues related to accreditation. It elaborates on the JC and other accreditation models, provides information generally applicable to quality management, peer review, credentialing, and privileging and on how to be successful in handling difficulties during an accreditation survey. Knowledge of the contents of this chapter strengthens one's ability to be successful in a performance-driven world where requirements for reimbursement and patients' expectations and those of our regulators are increasingly dependent on how we measure and manage quality.

References

1. Paine T. *Common Sense.* 1775.
2. Joint Commission on the Accreditation of Health Organizations: Task forces lay groundwork for new survey process. *Agenda for Change Update.* 1984;1:1–6.
3. Joint Commission on Accreditation of Hospitals: Medical Staff Issues in the Changing Hospital Environment. Chicago, IL: Joint Commission on Accreditation of Hospitals; 1987.
4. Cohen JA. Quality assurance and risk management. In: Gravenstein N, ed. *Manual of Complications During Anesthesia.* Philadelphia, PA: JB Lippincott; 1991:1–44.
5. Joint Commission on Accreditation of Healthcare Organizations. *Comprehensive Accreditation Manual for Hospitals.* Oakbrook Terrace, IL: Joint Commission Resources, Inc.; 2005.
6. Lagasse R. Relationship between adverse perioperative outcome, severity of illness, and human error. 49th Postgraduate Assembly in Anesthesiology. New York, NY: The New York Society of Anesthesiologists (NYSA); 1995.
7. Organizational Dynamics, Inc. *CQI for Physicians: Facilitator Manual.* Burlington, MA: Organizational Dynamics, Inc.; 1993.
8. Joint Commission Perspectives: The Joint Commission Announces the 2006 National Patient Safety Goals and Requirements. Oakbrook Terrace, IL: Joint Commission Resources, Inc.; 2005;25:7,1–10.
9. AAAHC Accreditation Handbook for Ambulatory Health Care 2006. Wilmette, IL: AAAHC, Inc.; 2006.
10. American Society of Anesthesiologists Committee on Ambulatory Surgical Care and Task Force on Office Based Anesthesia. Outcome indicators for office-based and ambulatory surgery (2003). Available at: http://www.asahq.org/publications AndServices/outcomeindicators.pdf. Accessed July 22, 2007.
11. Joint Commission on Accreditation of Healthcare Organizations (JCAHO). Sentinel Event Newsletter 32. Oakbrook Terrace, IL: JCAHO; 2004.

12. Sebel PS, Bowdle TA, Ghoneim MM, et al. The incidence of awareness during anesthesia: a multicenter United States study. *Anesth Analg.* 2004;99:833–839.

13. Osterman JE, Hopper J, Heran WJ, Keane TM, van der Kolk BA. Awareness under anesthesia and the development of posttraumatic stress disorder. *Gen Hosp Psychiatry.* 2001;23:198–204.

14. American Society of Anesthesiologists. Practice advisory for intraoperative awareness and brain function monitoring (2005). Available at: http://www.asahq.org/publicationsAndServices/practiceparam.htm#brain. Accessed July 22, 2007.

15. American Society of Anesthesiologists Task Force on Sedation and Analgesia by Non-Anesthesiologists. Practice guidelines for sedation and analgesia by non-anesthesiologists. *Anesthesiology.* 2002;96:1004–1017.

16. American Society of Anesthesiologists. Statement on granting privileges for administration of moderate sedation to practitioners who are not anesthesia professionals (2006). Available at: http://www.asahq.org/publicationsAndServices/standards/40.pdf. Accessed July 22, 2007.

17. American Society of Anesthesiologists. Guidelines for the ethical practice of anesthesiology (2003). Available at: http://www.asahq.org/publicationsAndServices/sgstoc.htm. Accessed July 22, 2007.

18. Department of Health and Rehabilitative Services, Centers for Medicare and Medicaid Services; Hospital Conditions of Participation: Requirements for History and Physical Examinations; Authentication of Verbal Orders; Securing Medications; and Post-anesthesia Evaluations, Proposed Rule. *Fed Regist.* 2005;70(57):15266–15274.

19. Clark SK, Leighton BL, Seltzer JL. A risk-specific anesthesia consent form may hinder the informed consent process. *J Clin Anesth.* 1991;3:11–13.

20. Bierstein K. Locked anesthesia carts: CMS proposes to change the rule (at last!). *ASA Newsletter.* 2006 69:5:28–29.

21. Department of Health and Rehabilitative Services, Centers for Medicare and Medicaid Services; Hospital Conditions of Participation: Requirements for History and Physical Examinations; Authentication of Verbal Orders; Securing Medications; and Post-anesthesia Evaluations, Final Rule. *Fed Regist.* 2006;71(227):68688–68691.

22. Cohen JA, Philip BK. How to prepare for a Joint Commission survey. *ASA Newsletter.* 2001;65:25–29.

15. Ambulatory surgery center profitability, efficiency, and cost containment

Tom Archer, MD, MBA
Steve Mannis, MD, MBA
Alex Macario, MD, MBA

Ambulatory surgery and anesthesia should be:
- Safe and effective
- Friendly and compassionate
- Profitable

Unless we are an ambulatory surgery center (ASC) owner, why should we care about the financial aspects of ASC management? Why not just give safe, effective, friendly, and compassionate care and not worry about ASC finances?

By understanding and promoting ASC profitability, we:
- Increase our value to the ASC
- Increase the value of the ASC to its owners
- Protect our ability to practice in the ASC

Recognizing that clinicians often do not fully understand the economic implications of our practices, this chapter will address the role of the anesthesiologist in contributing to the financial success of the ASC and discuss basic economic principles related to ASC management.

Role of the anesthesiologist in making the ASC a financial success

Anesthesiologists may help the ASC to be a financial success by reducing labor and supply costs per case. This may be done by engaging in the activities shown in Table 15-1. The anesthesia literature has focused on these activities since these are the only activities over which the anesthesiologist has significant control.

Table 15-1. Steps an anesthesiologist can take to reduce labor and supply costs per case

- Eliminating unnecessary preop testing
- Avoiding last-minute cancellations
- Shortening turnover times
- Performing tasks in parallel rather than in series
- Using less-expensive drugs
- Choosing between disposable and reusable supplies
- Bypassing the postanesthesia care unit (PACU) with rapid emergence general anesthesia, regional, or "local/monitored anesthesia care" techniques
- Minimizing PACU length of stay by minimizing pain and postoperative nausea and vomiting
- Limiting antiemetic use to at-risk patients
- Limiting monitors used in PACU (when appropriate)
- Omitting supplemental oxygen in PACU (when appropriate)

The anesthesiologist must realize, however, that the most important determinants of ASC profitability are *facility fees* and *case volume* and that she typically has no influence over either of these factors. Hence, the anesthesiologist must retain a sense of perspective and realism about how much impact she can really have on the overall profitability of the ASC. Managers and surgeons sometimes blame "anesthesia" for problems that really have nothing to do with the performance of the anesthesiologist, and we need to recognize when we are being criticized without justification.

On the other hand, we anesthesiologists are the only medical doctors who spend most of each workday in the operating room (OR) setting. If we keep our eyes and our minds open and if we bear in mind certain basic business principles, we can often come up with constructive suggestions for improving ASC efficiency.

What ASC problems are not under the clinical anesthesiologist's control?

To have a sense of perspective about how much impact anesthesiologists can have on overall ASC profitability, one needs to recognize those aspects of ASC function that are *not* normally under the clinician's control. These are shown in Table 15-2.

Table 15-2. What ambulatory surgery center problems are *not* under the anesthesiologist's control?

- Low case volume
- Slow surgeons
- Low facility fees
- Dysfunctional scheduling (unused block time, gaps in schedule, and unrealistic case duration estimates, leading to frequent compulsory overtime and employee discontent)
- Last-minute cancellations and no-shows
- Apathetic, unhappy, and burnt-out employees
- Inefficient use of "labor-saving" devices (fluoroscopy, endoscopy, and laparoscopy)
- Inefficient use of information technology for scheduling and billing
- High fixed costs ("overhead" such as mortgage interest, leases, utilities, insurance, and consultants and managers' salaries)

The anesthesiologist as a manager

Anesthesiologists, who work day-to-day on the front lines, have a unique understanding of how a surgery center functions, down to knowing which OR has the best air-conditioning in summer and which are the best sandwiches to order for lunch! Experienced anesthesiologists can be invaluable in helping the center negotiate the politics of disparate groups of busy surgeons who are trying to complete their cases in an efficient manner. The demands from surgeons are high, yet their presence is often ephemeral. Management looks for a stable, friendly face of an anesthesia leader who can help them solve day-to-day issues, such as setting policies, dealing with block time, developing new clinical programs, and handling quality of care or behavioral issues among staff members as part of peer review. An anesthesiologist is often best suited to become the medical director of the ASC, and, in this role, she leads the ASC along with the administrator.

The medical staff structure of a surgery center often calls for standing committees that include physician representatives. The anesthesiologist who shows even a modicum of interest is often a welcome addition to committees such as quality improvement, continuing education, or the medical executive committee.

An anesthesiologist's participation in management is important for two strategic reasons:

First, having a presence on committees allows the anesthesiologists to help shape policies and procedures in a manner that promotes high-quality patient care. The anesthesiologist-manager can work with surgery center staff, other anesthesiologists, and surgeons to shape expectations and achieve "buy-in" in a constructive manner.

Second, having a presence in the committee structure helps weave the anesthesia group into the fabric of the center, promoting a stable group of anesthesia practitioners and, along with it, helping to achieve job security for the anesthesia group. Excellent individual patient care is a baseline expectation for any anesthesiologist working at a surgery center. An important way to differentiate one anesthesia group from another is through value-added activities, such as working outside the OR with management.

An economic model of the ASC

The following ASC profit equation,[1] relating profit and case volume, is a simplified but useful model of how an ASC makes money. This model is taught in business schools as "break-even" analysis. An online presentation of "break-even" analysis from Harvard Business School (last accessed April 22, 2006) can be found at http://hbswk.hbs.edu/item.jhtml?id=1262&t=finance. For simplicity's sake, the model assumes that all cases have the same facility fees and variable labor and supply costs.

The ASC profit equation:

$$P = V \times (F - C_l - C_s) - C_f,$$

Where

P = profit / year

V = case volume / year

F = facility fee / case

C_l = variable labor costs / case

C_s = variable supply costs / case

C_f = fixed costs / year

Variable and fixed costs

In this simple model, all costs are either variable or fixed (Table 15-3). "Variable" refers to costs that vary directly with the volume of cases performed, and "fixed" refers to costs that do *not* vary with the volume of cases performed. It is important to realize that both "variable" and "fixed" costs can fluctuate widely from one ASC to another and that it is management's job to minimize both.

Particularly with respect to labor costs, this strict division into variable and fixed costs is somewhat inaccurate and unrealistic. Sometimes labor costs are only loosely tied to units of production,[2] and cost accountants talk about these nondivisible costs as being "semi-fixed" or "semi-variable." For example, on any given day, the ASC has to pay the employees scheduled to work that day,

Table 15-3. Variable and fixed costs

Variable labor costs	• Hourly wages paid per case (e.g., operating room and postanesthesia care unit nurses)
Variable supply costs	• Supplies used per case (e.g., intravenous lines, drapes, unit dose medications, sutures, disposable gas circuits, airway devices, implants, and waste disposal)
Fixed labor costs	• Employee salaries (e.g., administrators)
Other fixed costs	• Mortgage payments
	• Rents and leases
	• Contracted services (e.g., equipment maintenance)
	• Utilities
	• Insurance
	• Permits and licenses
	• Legal and consultant expenses
	• Regulatory compliance

even if all of the ASC's cases are cancelled. On the day of surgery, staff costs are fixed! Two other examples of how short-term labor costs can be nondivisible would be that one half of a nurse cannot be hired or if overtime can only be paid in 2-hour blocks for contractual reasons.

In the long run, however, the distinction between fixed and variable labor costs has a great deal of validity. If the ASC gets busier and decides to open another OR—or run longer workdays—then more hourly labor will have to be hired in order to staff the additional cases. Similarly, if the ASC loses cases to the competition, management may have to shorten the workday or close down an OR. Over the long run, in a well-managed ASC, variable hourly wages paid will be closely correlated with the volume of cases performed.

Contribution margin, fast surgeons, and profitability

The quantity $(F-C_1-C_s)$—the revenue per case (facility fee) minus the variable costs per case—is called the "contribution margin." Contribution margin is the revenue remaining after paying the variable costs of each case. Only contribution margin can pay the fixed costs, and—if anything is left over—it can be distributed to the ASC's owners as profit.

One of management's key functions is to maximize the total contribution margin for all of the cases performed at the ASC. A key insight into the profitability of an ASC (or any similar business) is the following: Performing cases more rapidly decreases labor costs per case, *even if the employees themselves do not change their behavior*. Hence, we may see a decrease in variable labor costs per case and an increase in contribution margin per case just by getting a fast surgeon to do cases at the ASC! Conversely, a slow surgeon who takes 3 or 4 hours to do cases that an average surgeon would do in 90 minutes may try to blame his low contribution margins per case on "slow anesthesia turnover times."

We can now see more clearly and analytically what is intuitively obvious: that a *large volume* of *high facility fee cases*, performed *rapidly*, is a recipe for large contribution margins and outstanding financial success.[3]

ASC profitability in greater detail

From the ASC profit equation, we can see that successful ASC managers will:
   a)   Maximize case volume
   b)   Maximize facility fees
   c)   Minimize variable labor costs per case
   d)   Minimize variable supply costs per case
   e)   Minimize fixed costs
We will now examine in greater detail how to achieve these five goals:

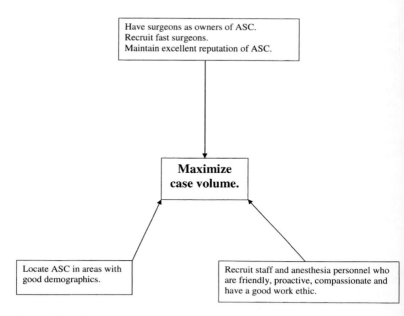

Figure 15-1. How to maximize case volume. ASC, ambulatory surgery center.

Maximize case volume

If a surgeon is an owner of an ASC, she will tend to bring her patients to her facility[4] (Figure 15-1). The surgeon's motive is not only to earn her part of the facility fee, but also to have more control over how care is given. As an owner of the facility, she will have a voice in all aspects of how the ASC functions and hence will want to bring her patients to that facility.

If the current owners of an ASC have unused OR capacity and want to increase their ASC's profits, they might invite a busy surgeon to buy an ownership stake in their facility, thereby offering the new partner a financial motive for bringing her cases to the ASC. There are, however, legal restrictions on the offering of financial incentives in return for patient referrals.

Maximize facility fee per case

Facility fees vary from procedure to procedure, from year to year, and from payer to payer (Figure 15-2). Provider groups negotiate with insurance compa-

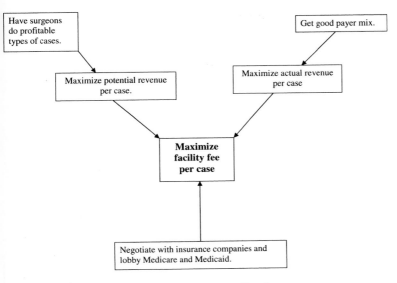

Figure 15-2. How to maximize facility fees per case.

nies and hire lobbyists to convince Medicare and Medicaid to raise facility fees—or at least not to reduce them! The strategy of the payers has been to offer lucrative facility fees initially for outpatient surgery procedures, in order to get a given type of surgical procedure to be performed outside the high fixed-cost environment of the hospital. Once the procedures have left the hospital, the payers try to ratchet facility fees downward, thus encouraging efficiency and cost containment on the part of providers in an ambulatory setting. For instance, facility fees for cataract surgery were generous in the 1980s, but have fallen considerably since then.

Facility fees change frequently in response to political and market forces. High facility fees attract new providers, which in turn will tend to lower facility fees in the future as a glut of providers develops. The facility fees that an ASC encounters depend on the payer mix in the community, the specific types of cases which the facility can attract, and the evolution of the health care market-place over time.

Minimize variable labor costs per case

Minimizing variable labor costs is the most complex and difficult part of the ASC management, since so many factors influence how much variable labor is needed per case (Figure 15-3). Managers and anesthesiologists should

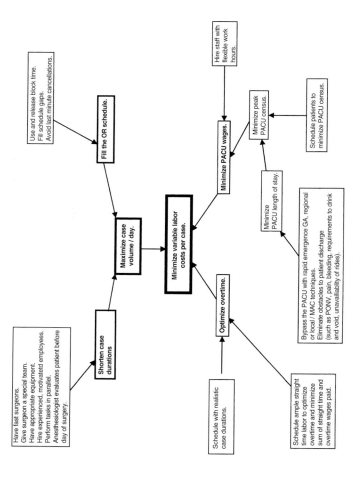

Figure 15-3. How to minimize variable labor costs per case. GA, general anesthesia; MAC, monitored anesthesia care; OR, operating room; PACU, postanesthesia care unit; PONV, postoperative nausea and vomiting.

focus on adopting specific techniques that promote the following general goals:

Shorten case durations (including turnover times)

Since labor costs accrue by the hour, one major determinant of variable labor costs per case is *how long the case lasts* (case duration).[5-7]

Interventions that decrease case duration decrease variable labor costs per case, increase contribution margin, and can also greatly increase ASC profit because *more cases can be performed per day*. Hence, interventions that decrease case duration can be extremely potent in terms of increasing ASC profitability.

Skilled nurses and technicians can make a surgeon's job easier by giving her exactly what she needs when she needs it. Hence, if possible, a surgeon should get her own special team who knows her equipment, needs, and idiosyncrasies.

To shorten turnover times, anesthesiologists could evaluate patients before the day of surgery, nurses can routinely start IVs and give antibiotics, anesthesiologists can use block rooms, surgical technicians can prepare their instrument tables during the induction of anesthesia, and housekeeping personnel can start cleaning the OR during the patient's emergence from anesthesia (personal communication, Steve Mannis). In other words, the ASC team should *perform as many activities as possible in parallel, rather than in series.*[8]

Fill the OR schedule to avoid OR staff downtime

Another major determinant of variable labor costs per case is how busy the ORs and the staff are throughout the day. In other words, to minimize variable labor costs per case, we have to keep the ORs and the employees generating revenue throughout the entire workday. Proper use of block time is one way of achieving this goal.[9]

Turnover time is a perennial sore point with surgeons, exemplified by reference 6. From the surgeon's point of view, turnover time is frustrating "downtime," even if its overall economic impact is minor.

Another approach is to use cost minimization analysis.[10] Labor and supply costs for a hypothetical ASC are shown in Figures 15-4 and 15-5, and we use

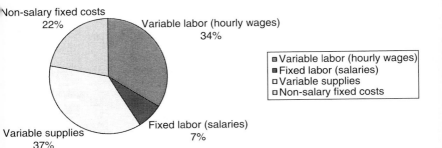

Figure 15-4. Ambulatory surgery center percentage costs.

4 ORs
10 hour workday
5 cases / OR / day
250 days / year
FTE assumes 8 hours / day for hourly workers

BUSINESS OFFICE	FTE	Salary	Wages $ / hr	Wages $ / yr
Business Office Manager	1	47000		
Surgery Scheduler	1.25		12	30000
Admissions Clerk	2.5		12.5	31250
Insurance Verifier	1.25		12.5	31250
Billing Clerk	1.25		15	37500
Collections Clerk	1.25		13.5	33750

CLINICAL STAFF

	FTE	Salary	Wages $ / hr	Wages $ / yr
RN Director of Operations	1	70000		
OR RN (Charge and Float)	1.25		24.5	61250
OR RN	5		24.5	61250
Holding Area (pre-op) RN	3.75		24.5	61250
PACU RN	5		24.5	61250
OR Technicians	5		18.5	46250
Anesthesia Technician	1.25		18.5	46250
Radiology Technician	1.25		18.5	46250
Orderly	1.25		12.5	31250

Total FTEs:	33.25			
Total salaries / yr		**117000**		
Variable labor / yr				**578750**
Total cases / yr				5000
Variable labor / case				116

SUPPLIES AND NON-SALARY FIXED COSTS

Variable supply costs / yr	**624575**
Variable supply costs / case	125
Non-salary fixed costs / yr	**375084**

Figure 15-5. Ambulatory surgery center dollar costs. FTE, full-time equivalent; OR, operating room; PACU, postanesthesia care unit; RN, registered nurse.

these data (personal communication, Diana Cooley, chief operating officer, and Elaine Morris, chief executive officer, Methodist Ambulatory Surgical Services, San Antonio, Texas) to construct several OR scheduling scenarios in Figure 15-6.[10] But before we proceed, we need to define the following metrics of OR efficiency:[10]

Traditional OR utilization (hereafter called "OR utilization"): Actual hours of surgery and associated turnover times divided by actual hours of straight time labor scheduled for the OR.

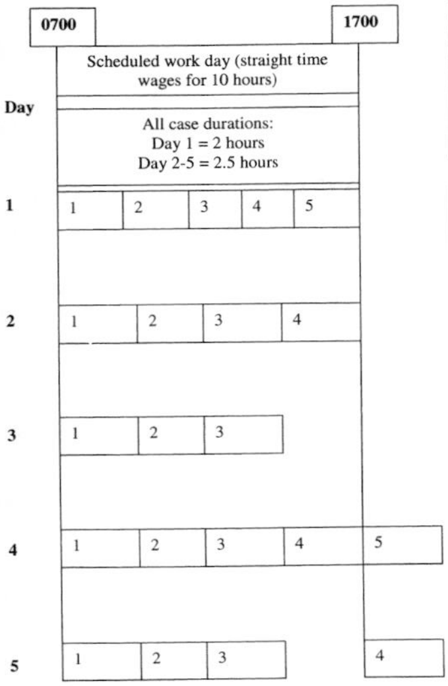

Day	0700 — Scheduled work day (straight time wages for 10 hours) — 1700	(A) OR utilization	(B) OR under-utilization "hours" (actual hours)	(C) OR over-utilization "hours" (actual hours x 1.75)	(D) OR inefficiency (B+C)	(E) Contribution margin / day (facility fees – variable costs)
1	1 2 3 4 5	100 %	0	0	0	$2795
2	1 2 3 4	100%	0	0	0	$2120
3	1 2 3	75%	2.5	0	2.5	$1445
4	1 2 3 4 5	125%	0	4.375	4.375	$2542
5	1 2 3 4	100%	2.5	4.375	6.875	$1866

(All case durations: Day 1 = 2 hours; Day 2-5 = 2.5 hours)

Figure 15-6. Operating room (OR) scheduling, efficiency, and profitability measures.

OR underutilization: Actual hours during the scheduled (straight time) workday for an OR, during which the OR is not occupied with surgery or turnovers.

OR overutilization: Actual hours of OR use during which overtime wages are paid, multiplied by the cost of overtime wages relative to straight time wages. OR overutilization will be expressed in this section as "hours."

OR inefficiency: The sum of OR underutilization and OR overutilization, expressed here as "hours."

The situation shown in Figure 15-6, day 1, is the ideal. On day 1, appropriate block scheduling and block time release have ensured that the workday will be full of cases. Last-minute cancellations are avoided by appropriate preoperative evaluation and by calling patients the day before to remind them of surgery and to rule out new illnesses that cause surgery to be cancelled. Case durations are estimated realistically to avoid overtime. On day 1, speedy surgeons perform high volumes of profitable cases. Turnover times are short and all of the employees are highly trained and motivated to help cases go as quickly as possible. There is no downtime (underutilized hours) and no overtime (overutilized hours). Employees are highly productive all day long and they get home on time because there is no overtime. OR utilization is 100%. Contribution margin per day is maximal at $2,795, since many short cases have been squeezed into a normal workday.

Days 2–6 in Figure 15-6 show the effects of longer case duration and less-than-ideal case scheduling on our metrics of OR efficiency.

Day 2 is similar to day 1 except that surgery proceeds more slowly and only four cases are performed in the 10-hour scheduled workday instead of the five cases performed on day 1. Day 2, like day 1, has a 100% OR utilization rate and it has zero "OR inefficiency" because underutilized and overutilized hours are both zero. On the negative side, however, total contribution margin for day 2, at $2,120, is not as high as for day 1, because less revenue is generated.

Day 3 shows the effect of a cancelled case (or OR time that goes unfilled for any reason). OR utilization is 75% and there are 2.5 hours of OR inefficiency due to underutilized time. Payroll expenses continue unabated despite OR downtime, and revenue generation is less than on days 1 or 2. Total contribution margin for day 3 is $1,445.

Day 4 shows the effect of an add-on case—or perhaps the effect of a surgeon who schedules more surgery than she can actually do during a normal workday. On day 4, OR utilization is 125%. OR inefficiency for day 4 is 4.375 "hours," calculated as the 2.5 actual overtime hours times their cost relative to straight time wages (1.75 times as expensive). This overtime is costly both in financial and emotional terms.

The revenues for days 1 and 4 are equal, but day 4 involves more wages being paid out because of the 2.5 hours of overtime wages paid. Hence, the contribution margin for day 4, at $2,542, is reduced relative to the $2,795 contribution margin for day 1.

Day 5 shows the effect of a gap in the regular daily schedule plus a case added on after regular work hours. In this example, OR utilization is 100%, but we have both 2.5 actual hours of underutilized time and 2.5 actual hours of overutilized time, leading to 6.875 total "hours" of OR inefficiency and to a total contribution margin for the day of $1,866.

Day 5 exemplifies the worst of both worlds, in that employees are idle during their regularly scheduled work hours but must nevertheless put in overtime that they do not want.

In summary, the goals of the ASC manager should be to completely fill normally scheduled OR time (when straight time wages are paid) and to reduce to a tolerable minimum the amount of overtime during which the employees are forced to work.

Minimize postanesthesia care unit wages

The next area that influences variable labor cost per case is the wages paid out for postanesthesia care unit (PACU) staffing. The anesthesia literature discusses three approaches to minimizing PACU wages:
1.   Scheduling techniques[11]
2.   Anesthetic, analgesic, and antiemetic techniques[12,13]
3.   Modifying ASC discharge criteria[14,15]
Since we have estimates of case duration, we could—at least in theory—schedule cases in such a way as to stagger PACU admissions and to prevent several ORs from coming out all at once and flooding the PACU with patients. This scheduling technique would minimize the peak PACU census and could minimize PACU wage costs. However, patients and surgeons may not, in practice, tolerate such restrictions on their scheduling flexibility, and these theoretical considerations may not have much significance in the setting of a small ASC.

Many anesthetic, analgesic, and antiemetic techniques can shorten an individual patient's length of stay in the PACU, thereby *possibly* reducing the peak

PACU census. In turn, a reduction in peak PACU census *may* enable the ASC's managers to pay less PACU wages, by allowing lower staffing levels.

Despite the fact that we can bypass the PACU in some cases and limit postoperative complications such as postoperative nausea and vomiting (PONV) that retard discharge, it is an open question whether shortened PACU stays for individual patients can be translated into overall cost savings for the ASC. This is due to the sometimes nondivisible nature of personnel costs.

As mentioned earlier, devices, medications, and techniques have been described and marketed in a way that suggests that they can increase patient "throughput" and hence decrease PACU staffing needs. These claims of cost savings have to be examined with skepticism.

In short, good anesthetic and analgesic care can certainly decrease postoperative complications and decrease a patient's length of stay postop in the ASC. What the entrepreneurial manager and anesthesiologist need to further attempt, however, is to translate a specific improvement in the quality of perioperative care into cost savings.

The third approach to improving patient care and minimizing PACU wages has been to individualize ASC discharge criteria so that selected patients no longer have to void or take fluids before they are allowed to go home from the ASC.

A fourth approach to minimizing PACU and other ASC wages is to employ people whose work hours are flexible (personal communication, D. Cooley). The ASC manager can call these employees the day before to ask them to come in for the time periods when they will be needed on the following day.

In the short term, labor costs are fixed. *Hence, making a superhuman effort to perform cases rapidly on any given day does not really save money; it just stresses people out.*

It is more important to understand the issues involved in these analyses than to be able to say that one technique will save money whereas another technique will not. The specific local circumstances of each health care facility will change over time, and the costs of the various techniques and medications will change as well, making it impossible to say, *a priori*, that one technique is cost-effective whereas another is not. Above all, the successful manager needs to understand that, in general, *businesses increase their efficiency by data-driven process redesign (continuous quality improvement) rather than by exhorting their workers to work harder or by punishing them.*[16]

Optimize overtime by realistically predicting case durations and scheduling ample amounts of straight time labor

Strum et al.[10] have described how to optimally schedule hourly labor in a way that will minimize financial costs and possibly limit staff burnout as well. In their technique, they describe OR efficiency as that state which is achieved when the combined costs of underutilized and overutilized time are minimized.

This line of reasoning leads to the intuitively attractive proposal to "schedule loose," that is, *to schedule somewhat generous and ample straight time labor so as to reduce to a tolerable minimum the amount of compulsory overtime that will be required from employees.*

Their useful insight is that *straight time labor is less expensive than overtime labor, both from a financial and an emotional point of view,* and that—while some overtime will occasionally be required—it should be held to an acceptable minimum by scheduling straight time labor generously, based on historical case durations.

Managers need to realize that ASC employees are people with their own families and interests who want generally predictable lives. Many nurses choose to work in ASCs because they hope to be able to get home on time as well as to avoid working weekends. When cost-conscious managers and hard-working surgeons combine to make their lives unpleasant and unpredictable, many nurses simply quit and go to work in another facility where their personal goals will be acknowledged and met. In the U.S., there is a nationwide nursing shortage and the nurse is in a strong position to pick and choose between employment options.

Minimize variable supply costs per case

Supply costs per case can be reduced by the following actions, when clinically appropriate (Figure 15-7):
1.   Reduce preop laboratory testing.[17–21]
2.   Only open supplies that will definitely be used.
3.   Use multiple-dose vials of medication.
4.   Use low gas flows.

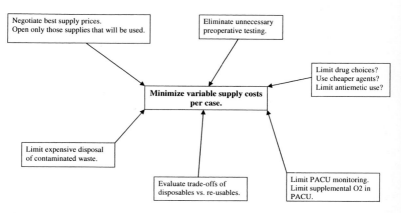

Figure 15-7. How to minimize variable supply costs per case. PACU, post-anesthesia care unit.

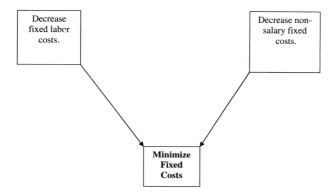

Figure 15-8. How to minimize fixed costs.

5. Use less expensive medications.[22]
6. Use less expensive disposable supplies (e.g., drapes, sutures, circuits, airways devices, IV supplies, and surgical implants).
7. Limit supplemental O_2 use in the PACU.
8. Limit monitor use in the PACU.
9. Limit expensive contaminated medical waste disposal (separate contaminated waste from noncontaminated waste).

If a manager promotes one or more of these techniques, she needs to make sure to do it in such a way as not to threaten the quality of care and not to antagonize physicians.

Minimize fixed costs

Fixed costs are not typically under the control of the anesthesiologist or the ASC manager (Figure 15-8). But if, for example, an unneeded administrator can be dispensed with, or if a cheaper equipment maintenance contract can be negotiated, it would be in the interests of the ASC's owners to do so.

A graphical portrait of an ASC's finances

Using the fixed costs and variable costs per case from Figures 15-4 and 15-5 (but varying the case volume per year), we can plot yearly ASC profit as a function of yearly case volume in Figure 15-9. The slopes of the ASC profit lines for situations A and B in Figure 15-9 are the contribution margins for each situation. The x-intercepts are the so-called "break-even points"—the volume of cases at which revenue just offsets the sum of variable and fixed costs and the profit for the ASC is zero. The y-intercepts are the yearly losses ("overhead")

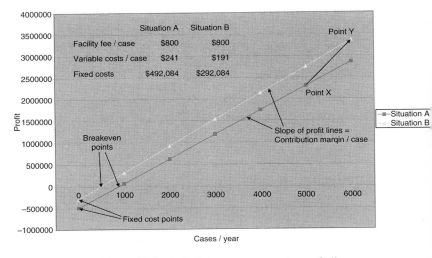

Figure 15-9. Ambulatory surgery center profit lines.

that would be associated with paying the ASC's fixed costs at zero case volume.

In Figure 15-9, situation B represents an improvement in ASC profitability with respect to situation A, due to a $200,000 per year reduction in fixed costs and a $50 reduction per case in variable labor and/or supply costs. In situation B, the ASC is operating more efficiently than in situation A and it has better "downside protection"; in situation B, the case volume can be lower than in situation A before the ASC starts to lose money. Conversely, the profit potential for situation B is higher than that for situation A; at any given case volume, situation B makes more money for the ASC's owners than does situation A.

As shown by Figure 15-9, it is management's job to move from point X on the profit line for situation A to point Y on the profit line for situation B, maximizing the contribution margin per case, minimizing fixed costs, and moving to as high a case volume as possible.

Priorities of the successful ASC manager

ASC manager's priority #1: hire and retain good people

People are the foundation of the ASC (Figure 15-10). Without good people, an ASC will be a failure, no matter where it is located or who owns it. People who take pride in their work and who treat patients well will help the facility

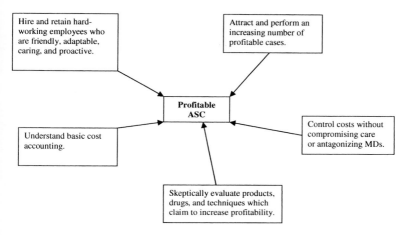

Figure 15-10. Five ambulatory surgery center (ASC) management priorities.

to run smoothly and to maintain an excellent reputation. The friendliness of the ASC staff may be the single most important determinant of patient satisfaction.[23]

Managers should also try to hire employees who are proactive. Will an employee take the initiative to help take better care of the patient, or will she do only what is absolutely necessary? Good employees frequently come up with excellent suggestions for improving the quality and efficiency of care.

The nationwide nursing shortage makes it particularly important that we *retain* good employees once hired. The following management actions keep employees happy and on the job:

1. To save costs per case, emphasize productivity enhancements rather than low wages.
2. Minimize compulsory overtime.
3. Do not tolerate abusive behavior by any personnel, including physicians.

ASC manager's priority #2: attract and perform an increasing number of profitable cases

Neither managers nor anesthesiologists have direct control over the most important determinants of case volume. The financial incentives implicit in a surgeon's ownership of the facility—plus the speed of the surgeon—are two of the most important factors in ensuring high case volume. Obviously, neither management nor the anesthesiologist can affect the ownership structure of the ASC or the speed of the surgeon as she operates. However, as anesthesiologists, we may be able to affect turnover times, and short turnover times may be able to marginally help the ASC to perform more cases within a scheduled workday.

Also, anesthesiologists are the "face" of the ASC in some respects (both for patients and for surgeons) and we can greatly influence the patient's and surgeon's experience of the ASC. Hence, anesthesiologists *do* affect the reputation of the ASC, both with patients and with surgeons, and an ASC's reputation may have some effect on its case volume.

ASC manager's priority #3: control costs

Anesthesia literature focuses on cost containment because this is an area over which there is some control. The goal—both for anesthesiologists and for ASC managers—should be *to minimize costs per dollar of ASC revenue*. This can be said in a more positive way by saying that the goal should be not to minimize costs *per se*, but rather to *maximize revenue per dollar of costs*.

In a manager's quest for controlling costs, she runs the risk of angering physicians who practice at the facility. Surgeons and anesthesiologists frequently have favorite equipment, disposable supplies, and medications that they are comfortable using, and they do not like to have to change their favorite tools in order to save a few pennies per case. The wise ASC manager will carefully "pick her battles" in the cost containment arena in order to avoid being perceived as a "penny pincher" who is interfering with patient care by insisting on the use of inferior—but cheaper—supplies.

ASC manager's priority #4: critically evaluate new devices, medications, and proposed changes in work processes

Many devices, medications, and techniques, such as the use of propofol and the BIS monitor, have been marketed by suggesting that their use will increase "throughput" or—in other words—shorten the PACU length of stay. The implication is that the marketed technique not only will contribute to a more satisfactory patient experience, but will save money as well. Increased throughput will save money only if it can cut down on PACU payroll costs, and this may not be the case. For example, if the use of PACU bypass techniques has enabled the ASC to reduce the maximum daily PACU census from four patients to three, there still may not be any money saved on PACU nursing labor, if the mandated minimum staffing ratio is one nurse for every two patients. PACU bypass efforts—while laudable in the sense of having achieved faster discharge and perhaps greater patient satisfaction—will not have saved any money. Similarly, PACU staff may need to be paid for their entire contracted shift, even if the patients all leave early. In short, innovations such as propofol and PACU bypass have been beneficial for patient care, but their overall effect on profitability is harder to evaluate and will depend on each specific situation.

ASC manager's priority #5: understand basic cost accounting

Similarly, the ASC manager must exercise appropriate skepticism when dealing with cost "information." For example, the ASC's accountant may tell the ASC manager that "OR time costs $20 per minute." From this cost "information," a naïve ASC manager might conclude that the OR team could save $60 if it could get the patient out of the OR 3 minutes more quickly at the end of surgery.

This conclusion would be completely wrong for at least two reasons:
1. The "$20 per minute" figure is an average based on hourly wages for OR personnel who will be paid whether or not the patient is actually in the OR.
2. The "$20 per minute" figure includes a portion of the facility's fixed costs which are allocated to the various profit-generating entities of the business, which, in the case of an ASC, consist of the ORs.

Hence, it should be apparent that simply coming out of the OR 3 minutes faster will not knock $60 off the ASC's monthly mortgage payment! Both the ASC manager and the anesthesiologist need to realize that business "costs" are not as simple or transparent as one might think. The discipline of management accounting is dedicated to teasing out the realities behind an apparently simple statement such as "the cost of OR time is $20 per minute."

Managers and physicians who work in ASCs need to be able to critically evaluate new devices, medications, and techniques to try to predict whether they will really result in substantive improvements in care or profitability.

Twelve key summary points

1. Besides giving safe and compassionate anesthesia care, it behooves the anesthesiologist to understand what she can—and cannot—do to support the financial success of the ASC.
2. "Anesthesia" is sometimes blamed for fundamental problems of scheduling and caseload in the ASC, which have nothing to do with the anesthesiologist.
3. Management's top priorities should be to:
   A. Hire and retain good people.
   B. Attract and perform an increasing number of profitable cases.
   C. Control costs.
   D. Skeptically evaluate new devices, medications, and proposed changes in work processes.
   E. Understand basic cost accounting.

4. High case volume and facility fees, and the avoidance of schedule gaps, are the cornerstones of ASC profitability. Anesthesiologists have minimal influence over these factors.

5. ASC profitability can be modeled as the following linear equation, which relates profit and case volume:

$$P = V \times (F - C_l - C_s) - C_f,$$

Where

P = profit / year

V = case volume / year

F = facility fee / case

C_l = variable labor costs / case

C_s = variable supply costs / case

C_f = fixed costs.

The slope of the "ASC profit line" is the contribution margin $(F - C_l - C_s)$, and the x-intercept is the "break-even" volume of cases, below which the ASC begins to lose money. It should be management's goals to increase the contribution margin $(F - C_l - C_s)$ for each case and to maximize the number of cases per year.

6. Contribution margin can be increased by increasing facility fees and by recruiting more profitable types of cases to the ASC.

7. Contribution margin can also be increased by reducing variable labor and supply costs with the techniques shown in Figures 15-3 and 15-7. This is an area in which managers and anesthesiologists can work together to increase contribution margins and ASC profitability.

8. Controlling variable labor and supply costs per case is important, but it is often not recognized that filling the OR schedule and surgeon speed are factors of overwhelming importance in determining both variable labor costs per case and overall ASC profitability. The anesthesiologist normally has no control over scheduling and she can affect case duration only by promoting teamwork and rapid turnover times.

9. Laudable innovations that increase the quality of care (such as PACU bypass, PONV prevention, multimodal pain control, and rapid patient discharge) do not *necessarily* also reduce variable labor costs. They may or may not, depending on each specific ASC setting. If the anesthesiologist or manager can simultaneously increase the quality of care and reduce costs, she will, in truth, be making both medical and economic progress.

10. Managers should attempt to decrease supply costs in a way that does not decrease quality of care and does not antagonize the medical staff.

11. Fixed costs are not normally under the anesthesiologist's control, but high fixed costs combined with low revenue generation can make the ASC lose money.

12. Allocation of fixed costs to ASC activities can artificially inflate the nominal "cost" of certain resources (e.g., OR time).

References

1. Archer TL, Mannis S, Macario A. Profit maximization for ambulatory surgery centers. In: Steele SM, Nielsen KC, Klein SM, eds. *Ambulatory Anesthesia and Perioperative Analgesia*. New York, NY: McGraw-Hill; 2005:123–133.

2. Dexter F, Coffin S, Tinker JH. Decreases in anesthesia-controlled time cannot permit one additional surgical operation to be reliably scheduled during the workday. *Anesth Analg.* 1995;81:1263–1268.

3. Macario A, Dexter F, Traub RD. Hospital profitability per hour of operating room time can vary among surgeons. *Anesth Analg.* 2001;93:669–675.

4. Lynk WJ, Longley CS. The effect of physician-owned surgicenters on hospital outpatient surgery. *Health Aff.* 2002;21:215–221.

5. Udelsman R. The operating room: war results in casualties. *Anesth Analg.* 2003; 97:936–937.

6. Dexter F, Epstein RH, Abouleish AE, Whitten CW, Lubarsky DA. Impact of reducing turnover times on staffing costs. *Anesth Analg.* 2004;98:872.

7. Dexter F, Abouleish AE, Epstein RH, Whitten CW, Lubarsky DA. Use of operating room information system data to predict the impact of reducing turnover times on staffing costs. *Anesth Analg.* 2003;97:1119–1126.

8. Sandberg WS, Daily B, Egan M, et al. Deliberate perioperative systems design improves operating room throughput. *Anesthesiology.* 2005;103:406–418.

9. Dexter F, Macario A, Traub RD, Hopwood M, Lubarsky DA. An operating room scheduling strategy to maximize the use of operating room block time: computer simulation of patient scheduling and survey of patients' preferences for surgical waiting time. *Anesth Analg.* 1999;89:7–20.

10. Strum DP, Vargas LG, May JH. Surgical subspecialty block utilization and capacity planning: a minimal cost analysis model. *Anesthesiology.* 1999;90:1176–1185.

11. Dexter F, Tinker JH. Analysis of strategies to decrease postanesthesia care unit costs. *Anesthesiology.* 1995;82:94–101.

12. Apfelbaum JL, Walawander CA, Grasela TH, et al. Eliminating intensive postoperative care in same-day surgery patients using short-acting anesthetics. *Anesthesiology.* 2002;97:66–74.

13. Song D, Chung F, Ronayne M, Ward B, Yogendran S, Sibbick C. Fast-tracking (bypassing the PACU) does not reduce nursing workload after ambulatory surgery. *Br J Anaesth.* 2004;93:768–774.

14. Jin F, Norris A, Chung F, Ganeshram T. Should adult patients drink fluids before discharge from ambulatory surgery? *Anesth Analg.* 1998;87:306–311.

15. Marshall SI, Chung F. Discharge criteria and complications after ambulatory surgery. *Anesth Analg.* 1999;88:508–517.

16. Archer T, Schmiesing C, Macario A. What is quality improvement in the preoperative period? *Int Anesthesiol Clin.* 2002;40:1–16.

17. Roizen MF. Preoperative evaluation. In: Miller RD, ed. *Anesthesia*. 6th ed. New York, NY: Churchill Livingstone; 2005:927–997.

18. Fleisher LA. Routine laboratory testing in the elderly: is it indicated? *Anesth Analg.* 2001;93:249–250.

19. Schein OD, Katz J, Bass EB, et al. The value of routine preoperative medical testing before cataract surgery. *N Engl J Med*. 2000;342:168–175.

20. Yuan H, Chung F, Wong D, Edward R. Current preoperative testing practices in ambulatory surgery are widely disparate: a survey of CAS members. *Can J Anaesth*. 2005;52:675–679.

21. Imasogie N, Wong DT, Luk K, Chung F. Elimination of routine testing in patients undergoing cataract surgery allows substantial savings in laboratory costs. A brief report. *Can J Anaesth*. 2003;50:246–248.

22. Kantor GS, Chung F. Anaesthesia drug cost, control and utilization in Canada. *Can J Anaesth*. 1996;43:9–16.

23. Tarazi EM, Philip BK. Friendliness of OR staff is top determinant of patient satisfaction with outpatient surgery. *Am J Anesthesiol*. 1998;25:154–157.

16. Administrative aspects of ambulatory surgery

William H. Beeson, MD

"Administration" of an ambulatory surgery center is an amalgamation of ownership and management responsibilities, which are an integration of both the clinical and business aspects of running an ambulatory surgery center. Effective, efficient, and profitable management of an ambulatory surgery center is a challenging task that rests on the shoulders of the administrative team. The late Peter Drucker, the "father of modern corporate management," is quoted as saying nearly half a century ago, "there is only one valid definition of business purpose: to create a customer."[1] He believed in an empowerment of people as an organization's most valuable business management strategy. In his 1950 book, *The Practice of Management*, he posed three seminal questions that should be asked by every manager: "what is our business, who is our customer, and what does our customer consider valuable?" This is the type of thinking that has spurred the development of ambulatory surgery centers. As one sets forth to establish an administrative framework for an ambulatory surgery center, it is important to realize that while structure is important, the key to success is an understanding that the physicians are the primary customers of any ambulatory surgery center, as well as an innate understanding of what motivates employees and retains patients. Effective management requires vision, sacrifice, integrity, and emotional intelligence. It is important that we not become "caught up" in the complicated and complex issues of daily management of a busy ambulatory surgery center and lose sight of these basic core concepts.

Development and management teams

A multitude of talents and expertise is required for the development and for the effective and efficient management of an ambulatory surgery center. One must put together both a "development team" (if one is starting an ambulatory surgery center "from the ground up," so to speak) and a "management team," both of which should consist of consultants, a lawyer, and an accountant. There are numerous tax, legal, and administrative issues that must be addressed in each phase of development and management.

The health care industry is a highly regulated industry that requires expertise in tax, corporate/partnership, securities, and administrative law issues. It is critical to have a health care attorney who is knowledgeable and proficient in surgery center development and management. Due to the fact that many centers are owned by physicians in combination with other partners such as hospitals, it is critical for the attorney to have knowledge of Stark laws, the Safe Harbor provisions, and the numerous state and federal laws governing for-profit joint ventures. There are many legal and regulatory road-blocks that must be navigated in order to both develop and manage a successful surgery center. It is imperative that the law firm selected have experience in all facets of health law pertinent to an ambulatory surgery center. In addition to the regulatory aspects, key tasks include the formation of the surgery center legal entity, drafting the operating agreement or limited partnership agreement, drafting the prospectus and related offering documents, and working with state regulatory agencies. Existing facilities need legal assistance in ensuring continued compliance with state and federal laws governing health care facilities as well as dealing with compliance issues, human resource issues, health privacy rules and regulations, and contracting issues. The importance of having a top-notch health care attorney as part of the administrative team cannot be overemphasized.[2]

An accountant with expertise in health care is a critical member of the administrative team. An ambulatory surgery center is a high fixed-cost business. The two variable costs associated with operating a surgery center are supply cost and staffing. The economic viability of a surgery center is very volume-sensitive because of the relatively high fixed cost. Successful ambulatory surgery centers are able to take advantage of significant economies of scale once the census exceeds the break-even point. An accountant can help the administrative team realize economy of scale by monitoring the various cost centers as well as by dealing with the complex tax issues inherent in any health care entity.

Because the various aspects of ambulatory surgery center development and management are so complex and technical, consultants are frequently used. This can vary from one individual with experience and expertise in ambulatory surgery centers to companies that specialize in management and development. In other instances, the entity will use a myriad of individuals within the community or region to obtain the technical advice and assistance they need in selected areas. Box 16-1 contains a checklist for areas of technical expertise required for ambulatory surgery center (ASC) management.

When looking at marketing, it is important to realize that there are two unique and distinct markets for the ambulatory surgery center. One market is the physician medical community, whereas the other market is the community at large and includes both the business and insurance sectors. It is important that both markets be addressed in an ongoing fashion by the management team.[3]

Box 16-1. Areas of technical expertise required for ambulatory surgery center management

- Infection control
- Medical records
- Environmental engineering
- Biomedical equipment
- Risk management/quality assurance
- Credentialing
- Human resources
- Marketing

Structure of organization: the governing body

Each ambulatory surgery center needs to have an organizational structure. That structure is a legally constituted entity that is constituted by a charter, articles of incorporation, a partnership agreement, a franchise agreement, or a legislative or executive act or that is a sole proprietorship.

The surgery center is controlled by the governing body. The governing body is legally responsible, both directly and indirectly, for the operation and performance of the ambulatory surgery center. The governing body has to determine the mission, goals, and objectives for the center. It has to establish the actual administrative organizational structure, which defines relationships among the various entities of the center. The governing body must adopt bylaws and the rules and regulations for the development and management of the surgery center as well as adopt polices and procedures relative to the clinical activities of the center. It is also charged with, and has the responsibility of, ensuring that the surgery center and facilities and personnel are adequate and appropriate to carry out the mission, goals, and objectives that have been selected.

The governing body also is responsible for ensuring that the quality of care at the center is evaluated and that problems are identified and addressed appropriately. It is responsible for all legal and ethical matters regarding the surgery center and its staff. The governing body is responsible for establishing and maintaining financial management and accountability for the surgery center. This includes approving and ensuring compliance with major contracts and arranging for appropriate services and support activities for the center.

The governing bodies also are responsible for ensuring that the surgery center is compliant with the various federal, state, and local rules and regulations applicable to an ambulatory surgery center. This includes developing polices that comply with all the applicable occupation, health, and safety regulations for health care workers. This would include ensuring compliance with the Occupational Safety and Health Administration rules on Occupational Exposure to Bloodborne Pathogens.

In recent years, promoting patient safety has become of paramount importance. For that reason, it is important for the governing body to establish a process for identifying, reporting, and preventing adverse events and developing an atmosphere that promotes patient safety. The governing body has ultimate responsibility in defining such a program and in delineating what events it feels are "adverse events." Numerous states have passed rules and regulations that define what they consider an adverse event, and some states require a reporting period. In addition, there are rules and regulations dealing with reporting and query of the National Practitioner Data Bank pertaining to physician performance, which would fall under the auspices of the governing body. Box 16-2 contains a checklist of major responsibilities of the governing body.

The organizational structure of a surgery center is such that the governing body is responsible for all administrative, fiscal, and legal activities of the entity, including granting of privileges to practitioners. The governing body may

---

Box 16-2. Major responsibilities of the governing body

- Developing mission, goals, and objectives for the ambulatory surgery center (ASC)
- Establishing organizational structure (i.e., outlining a chain of command and reporting relationships) as well as specifying functional responsibilities
- Adopting bylaws or regulations for management of the ASC
- Developing policies and procedures necessary for conducting the business of the ASC, including the clinical activities
- Ensuring that the facility is adequate and appropriate
- Ensuring that personnel hired by the ASC are adequate and appropriately trained
- Establishing appropriate financial management and accounting protocol for the ASC
- Approving all major contracts
- Possessing ultimate authority in approving employment or contracting of health care professionals
- Formulating long-range plans for the ASC in accordance with the adopted mission, goals, and objectives
- Developing an effective and appropriate quality assurance and risk management program for the ASC and developing policies and ensuring compliance with Occupational Safety and Health Administration rules and regulations applicable to ambulatory surgery centers
- Ensuring that the organization is compliant with local, state, and federal laws and regulations addressing ambulatory surgery centers (including ensuring that the entity is not in violation of anti self-referral regulations, fraud and abuse regulations, and health privacy rules and regulations and is compliant with reporting requirements to the National Practitioner Data Bank as applicable)
- Establishing process for identifying, reporting, and preventing adverse patient safety events and developing an appropriate patient safety program for the ASC
- Determining a policy on the rights of patients

subrogate much of the task work and management responsibility to the administrative staff, although the governing body still has the ultimate responsibility. There are various organizational structures that can be used. Frequently, the governing body will appoint an administrator and a medical director to carry out these functions for the governing body. In many small centers, the governing body and the administrator and medical director are often one in the same. The medical staff is governed by the medical staff bylaws. This governs how the medical staff and the governing body-administration interact. Legal counsel can advise as to what the appropriate medical bylaws should be and modify these to facilitate effective interaction and communication between that medical staff and governing body.

Regardless of the type of surgery that is performed in the ambulatory surgery center, each surgery center needs to have an administrative structure that addresses the following: the governance structure and activities of the governing body, the administrative structure and responsibilities, risk management and continuous quality improvement, medical records and health information, facilities and environmental issues, anesthesia services, surgical services, pathology and laboratory services (if applicable to the center), pharmaceutical services that are applicable to the surgery center, human resources, and research and educational services if the organization is involved in teaching medical students or residents, nurses, and allied health personnel or if they are involved in clinical research studies.[4]

Administrative staff

The governing body establishes the administrative policies, protocols, procedures, and controls for the ambulatory surgery center. The governing body then subrogates to the administrative staff the management responsibilities (Box 16-3), which include enforcing the policies delegated by the governing body, employing qualified management personnel, taking responsibility to ensure

---

Box 16-3. Administrative tasks
- Carrying out policies adopted by governing body
- Meeting short-range and long-range needs determined by governing body
- Ensuring compliance with applicable laws and regulations
- Employing qualified personnel
- Implementing financial controls, including billing, accounts payable, etc.
- Purchasing
- Collections
- Purchasing and equipment maintenance
- Establishing lines of authority, accountability, and supervision of personnel

- Maintaining appropriate documents and records for the surgery center
- Maintaining confidentiality, security, and safety for patients
- Ensuring compliance with clinical protocols approved by governing body
- Maintaining appropriate health information systems, including appropriate confidentiality and security
- Implementing appropriate quality assurance, continued quality improvement, risk management, and patient safety programs

compliance with applicable laws and regulations affecting the ambulatory surgery center, protecting the fiscal assets of the organization and ensuring that there are proper fiscal controls, implementing policies and procedures for collecting accounts and appropriate cash management, purchasing and maintaining equipment and supplies, and maintaining an appropriate health information system for the center. The administrative staff is also responsible for ensuring that the organization meets the long-range and the short-range planning needs as set forth by the governing body.

There are several key areas that are so critical to the success of the ambulatory surgery center that they deserve special attention and highlight. These include quality improvement and risk management.[5]

Quality improvement

In striving to improve the quality of care and to promote more effective and efficient use of facilities and services, it is critical that the governing body and administration have a very active and effective quality assurance and risk management program. It is also important that the program be an integrated, organized, peer-based program of quality management and improvement that links peer review, quality improvement activities, and risk management in an organized, systematic way. Such a program would be able to identify areas of significant problems or potential problems (near misses) and areas where there could be continued quality improvement. That is, "problems" are not limited to unacceptable or unexpected outcomes but could be areas that are critically important to quality of care and deserve to be frequently analyzed to identify areas where there can be additional improvement on an ongoing, continuous basis. Examples of "problems" that can be used as topics for quality assurance studies are outlined in Box 16-4.

The basic component of a quality assurance study is to identify a performance issue. Again, this does not necessarily have to be a problem but can be an area that is so critical that additional improvement would be beneficial to the surgery center. After the problem is selected, additional information is obtained related to exactly what the problem is, why it occurs, and the frequency, severity, and source of the suspected problem or concern. This information is then used to implement corrective actions for interventions, which could be used to resolve

Box 16-4. Quality assurance topics

- Unacceptable or unexpected outcomes
- Practice patterns or specific clinical performance of specific doctors
- Variances from expected outcomes identified through clinical record audits
- Information from patient satisfaction surveys
- Incident reports
- Staff concerns
- Medical/legal issues
- Overutilization or underutilization of services
- Wasteful practices
- Look at critical functions and try to identify "best practices" and benchmark against them

the problem or areas of concern. The steps necessary for the corrective action are delineated, and it is noted how the process will be implemented and by whom. The next step is taken after implementation of the corrective actions. After an appropriate period of time, the "problem" is re-measured to determine objectively whether the corrective actions have achieved and sustained the improvement that was desired. If it is determined that the problem still remains, there should be identification, analysis, and interpretation of any additional corrective actions that are necessary. If the initial corrective action sufficed, that is noted. All this information is then communicated to the governing body and disseminated to the appropriate members of the medical staff. It should be noted that the information obtained in these quality assurance studies should become part of the organization's overall educational opportunities and programs that foster continual quality improvement.

A performance measure is a clearly defined statement or question describing information to be collected for purposes of improving processes and outcomes of care. Performance benchmarking is an activity that looks at performance in a certain area and then compares that to key performance measures of similar organizations with recognized best practices of national or professional targets or goals. Many specialty societies have established performance measures in various areas for "benchmarking." These can be used, as well as information reported in the medical literature or comparison to other facilities, which management feels are high-quality organizations that they would like to emulate. Results of benchmarking activities should be incorporated into other quality improvement activities of the organization.

Risk management

Risk management is a subsection of quality assurance. It is important for the surgery center to develop and maintain a program of risk management that is directed to protect the life and welfare of both patients and employees. Typically,

Box 16-5. Commonly accepted definitions of adverse incidents

- Unexpected occurrence involving patient death or serious physical or psychological injury or illness, including loss of limb or function not related to the natural course of the patient's illness or underlying condition
- Any process variation for which a recurrence carries a significant chance of a serious adverse outcome
- Breaches in medical care resulting in a negative impact on patient even where death or loss of limb or function does not occur

such a program would at a minimum have reporting, reviewing, and appropriate analysis of incident reports from employees, patients, and physicians using the surgery center. It should also include a review of all litigation involving the surgery center and its staff. Any death, trauma, or adverse incidents such as sentinel events should be reviewed on a regular basis as would any patient complaint. Many states have established requirements for reporting of what they define as "adverse events" (Box 16-5).

The risk management program should also include review of reactions to drugs and materials, review of patient complaints, and review of processes and policies established to identify or designate the surgical site and involve the patient in those processes. The Joint Commission's Sentinel Event Program is an excellent process to incorporate into the surgery center risk management protocol (Chapter 14).

Job descriptions and functions

Responsibility for planning, organizing, and directing all activities of the surgery center according to the tenets established by the governing body falls upon the administrator. In some entities, the administrative functions dealing with business aspects are handled by one individual, and the medical aspects or clinical functions are under the direction of another, the "medical director." In some smaller facilities, these functions are combined under the direction of the medical director. Typical areas for delineation of specific individual functions in ambulatory surgery centers are the administrator, medical director, internal compliance officer, privacy officer (dealing with health information Health Insurance Portability and Accountability Act [HIPAA] issues), clinical director (director of nursing), risk management-safety director, and quality assurance-continuous performance improvement coordinator. These individuals all deal with the clinical issues associated with the surgery center operations. Business-related aspects are typically handled and assigned to individuals in the following areas: business office manager, medical records director, billing-insurance specialist, surgery scheduler, and admitting receptionist coordinator. Again, these functions can be amalgamated and assigned differently depending upon the size, scope, and volume of the facility.[6,7]

Administrator

The administrator has the responsibility for planning, organizing, and directing all activities of the facility according to the policies, procedures, and mission statement adopted by the governing body. The administrator is responsible for the financial and cost containment decisions, which ultimately have to be approved by the governing body. He or she is responsible that the facility meets all local, state, federal, and accrediting body rules and regulations applicable to the surgery center. They are also responsible for management of all aspects of environment of care, personnel materials/equipment, personnel education and in-service training, and administrative duties. They are also in charge of promoting a favorable image of the facility to physicians, patients, insurance companies, the medical community, and the general public. Obviously, many of these duties are delegated but are under the overall supervision and responsibility of the surgery center administrator.

Philosophy

The administrator has duties and responsibilities in approximately 12 key areas (Box 16-6). It is important that they have a philosophy that supports the surgery center's mission, goals, and objectives as set forth by the governing body. They must be a "team player" and be a positive role model.

General functions

General overall administrative responsibilities require participation at facility meetings, committee meetings, in-service training activities, and other edu-

---

Box 16-6. Key function areas of the facility administrator

- Overall administrative responsibilities: meetings and educational sessions, achieving facility goal, and monitoring environment of care
- Communications: internal and external
- Financial: cost containment, payroll and benefits, budgets, and contracts
- Compliance program
- Performance improvement
- Professional competence
- Personnel
- Medical staff
- Regulatory requirements
- Marketing

cational sessions. Administrators also are responsible for short- and long-term goals of the facility as recommended by the governing body. They have the responsibility of ensuring that the facility maintains cleanliness, sterility, and operation ability that is appropriate at all times and of monitoring the environment of care provided by the facility.

Communications

The administrator is also responsible for effective communications with patients, visitors, physicians, and coworkers. They need to ensure that effective communications between the clinical areas of the business offices and the physician's practice is maintained.

Financial

The administrator promotes cost containment and monitors office functions to maintain efficiency but also is responsible for monitoring payroll and benefits programs, as well as capital and operating budgets. Included in their function would be negotiation of any managed care contracts and purchasing contracts.

Compliance program

The administrator is responsible for ensuring that the organization has an appropriate compliance program that adheres to those policies and procedures. This program would be coordinated with appropriate legal counsel.

Performance improvement

The administrator oversees the quality assurance and risk management programs in conjunction with the medical staff. He or she ensures that the established performance improvement policy and procedures are being adhered to and appropriate monitoring programs are in place. He or she would evaluate suggestions, grievances, and incident reports to be sure that they are objectively evaluated and help to identify ways to improve patient care and performance standards.

Professional competence

The administrator oversees development and implementation of continuing education and in-service training programs for staff. They are in charge of being sure that a relevant professional environment appropriate to quality of care and patient safety is maintained. They are also responsible for maintaining appropriate personnel records.

Personnel

The administrator is in charge of implementing approved personnel policies according to state and federal laws. They oversee evaluation process for all employees as well as hiring, orientation, and mandatory education programs. They also are responsible for being sure appropriate in-service education programs are conducted in regard to demonstrated needs as well as state and federal rules and regulations and accrediting rules and regulations. They also are responsible for maintaining confidential personnel files according to state and federal guidelines.

Medical staff

The administrator communicates with the medical director and oversees medical staff credentialing programs and oversees quality assurance monitoring activities.

Regulatory

An important aspect of the administrator's job is being current on all applicable state and federal laws, rules, and regulations as well as professional accrediting body standards applicable to an ambulatory surgery center. They would also implement policies and procedures to meet those regulatory and accrediting guidelines as well as the routine functions and reporting requirements of regulatory and accrediting organizations to which the surgery center may be involved.

Marketing

Marketing is an important component for an ambulatory surgery center. Realizing that there is both a medical market and a general market, the administrator is responsible for developing and maintaining an appropriate marketing plan directed to physicians and their staff as well as for maintaining awareness of the medical community and the general community regarding the services and the activities of the facility.

Medical Director

The medical director is responsible for establishing, maintaining, and enforcing professional and ethical standards for the surgery center in accordance with policies and procedures adopted by the governing body and reflected in the medical staff bylaws. The medical director assists the administrator in ensuring that the facility meets all local, state, federal, and accrediting body rules and regulations pertinent to the surgery center. They also assist in coordinating and directing patient care in being sure that patient care is delivered in accordance with policies and procedures that the facility has adopted. The medical director serves as the liaison between the medical staff and the governing body/administration. Duties and responsibilities for the medical director are multiple but include responsibilities in the areas discussed below.

Philosophy

It is important that the medical director have a positive attitude and philosophy that reflect the mission statement, goals, and objectives delineated by the governing body. The medical director also needs to have strong ethical and professional tenets and serve as a positive role model for the medical staff as well as the administrative team. They need to be a strong clinician who advocates for quality of care, patient safety, and patient rights and has good communicative skills since they serve as a liaison between the medical staff and the governing body/administration.

In general, the medical director is responsible for establishing, maintaining, and enforcing the professional and ethical standards and performance of the medical staff (Box 16-7). They report to the governing body regarding quality and efficiency of the medical care that is being provided and oversee the day-to-day operations from a medical-issue standpoint. They work with the administrator to review activities for adherence to facility policies and ensure that the policies and procedures are in accordance with federal, state, and accrediting body standards and guidelines and that they are maintained.

Box 16-7. Responsibilities of the Medical Director
- Maintaining and enforcing professional and ethical standards of medical staff
- Report to governing body on quality of medical care
- Supervise day-to-day operations from a medical issue standpoint
- Review policies and procedures and adherence to facility policies

Medical staff

The medical director serves as a liaison between the medical staff and the governing body/administration. He or she investigates any breaches of quality of care and ethical conduct by medical staff members or patient/care personnel and reports those breaches to the governing body. They are also responsible for enforcing medical staff bylaws, rules, and regulations as well as facility policies and procedures. They are a critical component in reviewing the performance of medical staff members and oversee the reappointment recommendation process.

Patient care

One of the most important aspects, if not the most important aspect, of the medical director's job is to ensure that the quality of patient care is in accordance with established policies and procedures. They work up, identify, and solve any patient care-related problems and coordinate the continuity of patient care with physicians and the nursing staff.

Financial practices

The medical director works with the administrator and administrative staff to promote cost containment and effective use of surgery center resources. They may make recommendations to staff and administration regarding more cost-effective improvements. They work with medical staff regarding in-service and education regarding cost-containment and quality-of-care issues.

Quality improvement/risk management

The medical director contributes to the performance/improvement policies and procedures adopted by the facility and monitors to ensure they are being implemented. They are in charge of monitoring medical staff participation in quality assurance activities and assist with the credentialing and re-credentialing process as a part of the performance improvement activities of the facility. They are also responsible for ensuring that the facility adheres to the safety policies and procedures in performing job duties and responsibilities and in carrying out the clinical functions of the facility. They help to identify suspected safety violations, near misses, and policy/procedure noncompliance and address these issues in a multitude of ways, including developing in-service training and other educational programs that help to promote an atmosphere of patient safety.

Clinical Director

The clinical director is responsible for supervising and directing nursing care in all clinical areas of the facility and ensuring that the policies and procedures adopted by the governing body are adhered to. They work up, coordinate, and direct patient care and oversee patient scheduling and coordinating clinical activities. They are responsible for working with the medical director to analyze and evaluate nursing care to improve quality of care and work to ensure that the nursing aspects of clinical care are appropriate and consistent with accepted guidelines as well as local, state, federal, and accrediting body rules and regulations.

The duties and responsibilities of the nursing director/clinical director include participating in facility meetings, in-service, and other clinical activities. He or she is responsible for helping to develop the short- and long-term goals for the facility. They are directly involved in helping to maintain facility equipment and maintain the facility to ensure cleanliness, sterility, and operational ability at all times.

Communication

Clinical directors facilitate the communication between the nursing staff, the medical director, and the administration and foster good communication between patients, visitors, physicians, and nursing staff. They also promote effective communication between the clinical areas, the business office, the physicians, individual practices, and the nursing staff.

Fiscal practice

The clinical director has an important role in promoting cost containment and effective use of facility resources. In a surgery center, the cost of supplies and the staffing costs are the two critical areas. The clinical director is responsible for monitoring full-time equivalent (FTE) use and makes recommendations that are most cost-effective manpower practices. They work to develop and implement capital and operating budgets and help to conduct cost analysis to promote more cost-effective practices. They also assist in purchasing equipment and supplies to ensure the organization stays within budget allowances.

Typically, staffing costs for an ASC amount to approximately 46% of expenses, whereas supply costs can account for 15%-20% of expenses. It is typical to benchmark the hours of staff time per case. Generally, multispecialty cases will entail between 13 and 15 hours per case and single-specialty cases 6 to 8 hours per case. A general rule of thumb is 5 FTEs per 1,000 patients. It is critical for the clinical director to be able to control staffing costs. One way this can be done is to use staff efficiently by crosstraining where appropriate and by staffing to the exact needs of the facility and not overstaffing.

Quality improvement program

The clinical director/nursing director assists with implementation and maintenance of the organization's quality assurance continuous quality improvement programs and procedures. They help to establish policies and procedures to ensure quality of care and work to monitor patient care programs. They perform performance reviews, review outcome standards, and analyze reports to identify areas of concern and areas for potential improvement. They also help to maintain the patient safety/risk management programs by monitoring the facility environment for comfort, cleanliness, and compliance with policies and procedures. They ensure that Occupational Safety and Health Administration requirements are met by the clinical staff and that supplies are readily available. They ensure that the facility adheres to safety policies and procedures and performing job duties and responsibilities.

Professional education

The nursing director participates in continuing education programs and is responsible for developing appropriate in-service training programs to ensure that the nursing staff maintains competency and appropriateness in the medical care they deliver. The clinical director is responsible for administering the medical education program and assisting with orientation programs for new employees in all clinical areas.

Patient care

The clinical director is responsible for being sure that the facility applies acceptable clinical nursing principles and practices to patient care activities. They coordinate patient activities with surgeons and the anesthesiologist to ensure continuity of care. They assist in identifying problems and solving problems with nursing care. They oversee all nursing activities. They enforce nursing standards and ensure that licensing and accreditation rules and regulations are maintained. They make recommendations to revisions in patient care policies and procedures as necessary to conform to accepted principles. They supervise the care in the operating room area and ensure that the operating room area and equipment are clean, sterile, and in operation at all times. They also help to control patient/staff traffic and other practices to help prevent infections.

Daily operations

The clinical director coordinates and monitors the daily activities of the facility and is responsible for preparing staffing schedules. They also make daily personnel assignments and delegate duties according to experience and skill level to provide quality patient care. They also oversee crosstraining of clinical staff to make the staff more productive and efficient. They maintain attendance sheets and attendance logs. They evaluate the performance of clinical personnel and are involved in the continuous quality improvement and quality assurance programs as well as those of patient safety and risk management. They work as a liaison between patients, families, nurses, and medical staff as well as administrative staff to promote quality patient care.

Materials management

They help to promote cost-effective procedures and implement procedures to control waste. They review inventories for available supplies and equipment necessary for the daily function of the surgery center and initiate requests to replenish inventory and order new products. They oversee inventory, maintaining adequate supplies and equipment. They also monitor and verify purchases. They are responsible for maintaining records on equipment maintenance and reports needed for accreditation.

Business office manager

The business office manager has the function of supervising the business office personnel in the areas of insurance verification, compliance, scheduling for surgical procedures, transcription services, coordinating billing, coding, and accounts receivable with the billing company, maintaining accounts payable records, supervising payment of supplies and monitoring back orders, payroll monitoring, and maintaining computer services. He or she coordinates activities with other administrative personnel and is responsible for maintaining environmental services of the facility.

Duties and responsibilities of the business office manager include participating in surgery center committees, meetings, in-services, and other activities. He or she has the supervisory role of direct supervision of business office personnel, which includes orientation, performance appraisal, and maintenance of appropriate personnel records. The business office manager is also responsible for ensuring that the policies and procedures of the business office and administrative functions are carried out appropriately. The manager works with clinical administrative staff to ensure efficient and timely overall operations. An important aspect of the job is maintaining the regulatory compliance of the surgery center to be sure that it has an appropriate compliance monitoring program and that billing and coding are appropriate and commensurate with compliance policies and procedures set forth by the governing body. The business manager verifies that the facility is up to date on federal and state regulations regarding business office practices and participates where applicable in quality assurance and risk management programs as they apply to business operations.

The area of payroll is an important area the business office manager supervises. He or she maintains payroll and employee benefit records and verifies that appropriate documentation is maintained and that payroll checks are distributed as scheduled and according to policy. In addition, they would ensure timely deposits for payroll taxes.

The business office manager works with other administrative managers to be sure that the financial practices of the facility are cost-effective. The manager maintains appropriate records for the financial transactions and closely monitors insurance prequalification as well as timely and accurate billing for insurance and appropriate follow-up. This person is also responsible for reviewing delinquent accounts and dealing with them according to policies and protocols adopted by the governing body.

The business office manager is also responsible for evaluating the accuracy of accounts payable in terms of requester's purchasing procedures before approving payment. The manager is then responsible for monitoring accounts payable to see that any discounts or volume purchasing programs advantageous to the center are taken advantage of.

Also among the business office manager's duties is oversight of surgery scheduling to ensure that efficient patient flow is maintained. The manager monitors physician block time and makes recommendations for efficient use of operating room time to the administrator and the medical director.

As well as overseeing timely dispensation of completed charts when requests for information are received, the manager is an overseer of medical records for accuracy and completeness in compliance with federal and state rules and regulations. The manager verifies that records and patient information are being maintained according to strict HIPAA standards.

The business manager also assists with obtaining data regarding credentialing and re-credentialing of physicians and allied health personnel for the facility by working with the medical director to obtain current information on licensure, malpractice insurance, delineation of privilege, references, and other information pertinent to the credentialing of physicians and medical staff for the facility.

Medical records specialist

The medical records specialist is in charge of maintaining the surgery center's medical records and is responsible for their accuracy, safe storage, and use (e.g., the confidentiality of patient information). The medical records specialist is also responsible for ensuring that the medical records are kept in a manner consistent with HIPPA rules and regulations.

The duties of the medical records specialist include the collection, processing, filing, maintenance, storage, retrieval, and distribution of medical records according to the policies and procedures established by the governing body. The specialist is in charge of collecting and filing medical records for all laboratory pathology and other studies, for obtaining surgical operative dictations and the like, and for making sure that files are finally filed properly (including their inclusion of all appropriate correspondence regarding records and their maintenance in a manner consistent with federal and state guidelines and any accreditation body rules and regulations). The specialist also ensures that the signatures necessary in completing a chart are obtained (including contacting physician offices regarding necessary signatures and reports). The medical records specialist also works with outside monitoring consultants to verify appropriate compliance with policies and procedures and appropriate content of medical records.

Billing specialist

The billing specialist submits claims and statements to third-party payers regarding facility fees—maintaining correspondence regarding billing questions and responding to calls from patients regarding statements. The duties of the billing specialist also include insurance billing, which entails verifying the accuracy of the names and addresses of the patients' insurance companies (if applicable) and ensuring that proper data are maintained on the communications and dispensation involved in insurance filings per the correct patient record.

The billing specialist also has patient billing duties, which include verification of insurance payments received and posted and of adjustments as well as provision of statements to patients regarding balances due. The billing specialist is also responsible for calls and correspondence regarding patient bills, whether from patients or insurance companies. Whereas the billing specialist forwards requests for refunds and complex-problem questions to the business office manager, she generally handles most of these inquiries and documents them in the billing record system. The billing specialist also follows through on collections on overdue accounts for the surgery center.

Surgery scheduler

A critical area for a surgery center is the functioning of surgery scheduling. This is often done by a designated individual whose main function is to schedule all surgeries for the facility. It is important for this person to have a concept of the overall philosophy and mission of the facility and the policies and procedures applicable to surgery scheduling, including the types of procedures that can be performed at the center.

The scheduler follows the scheduling form to be sure that all pertinent patient demographic, health, and insurance information has been obtained from the physician's office. The scheduler also makes sure that scheduled procedures are consistent with the delineation of privileges for the physician as determined by the governing body and that appropriate equipment needs and supplies (such as implants) are available for the procedure (coordinating this with nursing and administrative staff). The scheduler also coordinates surgical and preoperative appointment schedules with the clinical director and perioperative nursing staff as well as with anesthesia personnel and the medical director. The scheduler distributes schedules to the appropriate areas to ensure that required staff and supplies are available for surgeries and follows through on notifications of changes in schedules (such as cancellations and rescheduling).

Admitting receptionist

The person handling the admitting and receptionist functions of the surgery center has an extremely critical function. It is important that patients and their families be handled in a courteous and professional manner commensurate with the ideals, missions, and goals of the surgery center. It is also important that all such interactions be done efficiently and effectively in order to enhance the experience and profitability of the center.

The duties of this individual include serving as telephone operator for the facility, triaging incoming calls, and taking accurate messages and information requests. This person also greets patients and provides the necessary paperwork for admission of the patient in the facility. The admitting receptionist also handles proper notification to the nursing staff and anesthesia personnel regarding the presence of the patient when paperwork is completed and ensures that appropriate records and information are obtained and maintained in accordance with confidentiality and professional protocols and guidelines established by the facility. This person also performs billing functions, including ensuring that appropriate collections of co-payments are obtained at the time of admission, making copies of all checks and credit card slips, logging cash received, maintaining appropriate billing records and supplying these to the accounting department in a timely fashion, and logging deposits for patient and insurance payments and maintaining these in an appropriate manner.

Twelve critical processes important to the success of an ambulatory surgery center

There are 12 critical processes essential to the success of an ambulatory surgery center which the administrative staff must address in a timely and effective manner according to *Becker's ASC Review*. Culberson et al.[2] point out that there are 12 key systems that must operate smoothly and effectively for a center to be efficient and financially sound. The 12 critical processes can be found in Box 16-8.

Scheduling

The scheduling function is critical. It should be delegated to a motivated and responsible individual because it is one of the most important functions

> **Box 16-8. Twelve critical processes for ambulatory surgical center success**
> - Scheduling
> - Insurance verification
> - Coding
> - Billing
> - Collections
> - Accounts payable
> - Cash management
> - Inventory management and purchasing
> - Staffing
> - Compliance
> - Risk management
> - Medical records

performed for the facility. The most effective ASC scheduling uses a medical information system to coordinate equipment used, block time, and staffing needs. Although this can be done manually, advanced electronic data processing systems are much more efficient and effective. They are well worth the expenditure.

Insurance verification

A system for precertification must exist that coordinates with the surgeon's office and gathers insurance and demographic information and identifies co-insurance and deductibles. This will ensure that surgical procedures will be reimbursed. Collection of co-insurance and deductibles before surgery is critical and is an important function to be performed by the admitting receptionist.

Coding

Correct coding is essential. If unable to hire certified coders, the surgery center should consider paying for employees to take a certification course. The surgery center should have regular coding audits by unaffiliated third-party personnel in order to ensure proper compliance with protocols and policies. The surgery center also needs to ensure that it is billing properly for implants and using correct modifiers. Coding should be coordinated with surgeons to review whether the surgeon's office is coding the case the same as the surgery center.

Billing

A sound billing system ensures proper oversight of third-party contracts and rates. The coder should report to the business manager on a daily basis regarding claims, submissions, and un-billed claims so that they can be processed within 3 days of surgery. One needs to ensure that the implants are billed properly and conform to third-party payer accounts.

Collections

Cash flow is critical for a surgery center. Co-payments and deductibles should be collected prior to surgery. There should be follow-up on open accounts after 30 days with insurance carriers and the use of letters from the patient to assist in collecting from the insurance companies. There should be analysis of accounts receivable to ensure that all claims over 30 days have been appropriately addressed. Although an appropriate benchmark would be to ensure collections are obtained within 45 days on average, most centers should try to strive for 25-day collection benchmark.

Accounts payable

It is important that ASC bills be addressed in a timely manner. It is recommended that payables be paid twice a month. Invoices should be recorded into the billing system each day (whether it be a computerized billing accounting program or a paper ledger book system). This ensures that you are able to see an accurate financial picture of the organization at any time and to more effectively manage your cash flow. Invoices should be logged so that the oldest invoices are paid first. A purchase order assistant should be in place whereby a separate employee issues the purchase order and the third party verifies receipt of goods. All invoices should be initialed by a third party and verified for accuracy. Checks should be in sequence and bank reconciliation reviewed by a third party each month. All checks should have stubs attached to paid invoices and all invoices should be approved by management by means of initialing the invoice or some other verification process. It is wise to consider having checks over a certain amount require dual signatures. A third party should perform the bank reconciliation each month.

Cash management

Three separate employees should control receipts or cash, checks, and credit card inflows to ensure effective checks and balances and avoid the possibility of fraud and embezzlement. Checks and cash should be logged by a separate employee who opens the mail, verifies accuracy of the entries, and initials the daily deposit log. This amount plus daily credit card slips should be reconciled with daily deposits in a log along with copies of amounts received. The second separate employee should make the deposit and a third separate employee should post the payments.

Inventory management and purchasing

It is critical to have the correct amount of inventory in place. Excess capital can be tied up in inventory. On the other hand, the surgery center needs to keep sufficient supplies, drugs, and implants on hand in order to conduct operations. Just-in-time inventory management can be advantageous, with deliveries scheduled to occur when inventory will be used use. A purchase order system should ensure that employees are submitting purchase orders and that there is proper checking of deliveries for accuracy. Medical information systems can facilitate better tracking and monitor purchases more effectively than manual systems and should be considered. The surgery center should also compare supply costs between physicians for similar cases. These results should be reported to the governing body in order to strive for a more cost-effective management.

Staffing

Staffing is a critical area since it is one of the two largest variables in cost for surgery centers. It is important to measure hours worked per patient, hours worked for the month, and overtime. These data should be benchmarked in order to effectively manage the center. Consideration should be given to crosstraining individuals for effective use of staff.

Compliance

The surgery center must have an active and ongoing regulatory compliance plan. The plan should be signed by all physicians and staff. There should be discussion at periodic times during the year and in-services for staff regarding updates pertaining to coding. There should also be regular legal review of compliance matters, including any problem areas identified by the surgery center. Operational audits should be periodically conducted to ensure proper coding and adherence to compliance policies and procedures.

Risk management

Promoting patient safety and appropriate risk management procedures is an important aspect of the surgery center. Consideration should be given to working with the medical liability carrier for internal and external audits. Consideration should be given to developing a patient safety program that integrates risk management, performance improvement, review of procedure functions, and consideration of implementation of sentinel events monitoring. Appropriate employee education regarding all of these areas should be implemented.

Medical records

Confidentiality of medical records is imperative. The medical records should be stored appropriately and there should be appropriate monitoring to ensure that the HIPAA is closely adhered to.

Performance improvement/best practice benchmarking

The Medical Group Management Association has identified better performing physician medical practices and has published these practices' quantitative performance results along with descriptive stories of how they achieved these performance outcomes. For medical practices, the study looked at four general areas and their corresponding matrix. These areas were productivity, capacity, and staffing; profitability and cost management; accounts receivable management; and managed care effectiveness. The first three of those areas likely relate to important performance concerns in ambulatory surgery centers.[8]

The study looked for groups' practices that produced more revenue while keeping their costs low. Once the organization identified these conditions, there was a process implemented to understand how these outcomes were achieved. Behaviors typically found in the better performing practices in the area of profitability were the following:

- Productivity-based physician compensation programs.
- Regular incentives (for employees) more often tied to timing of good performance rather than just as end-year bonuses.
- Higher staffing levels per FTE physician to better leverage the physician's time in patient care.
- Use of nonphysician providers such as nurse practitioners and physician assistants to expand patient base, offer new services, and allow physicians to focus on more complex patient issues.
- Implementation of new technologies to automate processes and increase efficiency.

Summary

Health care is highly specialized, so ambulatory surgery centers often view clinical and business functions as separate areas of expertise and activity. However, these are closely integrated. When you focus on quality and efficiency, the financial returns tend to follow.

It is important to remember that physicians are the primary customers of any ambulatory surgery center. It should be noted that physicians view the success of the surgery center based upon the quality of care the center provides, how easy it is for the physician to perform surgeries in the center, and the amount of return on any investment that they have. An effectively and efficiently managed surgery center is able to combine the clinical and business aspects in a manner that improves the quality of life for those practicing at the center, improves the quality of care for those receiving treatment at the ambulatory surgery center, and provides a quality of return on investment for those who have financially supported the facility.

References

1.   Drucker PF. *The Practice of Management*. New York, NY: HarperCollins Publishers; 1993.
2.   Culberson CA, et al. *Becker's ASC Review—Ambulatory Surgery Center Business and Legal Update*. March 2006, Vol. 2006 No. 3. Chicago, IL: McGuire Woods; 2006.
3.   Today's Surgery Center-Business and Clinical Aspects for the ASC. Volume 5, Issue 2, February 2006.
4.   *Accreditation Association for Ambulatory Healthcare Accreditation Handbook for Ambulatory Healthcare*. Wilmette, IL: Accreditation Association for Ambulatory Healthcare; 2005.
5.   Beeson W, Tobin H. *Development of an Ambulatory Surgical Facility*. New York, NY: Thieme Publishers; 1993.
6.   Serbin CA, English JL. *Essential Job Descriptions and Performance Evaluations for Ambulatory Surgery Centers*. Marblehead, MA: HCPro, Inc.; 2006.
7.   Personal Communication. L Conn RN, Director of Nursing and P. Blow, Administrator. Aesthetic Surgery Center, Carmel, Indiana.
8.   Steck D, Whitten B. *ASC Performance Improvement-Best Practice Benchmarking*. Aurora, CO: Medical Group Management Association Survey Operations Department, Medical Group Management Association; 2005.

Web resources

1.   American College of Medical Quality (ACMQ). Available at: http://www.acmq.org. Accessed July 21, 2007.

2. American College of Physician Executives (ACPE). Available at: http://www.acpe.
    org. Accessed July 21, 2007.
3. Association for Benchmarking Health Care™ (ABHC). Available at: http://www.
    abhc.org. Accessed July 21, 2007.
4. Fact Sheets, Agency for Healthcare Research and Quality (AHRQ). Available at:
    http://www.ahrq.gov/news/factix.htm. Accessed July 21, 2007.
5. Health Care Quality Resources—links to numerous QI, QA or PI resources. Available
    at: http://www.quality.org. Accessed July 21, 2007.
6. HIPAA—Health Insurance Portability and Accountability Act (information and
    resources from American Medical Association). Available at: http://www.ama-assn.
    org/ama/pub/category/4234.html. Accessed July 21, 2007.
7. Medical Group Management Association (MGMA). Available at: http://www.mgma.
    com. Accessed July 21, 2007.
8. HHS (U.S. Department of Health & Human Services) Office of Inspector General.
    Available at: http://www.oig.hhs.gov/authorities/regulatory.html. Accessed July 21,
    2007.

Recommended reading

Cohn KH. *Better Communication for Better Care: Mastering Physician-Administrator
    Collaboration*. Chicago, IL: Health Administration Press; 2005.
Hammon JL. *Fundamentals of Medical Management: A Guide for the New Physician
    Executive*. 2nd ed. Tampa, FL: American College of Physician Executives; 2000.
McLane-Kinzie DQ. *Scheduling Strategies for Ambulatory Surgery Centers*. Marblehead,
    MA: HCPro, Inc.; 2005.
Reeves CS. *Assessing and Improving Staffing and Organization*. American Medical Asso-
    ciation Press; 2000.
Reinertsen JL, Schellekens W. *10 Powerful Ideas for Improving Patient Care*. Chicago,
    IL: Health Administration Press; 2005.
Saxton JW. *Five-Star Customer Service: A Step-by-Step Guide for Physician Practices*.
    Marblehead, MA: HCPro, Inc.; 2005.
Serbin CA, English JL. *Essential Job Descriptions and Performance Evaluations for
    Ambulatory Surgery Centers*. Marblehead, MA: HCPro, Inc.; 2006.
Stubblefield A. *The Baptist Health Care Journey to Excellence: Creating a Culture that
    WOWs!* Hoboken, NJ: John Wiley & Sons, Inc.; 2005.

Appendices

Appendix 1

Table 1-10. Recommended laboratory testing for patients having ambulatory surgery

---

Age less than 50 years, Healthy
- No tests unless specified by surgeon for specific surgical issues

Electrocardiogram
- Age 50 or older
- Hypertension
- Current or past significant cardiac disease
- Current or past circulatory disease
- Cardiothoracic procedure

Chest x-ray
- Major respiratory condition with change of symptoms or acute episode within past 6 months
- Cardiothoracic procedure

Serum Chemistries
- Renal disease
- Adrenal, thyroid, or other major metabolic disorders
- Diuretic therapy

Urinalysis
- Genito-urological procedure

Complete blood count
- Hematological disorder
- Vascular procedure
- Chemotherapy

Coagulation studies
- Anticoagulation therapy
- Vascular procedure

Pregnancy testing
- Patients for whom pregnancy might complicate the surgery or anesthesia

---

These tests may be required for administration of anesthesia and are not intended to limit those required by surgeons for issues specific to their surgical management.

Appendix 2

Table 3-3. Antibiotic regimens for infective endocarditis prophylaxis for high risk adult patients undergoing dental procedures[+]

| Situation | Agent | Regimen: Single dose 30 to 60 minutes before dental procedure | |
		Adults	Children
Oral	Amoxicillin	2 g	50 mg/kg
Unable to take oral	Ampicillin	2 g IM or IV	50 mg/kg IM or IV
	OR		
	Cefazolin or ceftriaxone	1 g IM or IV	50 mg/kg IM or IV
Penicillin or ampicillin allergic–oral route	Cephalexin*[#]	2 g	50 mg/kg
	OR		
	Clindamycin	600 mg	20 mg/kg
	OR		
	Azithromycin or clarithromycin	500 mg	15 mg/kg
Penicillin or ampicillin allergic and unable to take oral medication	Cefazolin or ceftriaxone[†]	1 g IM or IV	50 mg/kg IM or IV
	OR		
	Clindamycin	600 mg IM or IV	20 mg/kg IM or IV

[+]Dental procedures involving manipulation of gingival tissue or the periapical region of teeth or perforation of the oral mucosa.
*Or other first- or second-generation oral cephalosporin in equivalent adult dosage.
[†]Cephalosporins should not be used in an individual with a history of anaphylaxsis, angioedema, or urticaria with penicillins or ampicillin.

Wilson W, Taubert KA, Gewitz M, et al. Prevention of infective endocarditis: Guidelines from the American Heart Association. A guideline from the American Heart Association Rheumatic Fever, Endocarditis and Kawasaki Disease Committee, Council on Cardiovascular Disease in the Young, and the Council on Clinical Cardiology, Council on Cardiovascular Surgery and Anesthesia, and the Quality of Care and Outcomes Research Interdisciplinary Working Group. JADA 2007;138(6):739–60. © 2007 American Dental Association. Excerpted by JADA with permission of Circulation. Circulation 2007 Apr 19;[Epub ahead of print]. © 2007 American Heart Association. Adapted 2008 with permission of The Journal of the American Dental Association.

Appendix 3

Table 6-9. Summary of major changes in updated American Heart Association infective endocarditis (IE) guidelines

---

- Bacteremia resulting from daily activities is much more likely to cause infective endocarditis (IE) than bacteremia associated with a dental procedure.
- Only an extremely small number of cases of IE might be prevented by antibiotic prophylaxis even if prophylaxis is 100% effective.
- Antibiotic prophylaxis is not recommended based solely on an increased lifetime risk of acquisition of IE.
- Limit recommendations for IE prophylaxis only to those high risk cardiac conditions listed in Table 6-7.
- Antibiotic prophylaxis is no longer recommended for any other form of CHD, except for the high risk cardiac conditions listed in Table 6-7.
- Antibiotic prophylaxis is recommended for all dental procedures that involve manipulation of gingival tissues or periapical region of teeth or perforation of oral mucosa only for patients with underlying cardiac conditions associated with the highest risk of adverse outcome from IE (Table 6-8).
- Antibiotic prophylaxis is recommended for procedures on incision or biopsy of respiratory tract mucosa or for procedures on infected skin, skin structures, or musculoskeletal tissue only for high risk patients (Table 6.8).
- Antibiotic prophylaxis solely to prevent IE is not recommended for GU or GI tract procedures (Table 6-8). High risk patients with established GI or GU infection at the time of procedure may be prophylaxed with an anti-enterococcal agent.
- Guidelines reaffirm the procedures noted in the 1997 prophylaxis guidelines for which endocarditis prophylaxis is not recommended and extends this to other common procedures, including ear and body piercing, tattooing, and vaginal delivery and hysterectomy.

Wilson W, Taubert KA, Gewitz M, et al. Prevention of infective endocarditis: Guidelines from the American Heart Association. A guideline from the American Heart Association Rheumatic Fever, Endocarditis and Kawasaki Disease Committee, Council on Cardiovascular Disease in the Young, and the Council on Clinical Cardiology, Council on Cardiovascular Surgery and Anesthesia, and the Quality of Care and Outcomes Research Interdisciplinary Working Group. JADA 2007;138(6):739–60. © 2007 American Dental Association. Excerpted by JADA with permission of Circulation. Circulation 2007 Apr 19;[Epub ahead of print]. © 2007 American Heart Association. Adapted 2008 with permission of The Journal of the American Dental Association.
Source: Antibiotics and your heart. American Dental Association Web site. Available at http://www.ada.org/public/topics/antibiotics.asp. © 2007 American Dental Association. All rights reserved.

Appendix 4

Table 3-8. Identification and assessment of obstructive sleep apnea (OSA)

Predisposing physical characteristics	Body mass index $>35\,\mathrm{kg/m^2}$
	Neck circumference >17 inches (men), 16 inches (women)
	Craniofacial abnormalities affecting the airway
	Anatomical nasal obstruction
	Tonsils nearly touching or touching in the midline
History of apparent airway obstruction during sleep (two or more)	Snoring (loud enough to be heard through closed door)
	Frequent snoring
	Observed pauses in breathing during sleep
	Awakens from sleep with choking sensation
	Frequent arousals from sleep
Somnolence (one or more)	Frequent somnolence or fatigue despite adequate "sleep"
	Falls asleep easily in a nonstimulating environment despite adequate "sleep"

Positive findings in two categories = moderate OSA, three categories = severe OSA.

Appendix 5

Table 3-12. Consultation with internist or cardiologists with specific questions

Medical issue	Specific question/request
Active cardiac conditions (American Heart Association/American College of Cardiology guidelines)	Can treatment lower risk and allow ambulatory procedure?
Poor or unclear exercise tolerance with one or more clinical risk factors scheduled for greater than low risk surgery.	Need for noninvasive cardiac testing? Need for beta blockers to lower perioperative risk?
Atrial fibrillation or angina on anticoagulant therapy.	Timing of anticoagulant discontinuation? Need for low-molecular-weight heparin?
Known coronary artery disease for intermediate surgical-risk procedure.	Need for beta blockers?
Myocardial infarction within 6 months.	Cardiac status stable? Cardiac function adequate for ambulatory surgery?
Recent percutaneous balloon angioplasty or cardiac stent placement, particularly drug-eluting stents.	Timing of ambulatory surgery? Timing of anticoagulation discontinuation? Need for low-molecular-weight heparin?
Pacemaker	Type and function? How to convert to fixed mode?
Automatic implantable cardioverter defibrillator	Plan for disabling, reenabling?
Active bronchospasm	Can therapy be augmented?
Undiagnosed, undertreated significant hypertension.	Begin or augment appropriate therapy.
Undiagnosed, undertreated significant diabetes.	Begin or augment appropriate therapy.
Long-acting psychiatric medications	Risk/benefit of discontinuation?
Bleeding disorder (hemophilia, factor deficiency)	Management strategy
Symptomatic hemoglobinopathy	Management strategy

Appendix 6

Box 4-5. Anesthesia machine preparation for malignant hyperthermia-susceptible patients

- Flush anesthesia machine for 20 minutes with high-flow oxygen 10 L/minute
- Disable or remove vaporizers
- Change disposables; consider changing soda lime
- Adequate supply of dantrolene to treat a crisis
- Nontriggering anesthetic technique
- Observe for 2.5 hours before discharge: minimum of 60 minutes in phase I plus 90 minutes in phase II
- Acceptable for outpatient status if no sequelae after nontriggering anesthetic

Appendix 7

Table 5-6. Pediatric adjunct agents

Agent	Dose	Route
Muscle relaxants:		
Succinylcholine	2 mg/kg	IV
	5–6 mg/kg	IM
Mivacurium (not currently available in the U.S.)	0.2 mg/kg	IV
Atracurium	0.5 mg/kg	IV
Vecuronium	0.1 mg/kg	IV
Rocuronium	0.6–1 mg/kg	IV
Opioids:		
Fentanyl	0.5–2 µg/kg	IV
Morphine	0.05–0.1 mg/kg	IV
Antiemetics:		
Metoclopramide	0.15 mg/kg	IV
Ondansetron	0.1 mg/kg (maximum 4 mg)	IV
	4 mg for children >20 kg	ODT
Dexamethasone	0.15 mg/kg (maximum 4 mg)	IV
Promethazine	12.5–25 mg	Rectally
Prochlorperazine	2.5–5 mg	Rectally

Doses should be titrated starting with the lower recommended dose. IM, intramuscular; IV, intravenous; ODT, oral disintegrating tablet.

Appendix 8

Table 5-8. Pediatric analgesic drug dosage

Drug	Route	Dose	Duration of action (hours)
Acetaminophen	Rectally	30–40 mg/kg*	4–6
	PO	10–15 mg/kg	4–6
Ketorolac	IV	0.5 mg/kg (maximum 30 mg)	6–8
	PO	1 mg/kg (maximum 10 mg)	4–6
Ibuprofen	PO	5 mg/kg	6–8
Codeine	PO	0.5–1 mg/kg	4–6
Naproxen	PO	10 mg/kg	6–8
Fentanyl	IV	1–2 μg/kg	0.5–1
Meperidine	IV/IM	0.5–1 mg/kg	2–4
Morphine	IV	0.05–0.1 mg/kg	2–4

Doses should be titrated starting with the lower recommended dose.
*Acetaminophen suppositories are available in sizes of 120, 325, and 650 mg. Usually, the calculated dose is rounded up or down to the nearest whole or half size suppository.
IM, intramuscular; IV, intravenous; PO, per os.

Appendix 9

Table 5-10. Oral sedation techniques in children

Drug	Usual dose
Chloral hydrate	25–50 mg/kg (for small infants up to 12 months) 25–75 mg/kg (for children older than 12 months)
Ketamine	5–10 mg/kg (above 1 year)
Midazolam	0.5–1.0 mg/kg orally 0.2–0.3 mg/kg intranasally (above 1 year)
Fentanyl (Oralet)	5–15 µg/kg transmucosally (for children weighing more than 15 kg)

Doses should be titrated starting with the lower recommended dose.

Appendix 10

Table 5-1. Fasting recommendations

Ingested material	Minimum fasting period (hours)
Clear liquids (*water, fruit juices without pulp, carbonated beverages*)	2
Breast milk	4
Infant formula	6
Nonhuman milk	6
Light meal	6
Heavy (high fat) meal	8

Appendix 11

Figure 6-4. American Society of Anesthesiologists difficult airway algorithm.

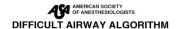

DIFFICULT AIRWAY ALGORITHM

1. Assess the likelihood and clinical impact of basic management problems:
   - A. Difficult Ventilation
   - B. Difficult Intubation
   - C. Difficulty with Patient Cooperation of Consent
   - D. Difficult Tracheostomy

2. Actively pursue opportunities to deliver supplemental oxygen throughout the process of difficult airway management

3. Consider the relative merits and feasibility of basic management choices:

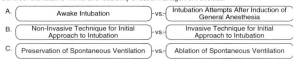

4. Develop primary and alternative strategies:

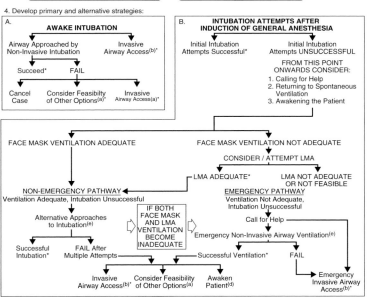

* Confirm ventilation, tracheal intubation, or LMA placement with exhaled CO_2

a. Other options include (but are not limited to): surgery utilizing face mask or LMA anesthesia, local anesthesia infiltration or regional nerve blockade. Pursuit of these options usually implies that mask ventilation will not be problematic. Therefore, these options may be of limited value if this step in the algorithm has been reached via the Emergency Pathway.

b. Invasive airway access includes surgical or percutaneous tracheostomy of cricothyrotomy.

c. Alternative non-invasive approaches to difficult intubation include (but are not limited to): use of different laryngoscope blades, LMA as an intubation conduit (with or without fiberoptic guidance), fiberoptic intubation, intubating stylet or tube changer, light wand, retrograde intubation, and blind oral or nasal intubation.

d. Consider re-preparation of the patient for awake intubation or canceling surgery.

e. Options for emergency non-invasive airway ventilation include (but are not limited to): rigid bronchoscope, esophageal-tracheal combitube ventilation, or transtracheal jet ventilation.

Source: American Society of Anesthesiologists Task Force on Management of the Difficult Airway.[31] Copyright © 2003, Lippincott Williams and Wilkins, Inc. Used with permission.

Appendix 12

Table 7-3. Adult sedative and analgesic drug doses administered as boluses or infusion technique[21–24]

Drugs	Bolus dosage	Infusion rate
Midazolam	25–50 µg/kg 1–2 mg (when used with propofol)	
Propofol	0.25–1 mg/kg	10–75 µg/kg per minute
Methohexital	0.25–1 mg/kg	10–75 µg/kg per minute
Dexmedetomidine		0.2–0.7 µg/kg per hour
Ketamine	0.3–0.6 mg/kg	300–600 µg/kg per hour
Fentanyl	25–50 µg	Not recommended
Alfentanil	5–10 µg/kg	0.25–1 µg/kg per minute
Remifentanil	0.1–0.3 µg/kg	0.025–0.1 µg/kg per minute

Doses should be titrated starting with the lower recommended dose.

Appendix 13

Table 8-3. Onset time, duration of effect, and maximum recommended dose of local anesthetic agents used for peripheral nerve blocks

	Onset (minutes)	Duration (hours)	Maximum dose (mg/kg) of solution with epinephrine
Chloroprocaine	10–20	1–2	14
Lidocaine	10–20	2–3	7
Mepivacaine	10–20	3–6	7
Bupivacaine	15–30	6–12	3
Ropivacaine	15–30	6–12	3.5

Appendix 14

Table 8-5. Dose of adjuvant in final solution according to site of administration

	Spinal	Epidural	Peripheral nerve block
Epinephrine	50–200 μg	2.5 μg/mL	2.5 μg/mL
Phenylephrine	1–5 mg		
Bicarbonate		0.1 mEq/mL	0.1 mEq/mL
Clonidine	150 μg	450 μg	50–100 μg

Appendix 15

Table 9-4. Perioperative analgesics in the ambulatory setting-adults

Analgesic	Dose	Duration of effect
Fentanyl	0.5–2 μg/kg	30 minutes
Remifentanil	0.015–0.2 μg/kg/min	5 minutes after end infusion
Acetaminophen	10–15 mg/kg PO 40 mg/kg PR	4 hours
Propacetamol	20–30 mg/kg IV	4 hours
Ketorolac	15–30 mg/IV 30–60 mg/IM	6–8 hours
Celecoxib	400 mg PO, then 200 mg PO	12 hours

Dose should be titrated starting with the lower recommended dose. IM, intramuscular; IV, intravenous; PO, per os; PR, per rectum.

Appendix 16

Table 9-5. Neuromuscular blocking agents and reversal agents in clinical practice

Agent	Intubation dose (2× ED95) mg/kg	Onset time (minutes)	Duration of action until train of four (TOF) > 0.9 after intubation dose (minutes)	Common side effects
Rocuronium	0.6	1.5–2.5	55–80	Mild vagolytic
Vecuronium	0.1	2–3	50–80	None
Mivacurium*	0.15–0.2	2.5–4.5	25–40	Histamine
Atracurium	0.5	2–3	55–80	Histamine
Cisatracurium	0.1–0.2	3–6	60–90	None
Neostigmine	0.05–0.07 µg/kg	2–5	60–90	Cholinergic
Edrophonium	0.5–1 mg/kg	1–2	60–90	Cholinergic
Glycopyrrolate	10 µg/kg	1–2	30	Tachycardia
Sugammadex	2–4 mg/kg	1.5–6.5	Unknown	No known side effects

*No longer available in the U.S.

Appendix 17

Table 11-6. Office anesthesia checklist

☑ **Facility design:**

	Date completed	Comments
• Sufficient space		
• Recovery area		
• Meets building codes		
• Sufficient electrical outlets		
• Backup power		
• Visual access to patient at all times during surgery/proper lighting		

☑ **Equipment and supplies:**

	Date completed	Comments
• Reliable O_2 source with backup		
• Adequate source of suction and catheters		
• Self-inflating (Ambu) resuscitation bag capable of administering at least 90% O_2 with backup bag		
• Emergency cart/airway equipment/ACLS drugs for population(s) served (i.e., adult, pediatric)		
• Communication device (telephone, intercom within reach)		
• Scavenging system for waste gas		
• Blood pressure, electrocardiogram, stethoscope, pulse oximeter, capnogram		
• Functioning resuscitation equipment and defibrillator		
• Appropriate-sized airways, laryngoscope blade, masks/laryngeal mask airways		
• Dantrolene when using triggering agents		

☑ **General preparedness:**

	Date completed	Comments
• Credentialed and licensed medical doctors		
• ACLS and/or pediatric ALS trained staff on premises until patient discharge		
• Hospital transfer agreement		
• Quality assurance policies/initiatives and peer reviews		

ACLS, advanced cardiac life support; ALS, advanced life support.

Appendix 18

Table 12-4. Postoperative antiemetic therapy-adults

Drug	Dose	Side effects
Serotonin (5HT$_3$) antagonists		
Ondansetron (Zofran)	4–8 mg IV	Headache, dizziness
Dolasetron (Anzemet)	12.5–25 mg IV	
Granisetron (Kytril)	0.35–1.0 mg IV	
Butyrophenones		
Droperidol	0.625–1.25 mg IV	Extrapyramidal effects, dysphoria, drowsiness, dizziness
Neurokinin (NK-1) antagonists		
Aprepitant (Emend)	40 mg PO	Headache, constipation, pruritis
Steroids		
Dexamethasone	4–10 mg IV	Rare with single dose
Phenothiazines		
Prochlorperazine (Compazine)	5–10 mg IV, IM, PO 25 mg PR suppository	Sedation, drowsiness, hypotension
Antihistamines (H-1) antagonists		
Promethazine (Phenergan)	6.25–12.5 mg IV 12.5–50 mg PR suppository	Sedation
Hydroxyzine (Vistaril)	12.5–25 mg IV, IM	
Benzamides		
Trimethobenzamide (Tigan)	100–200 mg IV, IM 200 mg PR suppository	Extrapyramidal effects, dysphoria, drowsiness, anxiety, dizziness
Anticholinergics		
Scopolamine patch (Transderm Scop)	1.5 mg transdermal	Dry mouth, blurred visions, hallucinations

IM, intramuscular; IV, intravenous; PO, per os; PR, per rectum.

Appendix 19

Figure 12-2. Algorithm for prophylactic antiemetic treatment.

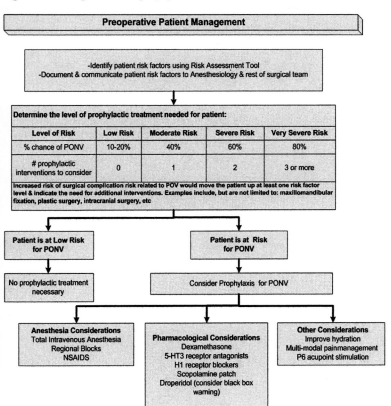

Appendix 20

Table 12-5. Treatment modalities for postoperative hypertension

Drug	Dose range	Half-life
Beta blockers		
Propranolol (Inderal)	0.5–1.0 mg IV	2–4 hours
Labetalol (mixed alpha and beta) (Trandate, Normodyne)	5–10 mg bolus IV	4–6 hours
Esmolol (beta 1-selective) (Brevibloc)	0.25–0.5 mg/kg bolus IV 50–200 µg/kg per minute infusion	9 minutes
Metoprolol (beta 1-selective) (Lopressor)	5–25 mg IV increments	2.5–4.5 hours
Vasodilators		
Hydralazine (Apresoline)	2.5–5.0 mg IV increments	4–6 hours
Nitroglycerin	50–100 µg IV bolus 0.1 µg/kg per minute	4–6 hours
Calcium channel blockers		
Nicardipene (Cardene)	2.5 mg IV	6 hours
ACE Inhibitors		
Enalapril (Vasotec)	2.5 mg IV	4–6 hours

IV, intravenous.

Index

Printed in the United States